Psychotherapeutic Drug Identification Guide

This guide contains color reproductions of some commonly prescribed major psychotherapeutic drugs. This guide mainly illustrates tablets and capsules. A † symbol preceding the name of the drug indicates that other doses are available. Check directly with the manufacturer. *(Although the photos are intended as accurate reproductions of the drug, this guide should be used only as a quick identification aid.)*

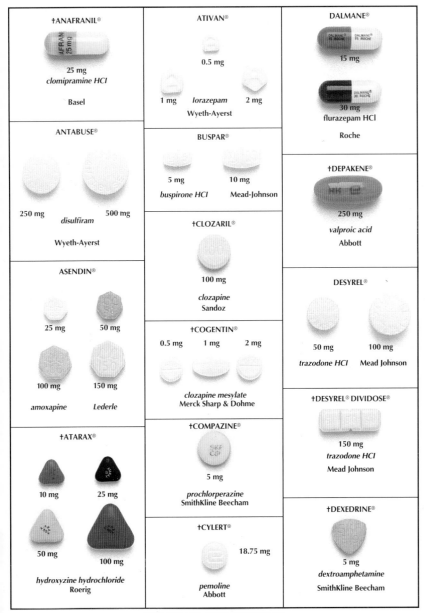

†ANAFRANIL®

25 mg
clomipramine HCl

Basel

ANTABUSE®

250 mg   500 mg
disulfiram

Wyeth-Ayerst

ASENDIN®

25 mg   50 mg

100 mg   150 mg

amoxapine   Lederle

†ATARAX®

10 mg   25 mg

50 mg   100 mg

hydroxyzine hydrochloride
Roerig

ATIVAN®

0.5 mg

1 mg   *lorazepam*   2 mg
Wyeth-Ayerst

BUSPAR®

5 mg   10 mg

buspirone HCl   Mead-Johnson

†CLOZARIL®

100 mg

clozapine
Sandoz

†COGENTIN®

0.5 mg   1 mg   2 mg

clozapine mesylate
Merck Sharp & Dohme

†COMPAZINE®

5 mg

prochlorperazine
SmithKline Beecham

†CYLERT®

18.75 mg

pemoline
Abbott

DALMANE®

15 mg

30 mg
flurazepam HCl

Roche

†DEPAKENE®

250 mg

valproic acid
Abbott

DESYREL®

50 mg   100 mg

trazodone HCl   Mead Johnson

†DESYREL® DIVIDOSE®

150 mg
trazodone HCl
Mead Johnson

†DEXEDRINE®

5 mg
dextroamphetamine
SmithKline Beecham

WILLIAMS AND WILKINS©

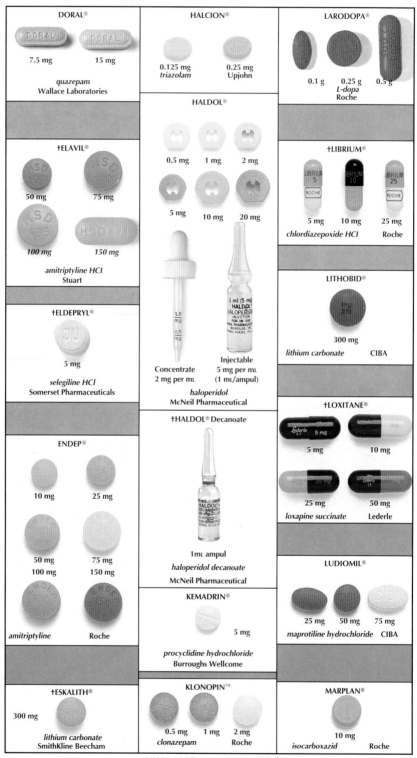

DORAL®

7.5 mg   15 mg

quazepam
Wallace Laboratories

HALCION®

0.125 mg   0.25 mg
triazolam   Upjohn

LARODOPA®

0.1 g   0.25 g   0.5 g
L-dopa
Roche

†ELAVIL®

50 mg   75 mg

100 mg   150 mg

amitriptyline HCl
Stuart

HALDOL®

0.5 mg   1 mg   2 mg

5 mg   10 mg   20 mg

1.0 mg
0.5 mg

Concentrate
2 mg per mL

1 ml (5 mg)
HALDOL®
HALOPERIDOL
INJECTION
FOR IM USE
McNEIL PHARMACEUTICAL
McNEILAB, INC.
SPRING HOUSE, PA

Injectable
5 mg per mL
(1 mL/ampul)

haloperidol
McNeil Pharmaceutical

†LIBRIUM®

LIBRIUM
5
ROCHE

LIBRIUM
10

LIBRIUM
25
ROCHE

5 mg   10 mg   25 mg

chlordiazepoxide HCl   Roche

LITHOBID®

300 mg

lithium carbonate   CIBA

†ELDEPRYL®

5 mg

selegiline HCl
Somerset Pharmaceuticals

†HALDOL® Decanoate

1mL ampul
haloperidol decanoate
McNeil Pharmaceutical

†LOXITANE®

Lederle
LT   5 mg

5 mg   10 mg

25 mg   50 mg

loxapine succinate   Lederle

ENDEP®

10 mg   25 mg

50 mg   75 mg
100 mg   150 mg

amitriptyline   Roche

LUDIOMIL®

25 mg   50 mg   75 mg

maprotiline hydrochloride   CIBA

KEMADRIN®

5 mg

procyclidine hydrochloride
Burroughs Wellcome

†ESKALITH®

300 mg

lithium carbonate
SmithKline Beecham

KLONOPIN™

0.5 mg   1 mg   2 mg
clonazepam   Roche

MARPLAN®

10 mg

isocarboxazid   Roche

WILLIAMS AND WILKINS©

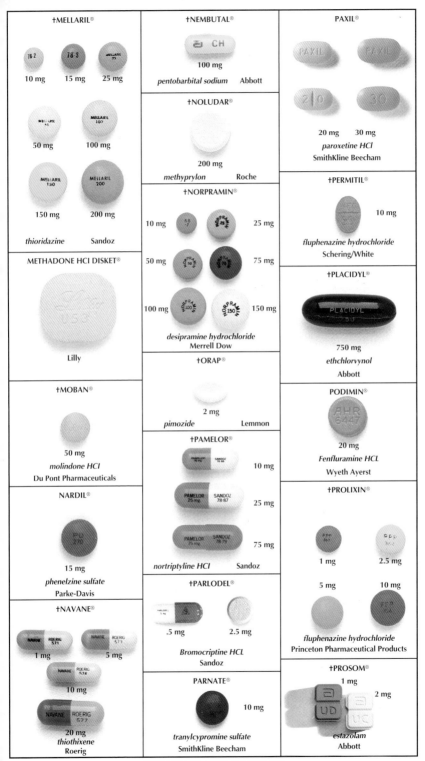

†MELLARIL®

78-2   78-3   MELLARIL 25

10 mg   15 mg   25 mg

MELLARIL 50   MELLARIL 100

50 mg   100 mg

MELLARIL 150   MELLARIL 200

150 mg   200 mg

thioridazine   Sandoz

METHADONE HCl DISKET®

U53

Lilly

†MOBAN®

50 mg

molindone HCl
Du Pont Pharmaceuticals

NARDIL®

P-D 270

15 mg

phenelzine sulfate
Parke-Davis

†NAVANE®

NAVANE ROERIG 571   NAVANE ROERIG 573

1 mg   5 mg

NAVANE ROERIG 574

10 mg

NAVANE ROERIG 577

20 mg
thiothixene
Roerig

†NEMBUTAL®

CH

100 mg

pentobarbital sodium   Abbott

†NOLUDAR®

200 mg

methyprylon   Roche

†NORPRAMIN®

10 mg   68-7   25 mg

50 mg   NORPRAMIN 50   NORPRAMIN 75   75 mg

100 mg   NORPRAMIN 100   NORPRAMIN 150   150 mg

desipramine hydrochloride
Merrell Dow

†ORAP®

2 mg

pimozide   Lemmon

†PAMELOR®

PAMELOR 10 mg   SANDOZ 78-86   10 mg

PAMELOR 25 mg   SANDOZ 78-87   25 mg

PAMELOR 75 mg   SANDOZ 78-79   75 mg

nortriptyline HCl   Sandoz

†PARLODEL®

PARLODEL 1 mg   2.5 mg

.5 mg   2.5 mg

Bromocriptine HCL
Sandoz

PARNATE®

SKF 10 mg

tranylcypromine sulfate
SmithKline Beecham

PAXIL®

PAXIL   PAXIL

2 | 0   30

20 mg   30 mg

paroxetine HCl
SmithKline Beecham

†PERMITIL®

PPP 3   10 mg

fluphenazine hydrochloride
Schering/White

†PLACIDYL®

PLACIDYL 750

750 mg

ethchlorvynol
Abbott

PODIMIN®

AHR 6447

20 mg

Fenfluramine HCL
Wyeth Ayerst

†PROLIXIN®

PPP 861   PPP 862

1 mg   2.5 mg

5 mg   PPP 864   10 mg

fluphenazine hydrochloride
Princeton Pharmaceutical Products

†PROSOM®

1 mg

2 mg

a UD   a UC

estazolam
Abbott

WILLIAMS AND WILKINS©

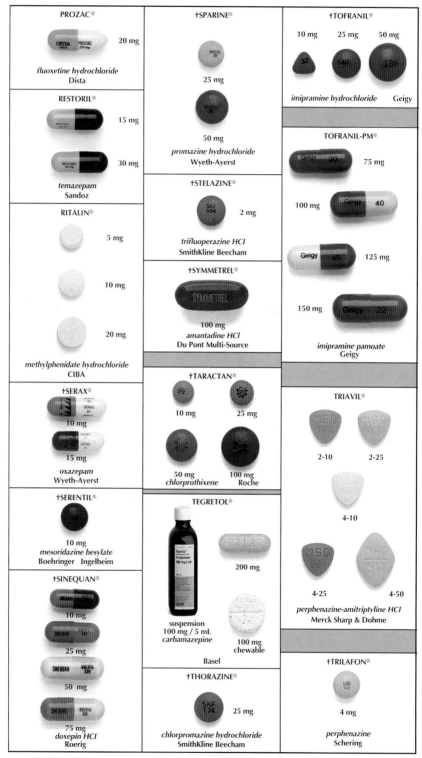

PROZAC®
20 mg
fluoxetine hydrochloride
Dista

RESTORIL®
15 mg
30 mg
temazepam
Sandoz

RITALIN®
5 mg
10 mg
20 mg
methylphenidate hydrochloride
CIBA

†SERAX®
10 mg
15 mg
oxazepam
Wyeth-Ayerst

†SERENTIL®
10 mg
mesoridazine besylate
Boehringer Ingelheim

†SINEQUAN®
10 mg
25 mg
50 mg
75 mg
doxepin HCl
Roerig

†SPARINE®
25 mg
50 mg
promazine hydrochloride
Wyeth-Ayerst

†STELAZINE®
2 mg
trifluoperazine HCl
SmithKline Beecham

†SYMMETREL®
SYMMETREL
100 mg
amantadine HCl
Du Pont Multi-Source

†TARACTAN®
10 mg   25 mg
50 mg   100 mg
chlorprothixene   Roche

TEGRETOL®
200 mg
suspension
100 mg / 5 mL
carbamazepine
100 mg
chewable
Basel

†THORAZINE®
25 mg
chlorpromazine hydrochloride
SmithKline Beecham

†TOFRANIL®
10 mg   25 mg   50 mg
imipramine hydrochloride   Geigy

TOFRANIL-PM®
75 mg
100 mg
125 mg
150 mg
imipramine pamoate
Geigy

TRIAVIL®
2-10   2-25
4-10
4-25   4-50
perphenazine-amitriptyline HCl
Merck Sharp & Dohme

†TRILAFON®
4 mg
perphenazine
Schering

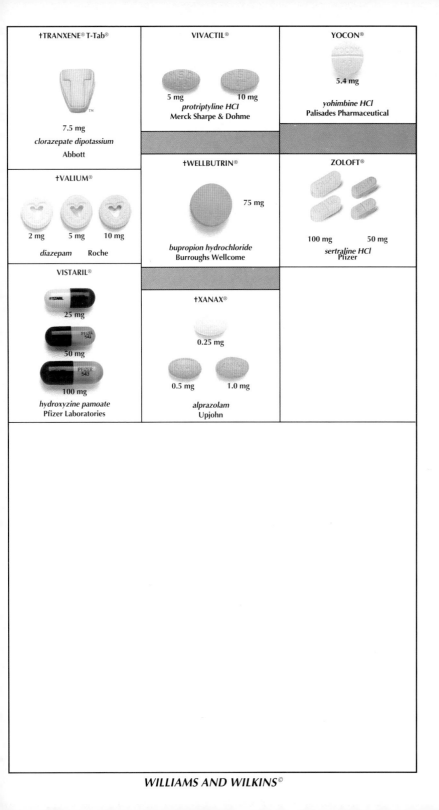

†TRANXENE® T-Tab®

7.5 mg

clorazepate dipotassium
Abbott

†VALIUM®

2 mg   5 mg   10 mg

diazepam   Roche

VISTARIL®

25 mg

50 mg

100 mg

hydroxyzine pamoate
Pfizer Laboratories

VIVACTIL®

5 mg   10 mg

protriptyline HCl
Merck Sharpe & Dohme

†WELLBUTRIN®

75 mg

bupropion hydrochloride
Burroughs Wellcome

†XANAX®

0.25 mg

0.5 mg   1.0 mg

alprazolam
Upjohn

YOCON®

5.4 mg

yohimbine HCl
Palisades Pharmaceutical

ZOLOFT®

100 mg   50 mg

sertraline HCl
Pfizer

POCKET
HANDBOOK
OF
PSYCHIATRIC
DRUG TREATMENT

SENIOR CONTRIBUTING EDITOR

ROBERT CANCRO, M.D., MED.D.SC.

Professor and Chairman, Department of Psychiatry,
New York University School of Medicine;
Director, Department of Psychiatry, Tisch Hospital
of the New York University
Medical Center, New York, New York;
Director, Nathan S. Kline Institute for
Psychiatric Research, Orangeburg, New York

CONTRIBUTING EDITOR

NORMAN SUSSMAN, M.D.

Clinical Associate Professor of Psychiatry,
New York University School of Medicine;
Director of Psychiatry Residency Training,
New York University School of Medicine;
Assistant Attending Psychiatrist, Tisch Hospital
of the New York University Medical Center;
Attending Psychiatrist, Bellevue Hospital, New York, New York

POCKET HANDBOOK OF PSYCHIATRIC DRUG TREATMENT

Harold I. Kaplan, M.D.

Professor of Psychiatry, New York University School of Medicine;
Attending Psychiatrist, Tisch Hospital of the New York
University Medical Center;
Attending Psychiatrist, Bellevue Hospital, New York, New York

Benjamin J. Sadock, M.D.

Professor of Psychiatry and Vice-Chairman, New York University
School of Medicine;
Attending Psychiatrist, Tisch Hospital of the New York
University Medical Center;
Attending Psychiatrist, Bellevue Hospital, New York, New York

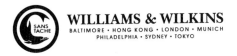

WILLIAMS & WILKINS
BALTIMORE · HONG KONG · LONDON · MUNICH
PHILADELPHIA · SYDNEY · TOKYO

Editor: David Retford
Managing Editor: Carol L. Eckhart
Copy Editors: Joan Welsh, S. Gillian Casey
Designer: Norman W. Och
Illustration Planner: Bob Och
Production Coordinator: Barbara Felton
Project Editor: Lynda Abrams Zittell, M.A.

Notice. The indications and dosages of all drugs in this book have been recommended in the medical literature and conform to the practices of the general medical community. The medications described do not necessarily have specific approval by the Food and Drug Administration for use in the diseases and dosages for which they are recommended. The package insert for each drug should be consulted for use and dosage as approved by the FDA. Because standards for usage change, it is advisable to keep abreast of revised recommendations, particularly those concerning new drugs.

Printed in the United States of America

Library of Congress Cataloging-in-Publication Data

Kaplan, Harold I.
    Pocket handbook of psychiatric drug treatment / Harold I. Kaplan, Benjamin J. Sadock.
        p.   cm.
    Includes bibliographical references and index.
    ISBN 0-683-04538-5
    1. Psychopharmacology—Handbooks, manuals, etc. 2. Psychotropic drugs—Handbooks, manuals, etc. I. Sadock, Benjamin J. II. Title.
    [DNLM: 1. Mental Disorders—drug therapy—handbooks.
    2. Psychopharmacology—handbooks.   WM 39 K17p]
RC483.K36   1993
616.89'18—dc20
DNLM/DLC
for Library of Congress   92-22846
                                                                                CIP

                                                      93   94   95   96
                                2   3   4   5   6   7   8   9   10

Dedicated
to our wives,
Nancy Barrett Kaplan
and
Virginia Alcott Sadock,
without whose help and sacrifice
this book would not have been possible

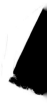

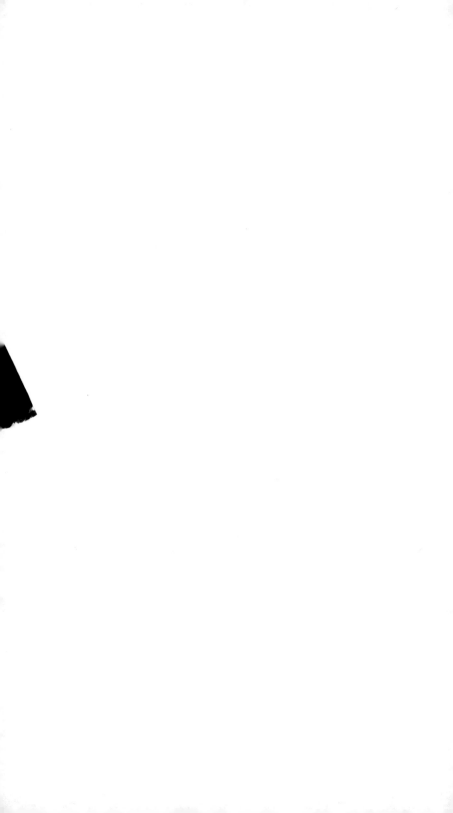

Preface

Pocket Handbook of Psychiatric Drug Treatment has been written for practicing psychiatrists, psychiatric residents, medical students, and mental health professionals who require a handy reference for the use of drugs in the treatment of psychiatric disorders in adults and children. It is especially useful for nonpsychiatric physicians, who often provide treatment for patients with emotional disturbances and who, in practice, dispense psychiatric drugs more often than do psychiatrists.

Pocket Handbook of Psychiatric Drug Treatment is one in a series of concise, practical guides dealing with specific issues in the treatment of patients with psychiatric disorders. This book covers the entire spectrum of drug therapy—also known as pharmacotherapy and psychopharmacology—which is the fastest growing field in psychiatry today.

The handbook is a companion to our encyclopedic fifth edition of *Comprehensive Textbook of Psychiatry* and to the sixth edition of *Synopsis of Psychiatry*, for which we were both editors and authors. Much of the content in this handbook derives from the material in those books; however, the handbook is more current than those books, since it covers drugs that were introduced after the publication of those books two years ago. It also contains new material that has appeared in the recent clinical literature.

ORGANIZATION

An introductory section describes the basic principles that govern the use of drugs in general and psychiatric drugs in particular. The issues covered include such topics as the choice of drug; combination drugs; patient education; the use of drugs in children, adults, geriatric patients, pregnant and nursing women, and medically ill patients; informed consent; the treatment of common adverse effects; and drug-drug interactions.

New Classification

The classification of the drugs presented here is a new approach that we first introduced in the sixth edition of *Synopsis of Psychiatry*. Drugs are classified according to their pharmacological activity and mechanism of action, rather than under the traditional format of antidepressants, antimanics, antipsychotics, and anxiolytics. The reasons for this arrangement are several: Many of the so-called antidepressant drugs are also used to treat anxiety; some anxiolytics are used as adjuncts in treating psychosis; drugs from all four categories are used to treat other clinical disorders, such as eating disorders, panic disorders, and impulse control disorders; and drugs such as carbamazapine (Tegretol) and propranolol (Inderal), among others, can effectively treat a variety of psychiatric disorders but do not fit into the traditional format. As an example of the new classification, the antipsychotics are discussed under two listings: (1) dopamine receptor antagonists, which include such drugs as chlorpromazine (Thorazine) and haloperidol (Haldol), and

(2) clozapine (Clozaril), which is listed alone because of its unique pharmacological qualities.

Alphabetized Drug Listing

Drugs are listed alphabetically for easy access, and each section provides a wealth of data about the drug. The data include (1) the drug's name and molecular structure; (2) its types of preparations and dosages; (3) its pharmacological actions, including its pharmacokinetics and pharmacodynamics; (4) the indications for its use and its clinical applications; (5) its use in children, elderly persons, and pregnant and nursing women; (6) its side effects and its adverse and allergic reactions; and (7) drug-drug interactions.

SPECIAL SECTIONS

Emergencies

We have included a special section in tabular form (Chapter 36) that lists the toxic and lethal doses of each drug, the signs and symptoms of overdose, and emergency management measures.

Indications

On the inside cover of the handbook and in Table 1–2 of the text, a chart of the drugs and the classes of drugs used in the treatment of major psychiatric disorders is found. This chart indicates the various medications that are used to treat a particular disorder and is completely up-to-date.

Combined Therapy

In many cases, pharmacotherapy is combined with psychotherapy to achieve maximum therapeutic results. The two therapies interact in that pharmacotherapy is oriented toward reducing the signs and symptoms of a disorder and psychotherapy is oriented toward understanding the causes of the signs and symptoms. A chapter written for this handbook discusses the use of the combined method in a succinct, thorough manner.

Laboratory Tests

A special section on laboratory tests is included to aid the clinician in understanding the relation of psychopharmacological agents and their effects on laboratory values and in monitoring baseline values necessary for effective drug treatment.

Investigational Drugs

A chapter covering drugs that are currently in various phases of investigation is included. It helps orient the reader to some of the new developments in the field of pharmacotherapy.

Illustrated Drug Identification Guide

As a unique aspect of this book, colored plates of all the major drugs used in psychiatry indicate both the forms in which they are commercially available and their dose ranges to help the physician recognize and prescribe the medications. The plates are completely up-to-date.

References

Each chapter ends with a list of several of the most current references about the drug, including reviews of the literature for the reader who requires more information than can be provided in a brief guide such as this book. The handbook cannot substitute for a major textbook; it is meant to serve as an easily accessible reference for busy doctors in training and for clinical practitioners.

ACKNOWLEDGMENTS

We thank Norman Sussman, M.D., Clinical Associate Professor of Psychiatry at New York University Medical Center, who served as Contributing Editor. He was most helpful in providing us with the most current information about the recently introduced pharmacological agents. Eugene Rubin, M.D., Fellow in Academic Psychiatry at New York University Medical Center, and Joseph Belanoff, M.D., were also of help.

Lynda Abrams Zittell, M.A., served as project editor, as she has for many of our other publications and for which we are deeply appreciative. She carries out her complex tasks with skill and enthusiasm. Laura Marino processed the manuscript, and we thank her for her prodigious efforts. We especially thank Joan Welsh, who is an outstanding, highly skilled editor and a much-valued friend. We also thank Dorice Horne, Head of Educational Services of the Frederick L. Ehrman Medical Library of the New York University School of Medicine, for her valuable assistance in this project.

Virginia Sadock, M.D., Clinical Professor of Psychiatry and Director of Graduate Education in Human Sexuality at New York University Medical Center, deserves special mention and thanks for her help in every aspect of this book, particularly in the area of drug effects on sexual behavior.

The authors also acknowledge Jack Grebb, M.D., for his outstanding contributions to the contents of the book. He served as Assistant to the Authors of the sixth edition of *Synopsis of Psychiatry* and is a distinguished educator, researcher, and clinician with special expertise in the area of psychopharmacology.

Finally, we thank Robert Cancro, M.D., Professor and Chairman of the Department of Psychiatry at New York University Medical Center, who served as Senior Contributing Editor. We are deeply grateful for the inspiration and the support he offers us in all our academic endeavors.

Harold I. Kaplan, M.D.
Benjamin J. Sadock, M.D.

October 1, 1992
New York University Medical Center
New York, New York

Contents

1

Basic Principles of Psychopharmacology

Drug therapy and other organic treatments of psychiatric disorders may be defined as an attempt to modify or correct pathological behaviors, thoughts, or moods by chemical or other physical means. The relations between, on the one hand, the physical state of the brain and, on the other hand, its functional manifestations (behaviors, thoughts, and moods) are highly complex, imperfectly understood, and at the frontier of biological knowledge. However, the various parameters of normal and abnormal behavior—such as perception, affect, and cognition—may be profoundly affected by physical changes in the central nervous system (for example, cerebrovascular disorders, epilepsy, legal and illicit drugs).

Because of incomplete knowledge regarding the brain and the disorders that affect it, the drug treatment of psychiatric disorders is somewhat empirical. Nevertheless, many organic therapies have proved to be highly effective and constitute the treatment of choice for certain psychopathological conditions. As such, organic therapies form a key part of the armamentarium for the treatment of psychiatric disorders.

The practice of pharmacotherapy in psychiatry should not be oversimplified—for example, a one diagnosis-one pill approach. Many variables impinge on the practice of pharmacotherapy, including drug selection, prescription, administration, psychodynamic meaning to the patient, and family and environmental influences. Some patients may view a drug as a panacea, and other patients may view a drug as an assault. The nursing staff and relatives, as well as the patient, must be instructed regarding the reasons, the expected benefits, and the potential risks of pharmacotherapy. In addition, the clinician often finds it useful to explain the theoretical basis for pharmacotherapy to the patient, the patient's caretakers, and psychiatric staff members. Moreover, the theoretical biases of the treating psychiatrist are critical to the success of drug treatment, since the psychiatrist prescribes pharmacotherapeutic drugs as a function of his or her theoretical beliefs about such treatments.

Drugs must be used in effective dosages for sufficient time periods, as determined by previous clinical investigations and personal experience. Subtherapeutic doses and incomplete trials should not be given to a patient simply because the psychiatrist is excessively concerned about the development of adverse effects. The prescription of drugs for psychiatric disorders must be made by a qualified practitioner and requires continuous clinical observation. Treatment response and the emergence of adverse effects must be monitored closely. The dosage of the drug should be adjusted accordingly, and appropriate treatments for emergent adverse effects must be instituted as quickly as possible.

Because the pharmacotherapy of psychiatric disorders is one of the most rapidly evolving areas in clinical medicine, any practitioner who prescribes such drugs must remain current with the research literature. The key areas for regular update are the emergence of new agents (for example, sertraline [Zoloft]), the demonstration of new indications for existing agents (for example, valproic acid [Depakene]), the clinical usefulness of plasma concentrations, and the identification and treatment of drug-related adverse events.

TERMINOLOGY

The numerous pharmacological agents used to treat psychiatric disorders are referred to by three general terms that are used interchangeably: psychotropic drugs, psychoactive drugs, and psychotherapeutic drugs. Traditionally, those agents were divided into four categories: (1) antipsychotic or neuroleptic drugs used to treat psychosis, (2) antidepressant drugs used to treat depression, (3) antimanic drugs used to treat bipolar disorder, and (4) antianxiety or anxiolytic drugs used to treat anxious states. That division, however, is less valid now than it was in the past for the following reasons: (1) Many antidepressant drugs are used to treat anxiety, and some antianxiety drugs are used adjunctively to treat psychosis. (2) Drugs from all four categories are used to treat other clinical disorders, such as eating disorders, panic disorders, and impulse control disorders. (3) Drugs such as clonidine (Catapres), propranolol (Inderal), and verapamil (Isoptin, Calan) can effectively treat a variety of psychiatric disorders and do not fit easily into the aforementioned classification of drugs. (4) Some descriptive psychopharmacological terms overlap in meaning. For example, anxiolytics decrease anxiety, sedatives produce a calming or relaxing effect, and hypnotics produce sleep. However, most anxiolytics function as sedatives and at high doses can be used as hypnotics, and all hypnotics at low doses can be used for daytime sedation.

For these reasons this book uses a classification in which each drug is discussed according to its pharmacological category. Each drug is described in terms of its pharmacological actions, including pharmacodynamics and pharmacokinetics. Indications, contraindications, drug-drug interactions, and adverse side effects are also discussed.

GUIDE TO USE

Table 1–1 lists the psychotherapeutic drugs according to the generic name, the trade name, and the chapter title and number in which it is discussed. Table 1–2 lists the major drugs used in the various psychiatric disorders.

HISTORY

Organic therapies such as electroconvulsive therapy (ECT) (pioneered by Ugo Cerletti and Lucio Bini), insulin coma therapy (developed by Manfred Sakel), and psychosurgery (introduced by António Egas Moniz) all began in the first third of the 20th century and heralded the biological revolution in psychiatry. In 1917 Julius von Wagner-Jauregg introduced malaria toxin to treat syphilis and is the only psychiatrist to have won a Nobel prize.

In the second half of the 20th century, chemotherapy as a treatment for mental illness became a major field of research and practice. Almost immediately after the introduction of chlorpromazine (Thorazine) in the early 1950s,

Table 1–1
Index to Book*

Generic Name	Trade Name	Chapter Title	Chapter Number
Acetophenazine	Tindal	Dopamine Receptor Antagonists	19
Alprazolam	Xanax	Benzodiazepines	7
Amantadine	Symmetrel	Amantadine	3
Amitriptyline	Endep. Elavil	Tricyclics and Tetracyclics	29
Amobarbital	Amytal	Barbiturates and Other Similarly Acting Drugs	6
Amoxapine	Asendin	Tricyclics and Tetracyclics	29
Atenolol	Tenoretic, Tenormin	β-Adrenergic Receptor Antagonists	2
Benztropine	Cogentin, Tremin	Anticholinergics	4
Biperiden	Akineton	Anticholinergics	4
Bromocriptine	Parlodel	Bromocriptine	8
Bupropion	Wellbutrin	Bupropion	9
Buspirone	BuSpar	Buspirone	10
Butabarbital	Butisol	Barbiturates and Other Similarly Acting Drugs	6
Butaperazine	Repoise	Dopamine Receptor Antagonists	19
Carbamazepine	Tegretol	Carbamazepine	12
Carisoprodol	Soma	Barbiturates and Other Similarly Acting Drugs	6
Carphenazine	Proketazine	Dopamine Receptor Antagonists	19
Chloral hydrate	Noctec	Chloral Hydrate	13
Chlordiazepoxide	Librium	Benzodiazepines	7
Chlorpromazine	Thorazine	Dopamine Receptor Antagonists	19
Chlorprothixene	Taractan	Dopamine Receptor Antagonists	19
Clomipramine	Anafranil	Tricyclics and Tetracyclics	29
Clonazepam	Klonopin	Benzodiazepines	7
Clonidine	Catapres	Clonidine	14
Clorazepate	Tranxene	Benzodiazepines	7
Clozapine	Clozaril	Clozapine	15
Cyproheptadine	Periactin	Antihistamines	5
Dantrolene	Dantrium	Dantrolene	16
Desipramine	Norpramin, Pertofrane	Tricyclics and Tetracyclics	29
Dextroamphetamine	Dexedrine	Sympathomimetics	26
Diazepam	Valium	Benzodiazepines	7
Diltiazem	Cardizem	Calcium Channel Inhibitors	11
Diphenhydramine	Benadryl	Antihistamines	5
Disulfiram	Antabuse	Disulfiram	17
L-Dopa	Larodopa	L-Dopa	18
Doxepin	Adapin, Sinequan	Tricyclics and Tetracyclics	29
Droperidol	Inapsine	Dopamine Receptor Antagonists	19
Estazolam	ProSom	Benzodiazepines	7
Ethchlorvynol	Placidyl	Barbiturates and Other Similarly Acting Drugs	6
Ethinamate	Valmid	Barbiturates and Other Similarly Acting Drugs	6
Ethopropazine	Parsidol	Anticholinergics	4
Fenfluramine	Pondimin	Fenfluramine	20
Flumazenil	Mazicon	Flumazenil	21
Fluoxetine	Prozac	Serotonin-Specific Reuptake Inhibitors	25
Fluphenazine	Permitil. Prolixin	Dopamine Receptor Antagonists	19
Flurazepam	Dalmane	Benzodiazepines	7
Fluvoxamine	Not available	Serotonin-Specific Reuptake Inhibitors	25
Glutethimide	Doriden	Barbiturates and Other Similarly Acting Drugs	6
Halazepam	Paxipam	Benzodiazepines	7
Haloperidol	Haldol	Dopamine Receptor Antagonists	19
Hydroxyzine	Atarax, Vistaril	Antihistamines	5
Imipramine	Tofranil	Tricyclics and Tetracyclics	29
Isocarboxazid	Marplan	Monoamine Oxidase Inhibitors	24
Lithium	Eskalith, Lithobid	Lithium	22
Lorazepam	Ativan	Benzodiazepines	7
Loxapine	Loxitane	Dopamine Receptor Antagonists	19
Maprotiline	Ludiomil	Tricyclics and Tetracyclics	29
Mephobarbital	Mebaral	Barbiturates and Other Similarly Acting Drugs	6
Meprobamate	Miltown, Equanil	Barbiturates and Other Similarly Acting Drugs	6
Mesoridazine	Serentil	Dopamine Receptor Antagonists	19
Methadone	Dolophine	Methadone	23
Methylphenidate	Ritalin	Sympathomimetics	26

(Continued)

Table 1–1
Index to Book (Continued)

*For antipsychotics, see dopamine receptor antagonists and clozapine.

psychotherapeutic drugs became a mainstay of psychiatric treatment, particularly for the seriously mentally ill patients.

In 1949 the Australian psychiatrist John Cade described the treatment of manic excitement with lithium. While conducting animal experiments, Cade had somewhat incidentally noted that lithium carbonate made the animals lethargic, thus prompting him to administer the drug to several agitated psychiatric patients.

In 1950 Charpentier synthesized chlorpromazine (an aliphatic phenothiazine antipsychotic) in an attempt to develop an antihistaminergic drug that would serve as an adjuvant in anesthesia. Laborit reported the ability of the

Table 1–2
Drugs and Classes of Drugs Used in the Treatment of Major Psychiatric Disorders

Major Psychiatric Disorder	Chapter Number
Aggression (see Episodic dyscontrol disorder)	
Akathisia (see Drug-induced extrapyramidal movement disorders)	
Alcohol-related disorders	
β-Adrenergic receptor antagonists	2
Benzodiazepines	7
Carbamazepine	12
Lithium	22
Anorexia nervosa (see Eating disorders)	
Anxiety (also see specific anxiety disorder)	
Antihistamines	5
Barbiturates and other similarly acting drugs	6
Benzodiazepines	7
Bipolar disorder	
Benzodiazepines (especially clonazepam)	7
Calcium channel inhibitors	11
Carbamazepine	12
Dopamine receptor antagonists	19
Lithium	22
L-Tryptophan	30
Valproic acid	31
Bulimia nervosa (see Eating disorders)	
Cyclothymia (see Bipolar disorder)	
Delusional disorder (see Schizophrenia)	
Depressive disorder	
Benzodiazepines (especially alprazolam)	7
Bupropion	9
Carbamazepine	12
Lithium	22
Monoamine oxidase inhibitors	24
Serotonin-specific reuptake inhibitors	25
Sympathomimetics	26
Thyroid hormones	27
Trazodone	28
Tricyclic and tetracyclic antidepressants	29
L-Tryptophan	30
Drug-induced extrapyramidal movement disorders	
β-Adrenergic receptor antagonists	2
Amantadine	3
Anticholinergics	4
Antihistamines	5
Benzodiazepines	7
Dysthymia (see Depressive disorder)	
Dystonias (see Drug-induced extrapyramidal movement disorders)	
Eating disorders	
Lithium	22
Monoamine oxidase inhibitors	24
Serotonin-specific reuptake inhibitors	25
Tricyclic and tetracyclic antidepressants	29
Episodic dyscontrol disorder	
β-Adrenergic receptor antagonists	2
Buspirone	10
Carbamazepine	12
Dopamine receptor antagonists	19
Lithium	22
Valproic acid	31
Generalized anxiety disorder	
β-Adrenergic receptor antagonists	2
Barbiturates and other similarly acting drugs	6
Benzodiazepines	7
Buspirone	10
Tricyclic and tetracyclic antidepressants	29

(Continued)

Table 1–2
Drugs and Classes of Drugs Used in the Treatment of Major Psychiatric Disorders (Continued)

Major Psychiatric Disorder	Chapter Number
Obsessive-compulsive disorder	
Serotonin-specific reuptake inhibitors	25
Tricyclic and tetracyclic antidepressants (especially clomipramine)	29
Opiate-related disorders	
Clonidine	14
Methadone	23
Panic disorder (with and without agoraphobia)	
β-Adrenergic receptor antagonists	2
Benzodiazepines (especially alprazolam and clonazepam)	7
Monoamine oxidase inhibitors	24
Serotonin-specific reuptake inhibitors	25
Tricyclic and tetracyclic antidepressants	29
Parkinsonism (see Drug-induced extrapyramidal movement disorders)	
Phobias (see also Panic disorder)	
β-Adrenergic receptor antagonists	2
Benzodiazepines	7
Posttraumatic stress disorder	
Monoamine oxidase inhibitors	24
Serotonin-specific reuptake inhibitors	25
Tricyclic and tetracyclic antidepressants	29
Psychosis (see Schizophrenia)	
Rabbit syndrome (see Drug-induced extrapyramidal movement disorders)	
Schizoaffective disorder (see Depressive disorder, Bipolar disorder, and Schizophrenia)	
Schizophrenia	
Benzodiazepines	7
Carbamazepine	12
Clozapine	15
Dopamine receptor antagonists	19
Lithium	22
Sleep disorders	
Antihistamines	5
Barbiturates and other similarly acting drugs	6
Benzodiazepines	7
Chloral hydrate	13
Sympathomimetics	26
L-Tryptophan	30
Violence (see Episodic dyscontrol disorder)	

drug to induce an "artificial hibernation." Reports by Paraire and Sigwald, Delay and Deniker, and Lehmann and Hanrahan described the effectiveness of chlorpromazine in treating severe agitation and psychosis. Chlorpromazine was quickly introduced into American psychiatry, and many similarly effective drugs have since been synthesized, including haloperidol (Haldol) (a butyrophenone antipsychotic) in 1958 by Janssen.

Imipramine (Tofranil) (a tricyclic antidepressant) is structurally related to the phenothiazine antipsychotics. While carrying out clinical research on chlorpromazinelike drugs, Thomas Kuhn found that, although imipramine was not very effective in reducing agitation, it did seem to reduce depression in some patients. The introduction of monoamine oxidase inhibitors (MAOIs) to treat depression evolved from the observation that the antituberculosis agent iproniazid had mood-elevating effects in some patients. In 1958 Nathan Kline was one of the first investigators to report the efficacy of MAOI treatment in depressed psychiatric patients.

By 1960, with the introduction of chlordiazepoxide (Librium) (a benzodiazepine antianxiety agent synthesized by Sternbach at the Roche laboratories in the late 1950s), the psychiatric armamentarium of drugs included antipsychotics (for example, chlorpromazine and haloperidol), tricyclics (for example, imipramine), and MAOIs (for example, iproniazid [Marsalid]), antidepressants, an antimanic agent (lithium [Eskalith]), and antianxiety agents (for example, the benzodiazepines in addition to the older drugs, such as the barbiturates). The next 30 years were devoted primarily to clinical studies demonstrating the efficacy of those drugs and to the development of related compounds in each category. The efficacy of each class of drugs for treating relatively specific psychiatric syndromes and for elucidating their pharmacodynamic effects provided the impetus to develop the various neurotransmitter hypotheses of mental disorders (for example, the dopamine hypothesis of schizophrenia, the monoamine hypothesis of mood disorders).

Since 1960 the major additions to the psychotherapeutic drugs have been the anticonvulsants, particularly carbamazepine (Tegretol) and valproic acid, which are effective in treating some patients with bipolar disorder. Buspirone (BuSpar), a nonbenzodiazepine anxiolytic, was introduced for clinical use in America in 1986. A number of new antidepressant and antiobsessive-compulsive drugs (fluoxetine [Prozac], bupropion [Wellbutrin], trazodone [Desyrel], clomipramine [Anafranil], sertraline [Zoloft]) and one new antipsychotic (clozapine [Clozaril]) have also been marketed. It is expected that the burgeoning knowledge of basic neuroscience and neuropharmacology will lead to the development of many new psychotherapeutic drugs during the next decade.

PHARMACOLOGICAL ACTIONS

Pharmacokinetic interactions describe how the body handles a drug; pharmacodynamic interactions describe the effects of a drug on the body. In a parallel fashion pharmacokinetic drug interactions refer to plasma concentrations of drugs, and the pharmacodynamic drug interactions refer to receptor activities of drugs.

Pharmacokinetics

The principal divisions of pharmacokinetics are drug absorption, distribution, metabolism, and excretion.

Absorption. A psychotherapeutic drug must first reach the blood on its way to the brain, unless it is directly administered into the cerebrospinal fluid or the brain. Orally administered drugs must dissolve in the fluid of the gastrointestinal (GI) tract before the body can absorb them. Drug tablets can be designed to disintegrate either quickly or slowly, the absorption depending on the drug's concentration and lipid solubility and the GI tract's local pH, motility, and surface area. Depending on the drug's pK and the GI tract's pH, the drug may be present in an ionized form that limits its lipid solubility. If the pharmacokinetic absorption factors are favorable, the drug may reach therapeutic blood concentrations more quickly if it is administered intramuscularly. If a drug is coupled with an appropriate carrier molecule, intramuscular administration can sustain the drug's release over a long period of time. Some antipsychotic drugs are available in depot forms that allow the drug to be administered only once every one to four weeks. Even though intravenous administration is the quickest route to achieve therapeutic blood levels, it also carries the highest risk of sudden and life-threatening adverse effects.

Distribution.   Drugs can be freely dissolved in the blood plasma, bound to dissolved plasma proteins (primarily albumin), or dissolved within the blood cells. If a drug is bound too tightly to plasma proteins, it may have to be metabolized and excreted before it can leave the bloodstream, thus greatly reducing the amount of active drug reaching the brain. The lithium ion is an example of a water-soluble drug that is not bound to plasma proteins. The distribution of a drug to the brain is determined by the blood-brain barrier, the brain's regional blood flow, and the drug's affinity with its receptors in the brain. Both high blood flow and affinity favor the distribution of the drug to the brain. Drugs may also reach the brain after passively diffusing into the cerebrospinal fluid from the bloodstream. The volume of distribution is a measure of the apparent space in the body available to contain the drug. The volume of distribution can also vary with the patient's age, sex, and disease state.

Metabolism and excretion.   Metabolism is somewhat synonymous with the term "biotransformation." The four major metabolic routes for drugs are oxidation, reduction, hydrolysis, and conjugation. Although the usual result of metabolism is to produce inactive metabolites that are more readily excreted than is the parent compound, many examples of active metabolites are produced from psychoactive drugs. The liver is the principal site of metabolism, and bile, feces, and urine are the major routes of excretion. Psychoactive drugs are also excreted in sweat, saliva, tears, and milk; therefore, mothers who are taking psychotherapeutic drugs should not breast-feed their children. Disease states or coadministered drugs that affect the ability of the liver or the kidneys to metabolize and eliminate drugs can both raise and lower the blood concentrations of a psychoactive drug.

Four important concepts regarding metabolism and excretion are time of peak plasma level, half-life, first pass effect, and clearance. The time between the administration of a drug and the appearance of peak concentrations of the drug in plasma varies primarily according to the route of administration and absorption. A drug's half-life is defined as the amount of time it takes for one half of a drug's peak plasma level to be metabolized and excreted from the body. A general guideline is that, if a drug is administered repeatedly in doses separated by time intervals shorter than its half-life, the drug will reach 97 percent of its steady-state plasma concentrations in a time equal to five times its half-life. The first pass effect refers to the extensive initial metabolism of some drugs within the portal circulation or liver, thereby reducing the amount of unmetabolized drug that reaches the systemic circulation. Clearance is a measure of the amount of drug excreted in each unit of time. If some disease process or other drug interferes with the clearance of a psychoactive drug, the drug may reach toxic levels.

Pharmacodynamics

The major pharmacodynamic considerations include receptor mechanism; the dose-response curve; the therapeutic index; and the development of tolerance, dependence, and withdrawal phenomena. The receptor for a drug can be defined generally as the cellular component that binds to the drug and initiates the drug's pharmacodynamic effects. A drug can be an agonist for its receptor, thereby stimulating a physiological effect; conversely, a drug can be an antagonist for the receptor, most often by blocking the receptor so that an endogenous agonist cannot

Examples of Dose-Response Curves

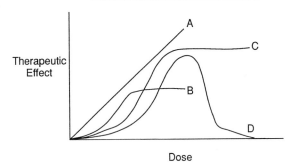

Dose

Figure 1–1. These dose-response curves plot the therapeutic effect as a function of increasing dose, often calculated as the log of the dose. Drug A has a linear dose response, drugs B and C have sigmoidal curves, and drug D has a curvilinear dose-response curve. Although smaller doses of drug B are more potent than are equal doses of drug C, drug C has a higher maximum efficacy than does drug B. Drug D has a therapeutic window, such that both low and high doses are less effective than are midrange doses.

affect the receptor. The receptor site for most psychotherapeutic drugs is also a receptor site for an endogenous neurotransmitter. For example, the primary receptor site for chlorpromazine is the dopamine receptor. However, for other psychotherapeutic drugs that may not be the case. The receptor for lithium may be the enzyme inositol-l-phosphatase, and the receptor for verapamil (Calan) (a calcium channel inhibitor) is a calcium channel.

The dose-response curve plots the drug concentration against the effects of the drug (Figure 1–1). The potency of a drug refers to the relative dose required to achieve a certain effect. Haloperidol, for example, is more potent than is chlorpromazine because approximately 5 mg of haloperidol is required to achieve the same therapeutic effect as 100 mg of chlorpromazine. Both haloperidol and chlorpromazine, however, are equal in their clinical efficacy—that is, the maximum clinical response achievable by the administration of a drug.

The side effects of most drugs are often a direct result of their primary pharmacodynamic effects and are better conceptualized as adverse effects. The therapeutic index is a relative measure of a drug's toxicity or safety. It is defined as the ratio of the median toxic dose (TD_{50}) to the median effective dose (ED_{50}). The TD_{50} is the dose at which 50 percent of patients experience toxic effects, and the ED_{50} is the dose at which 50 percent of patients have a therapeutic effect. Haloperidol, for example, has a very high therapeutic index, as evidenced by the wide range of doses in which it is prescribed. Conversely, lithium has a very low therapeutic index, thereby requiring careful monitoring of serum lithium levels when prescribing the drug. Both interindividual and intraindividual variation can be present in the response to a specific drug. An individual patient may be hyporeactive, normally reactive, or hyperreactive to a particular drug. For example, some patients with schizophrenia require 1 mg a day of haloperidol, others require a more typical 10 mg a day, and still others require 100 mg a day to achieve a therapeutic response. Idiosyncratic drug responses occur when a person experiences a particularly unusual effect from a drug. For example, some patients become quite agitated when given benzodiazepines, such as diazepam (Valium).

A person may become less responsive to a particular drug as it is administered over time, which is referred to as tolerance. The development of tolerance is associated with the appearance of physical dependence, which may be defined as the necessity to continue administering the drug to prevent the appearance of withdrawal symptoms.

CLINICAL GUIDELINES

The practice of clinical psychopharmacology requires skill as both a diagnostician and a psychotherapist, knowledge of the available drugs, and the ability to plan a pharmacotherapeutic regimen. The selection and the initiation of drug treatment should be based on the patient's past history, the patient's current clinical state, and the treatment plan. The psychiatrist should know the purpose or the goal of a drug trial, the length of time that the drug needs to be administered to assess its efficacy, the approach to be taken to reduce any adverse effects that may occur, alternative drug strategies should the current one fail, and whether long-term maintenance of the patient on the drug is indicated. In almost all cases the psychiatrist should explain the treatment plan to the patient and often to the family and other caretakers. The patient's reaction to and ideas about a proposed drug trial should be considered. However, if the psychiatrist believes that accommodating the patient's wishes would hinder treatment, that should be explained to the patient.

Choice of Drug

The first two steps in selecting drug treatment, the diagnosis and the identification of target symptoms, should be carried out when the patient has been in a drug-free state for one to two weeks. The drug-free state should include the absence of medications for sleep, such as hypnotics, as the quality of sleep can be both an important diagnostic guide and a target symptom. If a patient is hospitalized, however, insurance guidelines may make a drug-free period difficult or even impossible to obtain. Psychiatrists often evaluate symptomatic patients who are already receiving one or more psychoactive medications, and so it is usually necessary to wean the patient from the current medications and then to make an assessment. An exception to that practice occurs when a patient presents to the psychiatrist on a suboptimal regimen of an otherwise appropriate drug. In such cases the psychiatrist may decide to continue the drug at a higher dose to complete a full therapeutic trial.

From among the drugs appropriate to a particular diagnosis, the specific drug should be selected according to the patient's past history of drug response (compliance, therapeutic response, and adverse effects), the patient's family history of drug response, the profile of adverse effects for that drug with regard to a particular patient, and the psychiatrist's usual practice. If a drug has previously been effective in treating a patient or a family member, it should be used again unless there is some specific reason not to use the drug. A past history of severe adverse effects from a specific drug is a strong indicator that the patient would not be compliant with that drug regimen. It is unfortunate that patients and their families are often quite ignorant of what drugs have been used before, in what dosages, and for how long. That ignorance may reflect the tendency of psychiatrists not to explain drug trials to their patients, whereas psychiatrists should be encouraged to give their patients written records of drug trials for their personal medical records. A caveat to obtaining a past history of drug response from patients is that, because of their mental disorders, they may inaccurately report the effects of a previous drug trial. If possible, therefore, the patients' medical records should be obtained to confirm their reports. Most psychotherapeutic drugs of a single class have been demonstrated to be equally efficacious; however, the drugs do differ in their adverse effects on individual patients. A drug should be selected that minimally exacerbates any preexisting medical problems that a patient has.

Combination drugs.   Some combination drugs (Table 1–3) may increase the patient's compliance by simplifying the drug regimen. A problem with combination drugs, however, is that the clinician has less flexibility in adjusting the dosage of one of the components. That is, the use of combination drugs may cause two drugs to be administered when only one continues to be effective.

Nonapproved dosages and uses.   Under the federal Food, Drug, and Cosmetic (FDC) Act, the Food and Drug Administration (FDA) has authority to control the initial availability of a drug by approving only those new drugs that demonstrate both safety and effectiveness and then to ensure that the drug's proposed labeling is truthful and contains all pertinent information for the safe and effective use of that drug.

Before a new drug can be approved by the FDA, it must be studied in humans. For the drug ultimately to be approved for commercial use, the sponsor must justify the safety and the effectiveness of the drug by submitting a New Drug Application (NDA) to the FDA. The NDA is approved or disapproved, depending on the clinical data accumulated. For approval, the FDA requires that adequate tests be conducted showing that the drug "is safe for use under the conditions prescribed, recommended, or suggested." There must also be "substantial evidence that the drug will have the effect it purports under the conditions of use prescribed, recommended, or suggested in the proposed labeling." For additional information, see Chapter 35, "Investigational Drugs."

Use of FDA-approved drugs in private practice.   According to the Medical Liability Mutual Insurance Company (MLMIC), once a drug is approved for commercial use, the physician may, as part of the practice of medicine, lawfully prescribe a different dosage for a patient or otherwise vary the conditions of use from what is approved in the package labeling without notifying or obtaining the FDA's approval. Specifically, the FDC Act does not limit the manner in which a physician may use an approved drug. However, although physicians may treat patients with an approved drug for unapproved purposes—that is, indications not included on the drug's official labeling—without violating the FDC Act, the patient's right to redress for possible medical malpractice still remains. That is a significant concern because the failure to follow the FDA-approved label may create an inference that the physician was varying from the prevailing standard of care. Although the failure to follow the contents of the drug label does not impose liability per

Table 1–3
Combination Drugs Used in Psychiatry

Ingredients	Preparation	Manufacturer	Amount of Each Ingredient	Recommended Dosage	Indications	D.E.A.† Control
Perphenazine and amitriptyline	Triavil	Merck, Sharp & Dohme	Tablet—2:25, 4:25, 4:50, 2:10, 4:10	Initial therapy: tablet of 2:25 or 4:25 q.i.d. Maintenance therapy: tablet 2:25 or 4:25 b.i.d. or q.i.d.	Depression and associated anxiety	0
	Etrafon	Schering				
Meprobamate and benactyzine	Deprol	Wallace	Tablet—400:1	Initial therapy: one tablet q.i.d. Maintenance therapy: initial dosage may be increased to six tablets a day, then gradually reduced to the lowest levels that provide relief	Depression and associated anxiety	IV
Dextroamphetamine and amphetamine	Biphetamine‡	Pennwalt	Sustained release capsule—6.25:6.25	One capsule in the morning	Exogenous obesity Attention-deficit hyperactivity disorder (ADHD)	II
Chlordiazepoxide and clidinium bromide	Librax	Roche	Capsule—5:25	One or two capsules t.i.d. or q.i.d. before meals and at bedtime	Peptic ulcer, gastritis, duodenitis, irritable bowel syndrome, spastic colitis, and mild ulcerative colitis	0
Chlordiazepoxide and amitriptyline	Limbitrol	Roche	Tablet—5:12.5, 10:25	Tablet of 5:12.5 t.i.d. or q.i.d. Tablet of 10:25 t.i.d. or q.i.d. initially, then may increase to six tablets daily as required	Depression and associated anxiety	IV

†DEA, Drug Enforcement Administration.
‡The United States Food and Drug Administration recommends the use of amphetamine for weight reduction and ADHD.

Table 1–4
Characteristics of Drugs at Each DEA Level

DEA Control Level (Schedule)	Characteristics of Drug	Examples of Drugs
I	High abuse potential No accepted use in medical treatment in the United States at the present time and, therefore, not for prescription use Can be used for research	LSD, heroin, marijuana, peyote, PCP, mescaline, psilocybin, tetrahydrocannabinols, nicocodeine, nicomorphine
II	High abuse potential Severe physical dependence liability Severe psychological dependence liability No refills; no telephone prescriptions	Amphetamine, methamphetamine, opium, morphine, codeine, hydromorphine, phenmetrazine, cocaine, amobarbital, secobarbital, pentobarbital, methylphenidate
III	Abuse potential less than levels I and II Moderate or low physical dependence liability High psychological liability Prescriptions must be rewritten after six months or five refills	Glutethimide, methyprylon, nalorphine, sulfonmethane, benzphetamine, phendimetrazine, clortermine, mazindol, chlorphentermine; compounds containing codeine, morphine, opium, hydrocodone, dihydrocodeine, naltrexone, diethylpropion
IV	Low abuse potential Limited physical dependence liability Limited psychological dependence liability Prescriptions must be rewritten after six months or five refills	Phenobarbital, benzodiazepines,* chloral hydrate, ethchlorvynol, ethinamate, meprobamate, paraldehyde
V	Lowest abuse potential of all controlled substances	Narcotic preparations containing limited amounts of nonnarcotic active medicinal ingredients

*In New York State benzodiazepines are treated as schedule II substances, which require a triplicate prescription for a maximum of one month's supply.

se and should not preclude a physician from using good clinical judgment in the interest of the patient, the physician should be aware that the drug label represents important information regarding safe and effective use (as determined by the scientific data submitted to the FDA).

In summary, psychiatrists may prescribe medication for any reason that they believe to be medically indicated for the welfare of a patient. That clarification is important in view of the increasing regulation of physicians by federal, state, and local government agencies and the intimidation being experienced by many physicians in exercising their best medical judgment.

If clinicians are in doubt about a drug treatment plan, they should consult with a colleague or suggest that the patient obtain a second opinion. The Drug Enforcement Agency (DEA) has classified drugs according to abuse potential (Table 1–4), and clinicians are advised to be cautious when prescribing any controlled substances.

Therapeutic trials. A drug's therapeutic trial should last for a previously determined length of time. Because behavioral symptoms are more difficult to assess than are other physiological symptoms, such as hypertension, it is particularly important for specific target symptoms to be identified at the initiation of a drug trial. The psychiatrist and the patient can then assess the target symptoms over the course of the drug trial to help determine whether the drug has been effective. A number of objective rating scales, such as the Brief Psychiatric Rating Scale (BPRS) and the Schedule for Affective Disorders and Schizophrenia (SADS), are available to help assess a patient's progress over the course of a drug trial. If a drug has not been effective in reducing target symptoms within the specified length of time and if other reasons for the lack of response can be eliminated, the drug should be tapered and stopped. The brain is not a group of on-and-off neurochemical switches; rather, it is an interactive network of neurons in a complex homeostasis. Thus, the abrupt discontinuation of virtually any psychoactive drug is likely to disrupt further the brain's functioning. Another common clinical mistake is the routine addition of medications without the discontinuation of a prior drug. Although this practice is indicated in specific circumstances, such as lithium potentiation of an unsuccessful trial of antidepressants, it often results in increased noncompliance and adverse effects and the clinician's not knowing whether it was the second drug alone or the combination of drugs that resulted in a therapeutic success.

Therapeutic failures.   The failure of a specific drug trial should prompt the clinician to consider a number of possibilities. First, was the original diagnosis correct? That reconsideration should include the possibility of an undiagnosed organic mental disorder, including illicit drug abuse. Second, are the observed remaining symptoms actually the drug's adverse effects and not related to the original disease? Antipsychotic drugs, for example, can produce akinesia, which resembles psychotic withdrawal, or akathisia and neuroleptic malignant syndrome, which resemble increased psychotic agitation. Third, was the drug administered in sufficient dosage for an appropriate period of time? Patients can have vastly different drug absorption and metabolic rates for the same drug, and plasma drug levels should be obtained to assess that variable. Fourth, did a pharmacokinetic or pharmacodynamic interaction with another drug the patient was taking reduce the efficacy of the psychotherapeutic drug? Fifth, did the patient actually take the drug as directed? Drug noncompliance is a common clinical problem. Reasons for drug noncompliance are complicated drug regimens (more than one drug in more than one daily dose), adverse side effects (especially if unnoticed by the clinician), and poor patient education about the drug treatment plan (Table 1–5).

Special Considerations

Children.   Special care must be given when administering psychotherapeutic drugs to children. Although the small volume of distribution in children suggests the use of lower dosages than in adults, children's higher rate of metabolism suggests that higher ratios of milligrams of drug to kilograms of body weight should be used. In practice it is best to begin with a small dose and to increase the dosage until clinical effects are observed (Table 1–6). The clinician, however, should not hesitate to use adult dosages in children if the dosages are effective and there are no side effects.

Geriatric patients.   The two major concerns when treating geriatric patients with psychotherapeutic drugs are that elderly persons may be more susceptible to adverse side effects (particularly adverse cardiac effects) and may metabolize drugs

Table 1–5
Conditions That May Reduce Adherence to Recommended Treatment

Excessively complex regimen (multiple agents, multiple small doses)
Early onset and persistence of side effects
Slow onset of beneficial effects
Low apparent relapse risk experienced if treatment is interrupted
Psychosis, confusion, dementia, pseudodementia, low intelligence, impaired hearing or vision,
    illiteracy
Simple lack of information, need for patient education
Financial hardship, conflicting obligations of time or money
Resentment, lack of confidence or trust
Specific psychopathology: paranoid delusions, hopelessness, masochism, anxiety and fear,
    ambivalence, control, splitting, passive aggression, passive dependence, denial, sociopathy,
    substance abuse
Involvement of multiple clinicians
Poor clinician-patient relationship
Inevitable human error

Adapted from R J Baldessarini, J O Cole: Chemotherapy. In *The New Harvard Guide to Psychiatry*, A M
Nicholi, editor, p 530. Belknap Press, Cambridge, Mass, 1988. Used with permission.

more slowly, thus requiring lower dosages of medication (Tables 1–7 and 1–8).
Another concern is that geriatric patients are often taking other medications, thereby
requiring psychiatrists to consider possible drug interactions carefully. In practice,
psychiatrists should begin treating geriatric patients with a small dose, usually
about one half the usual dose. The dosage should be raised in small amounts more
slowly than in middle-aged adults until either a clinical benefit is achieved or
unacceptable adverse effects appear. Although many geriatric patients require a
small dosage of medication, many others require the usual adult dosage.

Pregnant and nursing women.   The basic rule is to avoid administering any
drug to a woman who is pregnant (particularly during the first trimester) or who
is breast-feeding a child. That rule, however, occasionally needs to be broken
when the mother's psychiatric disorder is severe. If psychotherapeutic medications
need to be administered during a pregnancy, the possibility of therapeutic abortion
should be discussed. The two most teratogenic drugs in the psychopharmacopeia
are lithium and anticonvulsants. Lithium administration during pregnancy is associated with a high incidence of birth abnormalities, including Ebstein's malformation, a serious abnormality in cardiac development. Other psychoactive drugs
(antidepressants, antipsychotics, and anxiolytics), although less clearly associated
with birth defects, should also be avoided during pregnancy if at all possible. The
most common clinical situation occurs when a pregnant women becomes psychotic.
If a decision is made not to terminate the pregnancy, it is preferable to administer
antipsychotics, rather than lithium.

The administration of psychotherapeutic drugs at or near delivery may cause
the baby to be overly sedated at delivery, requiring a respirator, or to be physically
dependent on the drug, requiring detoxification and treatment of a withdrawal
syndrome. Virtually all psychotropic drugs are secreted in the milk of a nursing
mother; therefore, mothers on these agents should be advised not to breast-feed
their children.

Medically ill patients.   Considerations in administering psychotropic drugs to
medically ill patients include a potentially increased sensitivity to side effects,
either increased or decreased metabolism and excretion of the drug, and interactions

Table 1–6
Common Psychoactive Drugs in Childhood and Adolescence

Drugs	Indications	Dosage	Adverse Reactions and Monitoring
Antipsychotics—also known as major tranquilizers, neuroleptics Divided into (1) high potency, low dosage, e.g., haloperidol (Haldol), trifluoperazine (Stelazine), Thiothixene (Navane) and (2) low potency, high dosage (more sedating), e.g., chlorpromazine (Thorazine), thioridazine (Mellaril)	In general, for agitated, aggressive, self-injurious behaviors in mental retardation (MR), pervasive development disorder (PDD), conduct disorder (CD), and schizophrenia Studies support following specific indications: haloperidol-PDD, CD, with severe aggression, Tourette's disorder	All can be given in two to four divided doses or combined into one dose after gradual buildup Haloperidol—0.5–16 mg a day Thiothixene—5–42 mg a day Chlorpromazine and thioridazine—10–400 mg	Sedation, weight gain, hypotension, lowered seizure threshold, constipation, extrapyramidal symptoms, jaundice, agranulocytosis, dystonic reaction, tardive dyskinesia Monitor; blood pressure, complete blood count (CBC), liver function tests (LFTs), electroencephalogram, if indicated; with thioridazine, pigmentary retinopathy is rare but dictates ceiling of 800 mg in adults and proportionately lower in children
Stimulants Dextroamphetamine (Dexedrine) FDA-approved for children 3 years and older Methylphenidate (Ritalin) and pemoline (Cylert) FDA-approved for children 6 years and older	In attention-deficit hyperactivity disorder (ADHD) for hyperactivity, impulsivity, and inattentiveness	Dextroamphetamine and methylphenidate are generally given at 8 AM and noon (the usefulness of sustained-release preparations is not proved) Dextroamphetamine—2.5–40 mg a day up to 0.5 mg per kg a day Methylphenidate—10–60 mg a day or up to 1.0 mg per kg a day Pemoline—37.5–112.5 mg given at 8 AM	Insomnia, anorexia, weight loss (and possibly growth delay), tachycardia, precipitation or exacerbation of tic disorders With pemoline, monitor LFTs, as hepatoxicity is possible
Lithium—considered an antipsychotic drug, also has antiaggressive properties	Studies support use in MR and CD for aggressive and self-injurious behaviors; can be used for same in PDD; also indicated for early-onset bipolar disorder	600–2,100 mg in two or three divided doses; keep blood levels to 0.4–1.2 mEq per L	Nausea, vomiting, headache, tremor, weight gain Experience with adults suggests thyroid and renal function monitoring
Antidepressants Imipramine (Tofranil) has been used in most child studies Clomipramine (Anafranil) is effective in child obsessive-compulsive disorder (OCD)	Major depressive disorder, separation anxiety disorder, bulimia nervosa, functional enuresis; sometimes used in ADHD, anorexia nervosa, somnambulism, and sleep terror disorder	Imipramine—start with dosage of about 1.5 mg kg a day; can build up to not more than 5 mg per kg a day Start with two or three divided doses;	Dry mouth, constipation, tachycardia, drowsiness, postural hypotension Electrocardiogram (ECG) monitoring is needed because of risk of

Drug	Indication	Dosage	Side effects/Comments
Fluoxetine (Prozac) may also be used in OCD	OCD—clomipramine, fluoxetine	Not FDA-approved for children except for functional enuresis; dosage is usually 50–100 mg before sleep, clomipramine—start at 50 mg a day; can raise to not more than 3 mg per kg a day or 200 mg a day. Fluoxetine dosage not established in children	consider lowering dosage if PR interval > 0.20 seconds or QRS interval > 0.12 seconds; baseline EEG is advised, as it can lower seizure threshold; blood levels of drug are sometimes useful
Carbamazepine (Tegretol)—an anticonvulsant	Aggression or dyscontrol in MR or CD	Start with 10 mg per kg a day, and can build to 20–30 mg per kg a day; therapeutic blood level range appears to be 4–12 mg per L	Drowsiness, nausea, rash, vertigo, irritability. Monitor: CBC and LFTs for possible blood dyscrasias and hepatotoxicity; blood levels are necessary
Anxiolytics—have been insufficiently studied in childhood and adolescence	Sometimes effective in parasomnias: somnambulism or sleep terror disorder; can be tried in overanxious disorder	Parasomnias: diazepam (Valium) 2–10 mg before bedtime	Benzodiazepines can cause drowsiness, dyscontrol, and can be abused
Fenfluramine (Pondimin)—an amphetamine congener	Well-studied in autistic disorder; generally ineffective, but some patients show improvement	Gradually increase to 1.0–1.5 mg per kg a day in divided doses	Weight loss, drowsiness, irritability, loose bowel movements
Propranolol (Inderal)—a β-adrenergic blocker	Aggression in MR, PDD, and organic brain dysfunction; awaits controlled studies	Effective dosage in children and adolescents is not yet established; range is probably 40–320 mg a day	Bradycardia, hypotension, nausea, hypoglycemia, depression; avoid in asthma
Clonidine (Catapres)—a presynaptic α-adrenergic blocking agent	Tourette's disorder	0.1–0.3 mg a day; 3–5.5 µg per kg a day	Orthostatic hypotension, nausea, vomiting, sedation, elevated blood glucose
Cyproheptadine (Periactin)	Anorexia nervosa	Dosages up to 8 mg four times a day	Antihistaminic side effects, including sedation and dryness of the mouth
Naltrexone (Trexan)	Self-injurious behaviors in MR and PDD; currently being studied in PDD	0.5–2.0 mg per kg a day	Sleepiness, aggressivity. Monitor LFTs, as hepatotoxicity has been reported in adults at high dosages

Table by Richard Perry, M.D.

Table 1–7
Pharmacokinetics and Aging

Phase	Change	Effect
Absorption	Gastric pH increases Decreased surface villi Decreased gastric motility and delayed gastric emptying Intestinal perfusion decreases	Little overall change Absorption is slower but just as complete
Distribution	Total body water and lean body mass decrease Increased total body fat, more marked in women Albumin decreases, gamma globulin increases, alpha₁ glycoprotein unchanged	Volume of distribution (Vd) increases for lipid-soluble drugs, decreases for water-soluble drugs The free or unbound percentage of albumin-bound drugs increases
Metabolism	Renal: renal blood flow and glomerular filtration rates decrease Hepatic: decreased enzyme activity and perfusion	Decreased metabolism leads to prolonged half-lives, if Vd remains the same
Total body weight	Decreases	Think on a mg-per-kg basis
Receptor sensitivity	May increase	Greater effect

Table from L B Guttmacher: *Concise Guide to Somatic Therapies in Psychiatry*, p 126. American Psychiatric Press, Washington, 1988. Used with permission.

with other medications. As with children and geriatric patients, the most reasonable clinical practice is to begin with a small dose, increase it slowly, and watch for both clinical and adverse effects. The testing of plasma drug levels may be particularly helpful in those patients.

ADVERSE EFFECTS

Most psychotherapeutic drugs do not affect a single neurotransmitter system, nor are their effects localized to the brain. The effects of psychotherapeutic drugs on neurotransmitter systems result in the wide range of adverse effects associated with their use. For example, some of the most common adverse effects of psychotherapeutic drugs are caused by the blockade of muscarinic acetylcholine receptors (Table 1–9). Many psychotherapeutic drugs antagonize dopaminergic, histaminergic, or adrenergic neurons, resulting in the adverse effects listed in Table 1–10. There are also several commonly observed adverse effects for which the neurotransmitters involved have not been specifically identified.

Patients generally have less trouble with adverse effects if they have previously been told to expect them. It is reasonable to explain the appearance of adverse effects as evidence that the drug is working. But clinicians should distinguish between probable or expected adverse effects and rare or unexpected adverse effects.

An extreme adverse effect of drug treatment is an attempt by a patient to commit suicide by overdosing on a psychotherapeutic drug. One psychodynamic theory of such behavior is that the patients are angry at their therapists for not having been able to help them. Whatever the motivation, psychiatrists should be aware of the

Table 1–8
Geriatric Dosages of Common Psychoactive Drugs

Monoamine Oxidase Inhibitors (MAOIs)

Generic Name	Trade Name	Geriatric Dosage Range (mg a day)
Isocarboxazid	Marplan	10–30
Phenelzine	Nardil	15–45
Tranylcypromine†	Parnate	10–20

†Persons taking MAOIs should be on a tyramine-free diet.
Not recommended in persons over 60 because of pressor effects.

Psychostimulants

Generic Name	Trade Name	Geriatric Dosage Range (mg a day)
Dextroamphetamine	Dexedrine	2.5–10
Pemoline	Cylert	18.75–37
Methylphenidate	Ritalin	2.5–20

Antipsychotics: Dopamine Receptor Antagonists

Generic Name	Trade Name	Geriatric Dosage Range (mg a day)
Phenothiazines		
Aliphatic		
Chlorpromazine	Thorazine	30–300
Triflupromazine	Vesprin	1–15
Piperazine		
Perphenazine	Trilafon	8–32
Trifluoperazine	Stelazine	1–15
Fluphenazine	Prolixin, Permitil	1–10
Piperidine		
Thioridazine	Mellaril	25–300
Mesoridazine	Serentil	50–400
Thioxanthenes		
Chlorprothixene	Taractan	30–300
Thiothixene	Navane	2–20
Dibenzoxazepine		
Loxapine	Loxitane	50–250
Dihydroindole		
Molindone	Moban	50–225
Butyrophenone		
Haloperidol	Haldol	2–20

Tricyclic, Tetracyclic, and Unicyclic Antidepressants

Generic Name	Trade Name	Geriatric Dosage Range (mg a day)
Imipramine	Tofranil	25–300
Desipramine	Norpramin, Pertofrane	10–300
Trimipramine	Surmontil	25–300
Amitriptyline	Elavil	25–300
Nortriptyline	Pamelor, Aventyl	10–150
Protriptyline	Vivactil	10–40

(Continued)

Table 1–8
Geriatric Dosages of Common Psychoactive Drugs (Continued)

Tricyclic, Tetracyclic, and Unicyclic Antidepressants (Continued)

Generic Name	Trade Name	Geriatric Dosage Range (mg a day)
Doxepin	Adapin, Sinequan	10–300
Maprotiline	Ludiomil	25–150
Bupropion	Wellbutrin	75–450

Exact range may vary among laboratories.

Serotonin-Specific Reuptake Inhibitors

Generic Name	Trade Name	Geriatric Dosage Range (mg a day)
Fluoxetine	Prozac	5–80
Sertraline	Zoloft	50–200
Paroxetine	Paxil	10–40

Drugs Used to Treat Bipolar Disorder

Generic Name	Trade Name	Geriatric Dosage Range (mg a day)
Lithium carbonate	Eskalith, Lithane, Lithotabs	75–900
Carbamazepine (an anticonvulsant)	Tegretol	200–1,200
Valproic acid (an anticonvulsant)	Depakene, Depakote	250–1,000
Clonazepam (a benzodiazepine)	Klonopin	0.5–1.5

Drugs Used to Treat Anxiety and Insomnia

Generic Name	Trade Name	Geriatric Dosage Range (mg a day)
Benzodiazepines		
Alprazolam	Xanax	0.5–6
Chlordiazepoxide	Librium	15–100
Chlorazepate	Tranxene	7.5–60
Diazepam	Valium	2–60
Flurazepam	Dalmane	15–30
Halazepam	Paxipam	60–160
Lorazepam	Ativan	2–6
Oxazepam	Serax	30–120
Prazepam	Centrax	20–60
Temazepam	Restoril	15–30
Triazolam	Halcion	0.125–0.25
Nonbenzodiazepines		
Buspirone	BuSpar	5–60
Secobarbital	Seconal	50–300
Meprobamate	Miltown	400–800
Chloral hydrate	Noctec	500–1,000
β-Adrenergic blocking agents		
Propranolol	Inderal	40–160
Atenolol	Tenormin	25–100

Table 1–9
Potential Adverse Effects Caused by Blockade of Muscarinic Acetylcholine Receptors

Blurred vision
Constipation
Decreased salivation
Decreased sweating
Delayed or retrograde ejaculation
Delirium
Exacerbation of asthma (through decreased bronchial secretions)
Hyperthermia (through decreased sweating)
Memory problems
Narrow-angle glaucoma
Photophobia
Sinus tachycardia
Urinary retention

Table 1–10
Potential Adverse Effects of Psychotherapeutic Drugs and Associated Neurotransmitter Systems

Antidopaminergic
  Endocrine dysfunction
    Hyperprolactinemia
    Menstrual dysfunction
    Sexual dysfunction
  Movement disorders
    Akathisia
    Dystonia
    Parkinsonism
    Tardive dyskinesia
Antiadrenergic (primarily α)
  Dizziness
  Postural hypotension
  Reflex tachycardia
Antihistaminergic
  Hypotension
  Sedation
  Weight gain
Multiple neurotransmitter systems
  Agranulocytosis (and other blood dyscrasias)
  Allergic reactions
  Anorexia
  Cardiac conduction abnormalities
  Nausea and vomiting
  Seizures

risk and attempt to prescribe the safest possible drugs. It is good clinical practice to write nonrefillable prescriptions for small quantities of drugs when suicide is a consideration. In extreme cases, attempts should be made to verify that patients are taking the medication and not hoarding the pills for a later overdose attempt. Patients may attempt suicide just as they are beginning to get better. Clinicians, therefore, should continue to be careful about prescribing large quantities of medication until the patient is almost completely recovered. Another consideration for psychiatrists is the possibility of accidental overdose, particularly by children in the household. Patients should be advised to keep psychotherapeutic medications in a safe place.

Treatment of Common Adverse Effects

Many adverse effects are seen with a great number of different psychotherapeutic drugs. The management of the adverse effects is similar, regardless of which psychotherapeutic drug the patient is taking.

Dry mouth. Dry mouth is caused by the blockade of muscarinic acetylcholine receptors. When patients attempt to relieve the dry mouth by constantly sucking on sugar-containing hard candies, they increase their risk of dental caries. They can avoid the problem by chewing sugarless gum or sucking on sugarless hard candies. Some clinicians recommend the use of a 1 percent solution of pilocarpine, a cholinergic agonist, as a mouth wash three times daily. Other clinicians suggest bethanechol (Urecholine, Myotonachol) tablets, a cholinergic agonist, 10 to 30 mg, once to twice daily. It is best to start with 10 mg once a day and to increase the dosage slowly. Adverse effects of cholinomimetic drugs, such as bethanechol, include tremor, diarrhea, abdominal cramps, and excessive eye watering.

Blurred vision. The blockade of muscarinic acetylcholine receptors causes mydriasis (pupillary dilation) and cycloplegia (ciliary muscle paresis), resulting in presbyopia (blurred near vision). The symptom can be relieved by cholinomimetic eyedrops. A 1 percent solution of pilocarpine can be prescribed as one drop four times daily. Bethanechol can be used as for dry mouth as an alternative.

Urinary retention. The anticholinergic activity of many psychotropics can lead to urinary hesitation, dribbling, urinary retention, and increased urinary tract infections. Elderly patients with enlarged prostates are at increased risk for that adverse effect. Ten to thirty milligrams of bethanechol three to four times daily is usually effective in the treatment of the adverse effect.

Constipation. The anticholinergic activity of psychotropic drugs can result in the particularly disturbing adverse effect of constipation. The first line of treatment involves the prescribing of bulk laxatives, such as Metamucil and Fiberall. If that treatment fails, cathartic laxatives, such as milk of magnesia, can be tried. Prolonged use of cathartic laxatives can result in a loss of their effectiveness. Bethanechol, 10 to 30 mg three to four times daily, can also be used.

Orthostatic hypotension. Orthostatic hypotension is caused by the blockade of α_1-adrenergic receptors. It is necessary to warn patients of that possible adverse effect, particularly if the patient is elderly. The risk of hip fracture from falls is significantly elevated in patients who are taking psychotropic drugs. With patients at high risk of experiencing orthostatic hypotension, the clinician should choose a drug with low α_1-adrenergic activity. Most simply, the patient can be instructed to get up slowly and to sit down immediately if dizziness is experienced. The patient can also try support hose to help reduce venous pooling. Specific adjuvant medications have been recommended for specific pharmacotherapeutic agents.

Sexual dysfunction. Psychotropic drug use can be associated with sexual dysfunctions—decreased libido, impaired ejaculation and erection, and inhibition of female orgasm. Warning a patient about those adverse effects may increase the patient's concerns. Alternatively, patients are not likely to report adverse sexual effects to the physician. Also, some sexual dysfunctions may be related to the primary psychiatric disorder. Nevertheless, if sexual dysfunctions emerge after pharmacotherapy has begun, it may be worthwhile to attempt to treat them. Neostigmine (Prostigmin), 7.5 to 15 mg orally 30 minutes before sexual intercourse, may help alleviate impaired ejaculation. Impaired erectile function may be helped with bethanechol given regularly. Cyproheptadine (Periactin), 4 mg every morning, can be used for the treatment of inhibited female orgasm or 4 to 8 mg orally one to two hours before anticipated sexual activity for the treatment of inhibited male orgasm secondary to serotonergic agents.

Weight gain.   Weight gain accompanies the use of many psychotropic drugs. The weight gain can be the result of retained fluid, increased caloric intake, or decreased exercise. Edema can be treated by elevating the affected body parts or by administering a thiazide diuretic. If the patient is taking lithium or cardiac medications, the clinician must monitor drug levels, blood chemistries, and vital signs. The patient should also be instructed to minimize the intake of fats and carbohydrates and to exercise regularly. If the patient has not been exercising, however, the clinician should recommend that the patient start an exercise program at a modest level of exertion.

Extrapyramidal side effects.   Neurological side effects—such as dystonias, parkinsonian effects, rabbit syndrome, and tardive dyskinesia—are discussed in Chapter 19, ''Dopamine Receptor Antagonists.''

DRUG-DRUG INTERACTIONS

Drug-drug interactions may be either pharmacokinetic or pharmacodynamic and vary greatly in their potential to cause serious problems. An additional consideration is one of phantom drug-drug interactions. The patient may be taking only drug A and then later receive both A and B. The clinician may notice some effect and attribute it to the induction of metabolism. What may have gone on is that the patient was more compliant at one point in the observation period than in another, or there may have been some other effect of which the clinician was unaware. Thus, the clinical literature contains reports of phantom drug-drug interactions, but such interactions probably did not really take place.

There may be other interactions that are true but unproved, although reasonably plausible. Still other interactions have some modest effect and are well-documented. There are also well-studied, well-proved, clinically important drug-drug interactions. However, clinicians must remember that (1) animal pharmacokinetic data are not always readily generalizable to humans; (2) in vitro data do not necessarily replicate results obtained under in vivo conditions; (3) single-case reports can contain misleading information; and (4) acute studies should not be uncritically regarded as relevant to investigations of chronic, steady-state conditions.

The informed clinician needs to keep those considerations in mind and to focus on the clinically important interactions—not on the ones that may be mild, unproved, or entirely phantom—and yet still maintain an open and receptive attitude toward drug-drug interactions.

References

Beardsley R S, Gardocki G J, Larson D B, Hidalgo J: Prescribing of psychotropic medication by primary care physicians and psychiatrists. Arch Gen Psychiatry 45: 1117, 1988.

Beers M, Avorn J, Sourmerai S B, Everitt D E, Sherman D S, Salem S: Psychoactive medication use in intermediate-care facility residents. JAMA 260: 3016, 1988.

Cahn C, editor: Pioneers in psychopharmacology. Psychiatr J Univ Ottawa *14*: 248, 1989.

Christison G W, Kirch D G, Wyatt R J: When symptoms persist: Choosing among alternative somatic treatments of schizophrenia. Schizophr Bull *17*: 217, 1991.

Grebb J A: Biological therapies: Introduction and overview. In *Comprehensive Textbook of Psychiatry*, ed 5, H I Kaplan, B J Sadock, editors, p 1574. Williams & Wilkins, Baltimore, 1989.

Hollister L E: Psychopharmacology: The bridge between psychiatry and biology. Clin Pharmacol Ther *44*: 123, 1988.

Jacobsen E: The early history of psychotherapeutic drugs. Psychopharmacology *89*: 138, 1986.

Jefferson J W, editor: Management of patients who are non-responders to or non-tolerators of initial antidepressant therapy. J Clin Psychiatry *10*(5, Monogr): 3, 1992.

Langer R: New methods for drug delivery. Science *249*: 1527, 1990.

Plaut E A: The ethics of informed consent: An overview. Psychiatry J Univ Ottawa *14*: 435, 1989.

Pollack M H, Rosenbaum J F: Management of antidepressant-induced side effects: A practical guide for the clinicians. J Clin Psychiatry *48*: 3, 1987.

Ray W A, Griffin M R, Schaffner W, Baugh D K, Melton L J: Psychotropic drug use and the risk of hip fracture. N Engl J Med *316*: 363, 1987.

Segraves R T: Effects of psychotropic drugs on human erection and ejaculation. Arch Gen Psychiatry *46*: 275, 1989.

Winer J A, Andriukaitis S M: Interpersonal aspects of initiating pharmacotherapy: How to avoid becoming the patient's feared negative other. Psychiatr Ann *19*: 318, 1989.

2

β-Adrenergic Receptor Antagonists

β-Adrenergic receptor antagonists (for example, propranolol [Inderal]), also known as β-blockers and β-adrenergic drugs, are most useful in psychiatric practice in treating drug-induced akathisia, lithium-induced tremor, aggression, and somatic symptoms of anxiety (Figure 2–1). The β-adrenergic drugs have also been reported to be third- or fourth-line drugs for a wide range of other psychiatric disorders.

PHARMACOLOGICAL ACTIONS

Many β-adrenergic drugs are available in the United States. The β-adrenergic drugs that have been studied with regard to neuropsychiatric disorders are presented in Table 2–1. The drugs differ in terms of ability to dissolve in lipids, routes of metabolism, half-lives, and relative selectivity for β_1 or β_2 receptors. The β-adrenergic drugs are readily absorbed from the gastrointestinal (GI) tract and are either metabolized by the liver or excreted unchanged by the kidneys. The agents that are more soluble in lipids (that is, lipophilic) are more likely to enter the brain; those that are less lipophilic (that is, more water-soluble than lipid-soluble) are less likely to enter the brain. When central nervous system (CNS) effects are desired, a lipophilic drug may be preferred; when only peripheral effects are desired, a less lipophilic drug may be indicated.

Peripheral β_1-adrenergic receptors modulate chronotropic and inotropic cardiac functions; peripheral β_2-adrenergic receptors modulate bronchodilation and vasodilation. There are more β_1-adrenergic receptors than β_2-adrenergic receptors in the CNS. The so-called β_1-specific drugs still have some β_2 activity, and their use should be carefully monitored in patients with pulmonary disease or asthma; β_1-specific drugs are preferable for such patients.

INDICATIONS

Drug-Induced Akathisia

Many studies have shown that β-adrenergic antagonists can be effective in the treatment of antipsychotic-induced akathisia, which can be particularly resistant to drug therapy. Other drugs used for the treatment of akathisia are the anticholinergics, benzodiazepines, and, perhaps, clonidine (Catapres). It is not yet possible to predict which patients will respond to a particular agent. The β-adrenergic antagonists are not effective at treating other antipsychotic-induced extrapyramidal symptoms, such as acute dystonia and parkinsonism. Propranolol is the drug that has been used most often in studies and seems to be the standard drug for that indication. Studies have not indicated whether peripheral-acting drugs are effective.

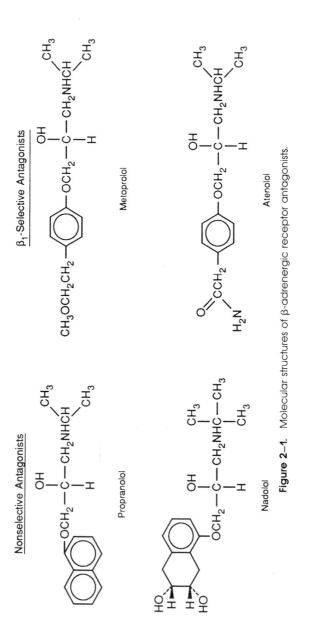

Figure 2–1. Molecular structures of β-adrenergic receptor antagonists.

Table 2–1
β-Adrenergic Drugs Used in Psychiatry

Generic Name	Trade Name	Lipophilic	Metabolism	Receptor Selectivity	Half-Life (hrs)	Usual Starting Dose (mg)	Usual Maximal Dose (mg)
Atenolol	Tenormin	No	Renal	β_1	6–9	50 once a day	50–100 once a day
Metoprolol	Lopressor	Yes	Hepatic	β_1	3–4	50 twice a day	75–150 twice a day
Nadolol	Corgard	No	Renal	$\beta_1–\beta_2$	14–24	40 once a day	80–240 once a day
Propranolol	Inderal	Yes	Hepatic	$\beta_1–\beta_2$	3–6	10–20 two or three times a day	80–140 three times a day

Lithium-Induced Tremor

Lithium can be associated with a tremor even when lithium concentrations are within normal therapeutic ranges. Propranolol (20 to 160 mg a day, two or three times a day) is effective treatment for the adverse effect. It is controversial whether nonlipophilic, peripherally acting β-adrenergic antagonists are as effective as propranolol.

Aggression and Violent Behavior

According to some studies, β-adrenergic antagonists are effective in treating the aggressiveness and violent behavior that can be associated with schizophrenia and organic mental diseases, such as trauma, tumor, anoxic injury, encephalitis, alcoholism, and Huntington's chorea. Most of the patients studied in the reports have been nonresponsive to antipsychotics, lithium, anticonvulsants, and benzo-diazepines. Approximately 50 percent of the patients in the studies improved with β-adrenergic antagonist treatment. The range of propranolol dosages is from 50 to 960 mg a day. Two lipophilic, centrally acting drugs, pindolol (Visken) and metoprolol (Lopressor), have also been successfully used for that indication in case reports and open trials.

Social Phobias

Propranolol has been reported to be useful in reducing the peripheral manifestations of anxiety (for example, tremor, tachycardia) associated with social phobia and the anxiety associated with performance, such as examinations and musical recitals. Propranolol (10 to 40 mg) taken 20 to 30 minutes before the performance is the usual dose.

Alcohol Withdrawal

Propranolol has been reported to be useful as an adjuvant to benzodiazepines but not as a sole agent in the treatment of alcohol withdrawal. One study used the following dose schedule: no propranolol for a pulse less than 50; 50 mg propranolol for a pulse between 50 and 79; 100 mg propranolol for a pulse equal to or greater than 80. The patients who also received propranolol had less severe withdrawal symptoms, more stable vital signs, and a shorter hospital stay than the patients who received only benzodiazepines.

Other Disorders

Various case reports found clinical uses for β-adrenergic antagonists in the treatment of mania, schizophrenia, and generalized anxiety disorder. The treatment of mania is promising; however, very high doses (1,000 mg a day) were required, and severe adverse effects were encountered. The data for schizophrenia are much more extensive and more contradictory. The β-adrenergic antagonists are useful,

Table 2–2
β-Adrenergic Receptor Antagonist Preparations

	Tablets	**Capsules (Extended Release)**	**Solution**	**Parenteral**
Atenolol	50, 100 mg	—	—	5 mg/10 mL ampules
Metoprolol	50, 100 mg	—	—	1 mg/mL
Nadolol	20, 40, 80, 120, 160 mg	—	—	—
Propranolol	10, 20, 40, 60, 80, 90 mg	60, 80, 120, 160 mg	20 mg/5 mL, 40 mg/ 5 mL, 80 mg/mL (concentrate)	1 mg/mL

however, in controlling aggressive behavior in schizophrenia; a trial of propranolol may be warranted in schizophrenic patients who have not responded to other drugs.

CLINICAL GUIDELINES

For the treatment of chronic disorders, propranolol is usually initiated at 10 mg orally (PO) three times a day or 20 mg PO twice a day. The dosage can be raised by 20 to 30 mg a day until a therapeutic effect begins to emerge. The dosage should be leveled off at the appropriate range for the disorder under treatment. The treatment of aggressive behavior sometimes requires dosages up to 800 mg a day, and therapeutic effects may not be seen until the patient has been receiving the maximal dosage for four to eight weeks. The patient's pulse and blood pressure should be taken regularly, and the drug should be withheld if the pulse is less than 50 or the systolic blood pressure is less than 90. The drug should also be temporarily withheld if the patient has severe dizziness, ataxia, or wheezing. Treatment with β-adrenergic antagonists should never be discontinued abruptly. Propranolol should be tapered at 60 mg a day until a dosage of 60 mg a day is reached, after which the drug should be tapered by 20 mg a day every three or four days. Available preparations of β-adrenergic antagonists are given in Table 2–2. The elderly are more sensitive than younger adults or children to the effects of β-receptor antagonists. Adverse effects in children are similar to those in adults.

ADVERSE EFFECTS

The use of β-adrenergic antagonists is relatively contraindicated in patients with bronchial asthma, chronic obstructive pulmonary disease, diabetes, congestive heart failure, persistent angina, hyperthyroidism, and peripheral vascular disease. β-Adrenergic antagonists can worsen atrioventricular (AV) conduction defects and lead to complete AV heart block and death. β-Adrenergic drugs elevate blood glucose by inhibiting insulin release and are capable of masking the signs and symptoms of hypoglycemia (except hyperhidrosis). The drugs should be used with caution in patients with renal or hepatic disease. The drugs should be used in pregnancy only if the benefit outweighs the risk.

Table 2–3
Side Effects and Toxicity of β-Blockers

Cardiovascular
  Hypotension
  Bradycardia
  Dizziness
  Congestive failure (in patients with compromised myocardial function)

Respiratory
  Asthma (less risk with β_1-selective drugs)

Metabolic
  Worsened hypoglycemia in diabetics receiving insulin or oral agents

Gastrointestinal
  Nausea
  Diarrhea
  Abdominal pain

Sexual function
  Impotence

Neuropsychiatric
  Lassitude
  Fatigue
  Dysphoria
  Insomnia
  Vivid nightmares
  Depression (possible)
  Psychosis (rare)

Other (rare)
  Raynaud's phenomenon
  Peyronie's disease

Withdrawal syndrome
  Rebound worsening of preexisting angina pectoris when β-blockers are discontinued

Table from G W Arana, S E Hyman: *Handbook of Psychiatric Drug Therapy*, ed 2, p 176. Little, Brown, Boston, 1991. Used with permission.

The most common adverse effects of the β-adrenergic antagonists are hypotension and bradycardia. In patients at risk for those adverse effects, a test dose of 20 mg a day of propranolol can be given to assess the patient's reaction to the drug. The results of early research that linked β-adrenergic antagonists with depression as a side effect were not replicated in recent studies. Nausea, vomiting, diarrhea, constipation, sexual dysfunction, dizziness, insomnia, and fatigue may also be caused by treatment with the agents. Serious CNS adverse effects (agitation, confusion, and hallucinations) are rare (Table 2–3). The agents do pass into breast milk. Although untoward effects have not been reported in nursing babies, cardiovascular effects are possible.

Intoxication is manifested as dizziness, dyspnea, bradycardia, arrhythmias, and convulsions.

DRUG-DRUG INTERACTIONS

Propranolol has been reported to increase dramatically the plasma concentrations of chlorpromazine (Thorazine), thioridazine (Mellaril), and theophylline. It is clinically indicated to monitor plasma concentrations of antipsychotics and anticonvulsants in patients who are taking β-adrenergic antagonists. Barbiturates increase the elimination of β-adrenergic antagonists that are metabolized in the liver. Several reports have associated hypertensive crises and bradycardia with the coadministration of β-adrenergic antagonists and monoamine oxidase inhibitors. Patients on those two drugs should be treated with low dosages of both drugs and have their blood pressure and pulse rates monitored regularly. Other interactions include those with oral antidiabetics and insulin (increased risk of hypoglycemia or hyperglycemia) and calcium channel blockers (depressed myocardial contractility and AV nodal conduction).

References

Bright R A, Everitt D E: β-Blockers and depression: Evidence against an association. JAMA 267: 1783, 1992.

Carney R M, Rich M W, Saini J, Clark K, Freedland K E: Prevalence of major depressive disorder in patients receiving β-blocker therapy versus other medications. Am J Med 83: 223, 1987.

Dupuis B, Catteau J, Dumon J-P, Libert C, Petit H: Comparison of propranolol, sotalol, and βxolol in the treatment of neuroleptic-induced akathisia. Am J Psychiatry 144: 802, 1987.

Fleischhacker W W, Roth S D, Kane J M: The pharmacologic treatment of neuroleptic-induced akathisia. J Clin Psychopharmacol 10: 12, 1990.

Gorman J M, Gorman L K: Drug treatment of social phobia. Special Issue: Drug treatment of anxiety disorders. Affective Disord 13: 183, 1987.

Jenkins S C, Maruta T: Therapeutic use of propranolol for intermittent explosive disorder. Mayo Clin Proc 62: 204, 1987.

Kaplan P M, Boggiano W E: Anticonvulsants, noradrenergic drugs, and other organic therapies. In Comprehensive Textbook of Psychiatry, ed 5, H I Kaplan, B J Sadock, editors, p 1681. Williams & Wilkins, Baltimore, 1989.

Liebowitz M: Phenelzine vs atenolol in social phobia: A placebo-controlled comparison. Arch Gen Psychiatry 49: 290, 1992.

Lipinski J F, Keck P E, McElroy S L: Beta-adrenergic antagonists in psychosis: Is improvement due to treatment of neuroleptic-induced akathisia? J Clin Psychopharmacol 8: 409, 1988.

Noyes R: Beta-adrenergic blocking drugs in anxiety and stress. Psychiatr Clin North Am 8: 119, 1985.

Schneier F R: Social phobia. Psychiatric Annals 21: 349, 1991.

Tyrer P: Current status of β-adrenergic drugs in the treatment of anxiety disorders. Drugs 36: 773, 1988.

Wells B G, Cold J A, Marken P A, Brown C S, Chu C-C, Johnson R P, Nasdahl C S, Ayubi M A, Knott D H, Arheart K L: A placebo-controlled trial of naldolol in the treatment of neuroleptic-induced akathisia. J Clin Psychiatry 52: 255, 1991.

3

Amantadine

Amantadine (Symadine, Symmetrel) is a dopamine agonist that is used primarily for the treatment of drug-induced extrapyramidal disorders, such as parkinsonism. Its chemical formula is $MgSO_4 7H_2O$.

PHARMACOLOGICAL ACTIONS

Pharmacokinetics

Amantadine is well absorbed from the gastrointestinal (GI) tract, reaches peak plasma levels in approximately two to three hours, has a half-life of about 24 hours, and attains steady-state plasma levels after approximately four to five days of therapy. Amantadine is excreted unmetabolized in the urine. Amantadine plasma concentrations can be as much as twice as high in elderly persons as in nonelderly adults. Patients with renal failure accumulate amantadine in their bodies.

Pharmacodynamics

Amantadine augments dopaminergic neurotransmission in the central nervous system (CNS); however, the precise mechanism for the effect is unknown. The mechanism may involve dopamine release from presynaptic vesicles, blocking reuptake of dopamine into presynaptic nerve terminals, or an agonist effect on postsynaptic dopamine receptors.

INDICATIONS

The primary indication for amantadine in psychiatry is for the treatment of extrapyramidal signs and symptoms, such as parkinsonism, akinesia, and rabbit syndrome (focal perioral tremor of the choreoathetotoid type) caused by the administration of antipsychotic drugs (for example, haloperidol [Haldol]). Amantadine is as effective as the anticholinergics (for example, benztropine [Cogentin, Tremin]) for those indications and results in improvement in approximately one half of all patients. Amantadine is not, however, generally considered as effective as the anticholinergics for the treatment of acute dystonic reactions. It may be the drug of choice when the clinician does not want to add additional anticholinergic drugs to a patient's treatment regimen. That may be particularly true if a patient is taking an antipsychotic with high anticholinergic activity (for example, chlorpromazine [Thorazine]) or is elderly; elderly patients are prone to anticholinergic adverse effects—both peripheral, such as urinary retention, and central, such as anticholinergic delirium. One study of patients being treated with antipsychotics reported that amantadine was associated with less memory impairment than the anticholinergics.

Amantadine is used in general medical practice for the treatment of parkinsonism with any cause, including idiopathic parkinsonism. It is also used for the prevention and symptomatic treatment of influenza type A infections.

CLINICAL GUIDELINES

Amantadine is available in 100 mg capsules and as a syrup (10 mg per mL). The usual starting dose of amantadine is 100 mg orally (PO) twice a day, although the dose can be cautiously increased up to 200 mg PO twice a day if indicated. Amantadine should be used in patients with renal impairment only in consultation with the physician treating the renal condition. If amantadine is successful in the treatment of the drug-induced extrapyramidal symptoms, it should be continued for four to six weeks and then discontinued to see if the patient has become tolerant to the neurological adverse effects of the antipsychotic medication. Amantadine should be tapered over one to two weeks once a decision has been made to discontinue the drug. Patients should not drink alcoholic beverages while taking amantadine.

ADVERSE EFFECTS

The most common CNS effects are mild dizziness, insomnia, and impaired concentration (dose-related), which occur in 5 to 10 percent of all patients. Irritability, depression, anxiety, and ataxia (tremor, hyperexcitability) occur in 1 to 5 percent of patients. More severe CNS adverse effects, including seizures and psychotic symptoms, have been reported. Nausea is the most common peripheral adverse effect of amantadine. Headache, loss of appetite, and blotchy spots on the skin have also been reported.

As stated above, amantadine is relatively contraindicated in patients with renal disease or a seizure disorder. Amantadine should be used with caution in patients with eczema or cardiovascular disease. Some evidence indicates that amantadine is teratogenic and, therefore, should not be given to pregnant women. Because amantadine is excreted in milk, women who are breast-feeding should not be given the drug.

Suicide attempts with amantadine overdoses are life-threatening. Symptoms can include toxic psychoses (confusion, hallucinations, aggressiveness) and cardiopulmonary arrest. Emergency treatment beginning with gastric lavage or induction of emesis is indicated.

DRUG-DRUG INTERACTIONS

There is one case report that amantadine coadministered with phenelzine (Nardil) resulted in a significant increase in resting blood pressure. Because of the dopaminergic activity of amantadine, the drug may augment the stimulatory effects of

CNS stimulant drugs, such as cocaine and sympathomimetics (for example, amphetamine).

The coadministration of amantadine with CNS stimulants can result in insomnia, irritability, nervousness, and possibly seizures or irregular heartbeat. Amantadine should not be coadministered with anticholinergics because unwanted side effects—such as confusion, hallucinations, nightmares, dryness of mouth, and blurred vision—may be exacerbated.

References

Davis J M, Barter J T, Kane J M: Antipsychotic drugs. In *Comprehensive Textbook of Psychiatry*, ed 5, H I Kaplan, B J Sadock, editors, p. 1591. Williams & Wilkins, Baltimore, 1989.

de Roin S, Winters S: Amantadine hydrochloride: Current and new uses. J Neurosci Nurs 22: 322, 1990.

Pimentel L, Hughes B: Amantadine toxicity presenting with complex ventricular ectopy and hallucinations. Pediatr Emerg Care 7: 89, 1991.

Snoey E R, Bessen H A: Acute psychosis after amantadine overdose. Ann Emerg Med 19: 668, 1990.

Weddington W W Jr, Brown B S, Haertzen C A, Hess J M, Mahaffey J R, Kolar A F, Jaffe J H: Comparison of amantadine and desipramine combined with psychotherapy for treatment of cocaine dependence. Am J Drug Alcohol Abuse 17: 137, 1991.

Wilcox J A, Tsuang J: Psychological effects of amantadine on psychotic subjects. Neuropsychobiology 23: 144, 1990.

4

Anticholinergics

Anticholinergic drugs are used in psychiatry for the treatment of drug-induced extrapyramidal symptoms, such as antipsychotic-induced parkinsonism. Five anticholinergic drugs are available in the United States for that indication (Table 4–1). The variations among the five drugs are of little significance except for local differences in price. The molecular structures of selected anticholinergic drugs are given in Figure 4–1.

PHARMACOLOGICAL ACTIONS

The pharmacokinetics of the anticholinergic drugs are not well studied, although all are well absorbed from the gastrointestinal (GI) tract. Only two of the preparations are available in parenteral forms. Benztropine (Cogentin, Tremin) is probably the most often used parenteral anticholinergic. Benztropine is absorbed equally rapidly by intramuscular (IM) and intravenous (IV) administration; therefore, IM is preferred because of a lower risk of adverse effects. Although all five drugs have their primary effects through the blockade of muscarinic acetylcholine receptors, benztropine and ethopropazine (Parsidol) also have some antihistaminergic effects. Of the five drugs, benztropine tends to be least stimulating, and trihexyphenidyl (Artane) tends to be most stimulating.

The major alternatives to the anticholinergic drugs are diphenhydramine (Benadryl) (an antihistamine) (Chapter 5) and amantadine (Symadine, Symmetrel) (Chapter 3). Amantadine has the advantage of not causing the adverse effects that are associated with the anticholinergics; however, it is a dopamine agonist that may exacerbate psychosis. Amantadine may also be associated with less memory impairment than the anticholinergics.

INDICATIONS

The anticholinergics are effective in the treatment of acute dystonic reactions, parkinsonism, akinesia, and rabbit syndrome. The anticholinergics are less effective for the treatment of akathisia, which is perhaps better treated with β-adrenergic receptor antagonists (for example, propranolol [Inderal]), (Chapter 2) or a benzodiazepine (for example, lorazepam [Ativan]) (Chapter 7).

CLINICAL GUIDELINES

For the treatment of acute dystonic reactions, benztropine, 1 to 2 mg, or its equivalent in another drug should be given IM. If the dose is not effective in 20 to 30 minutes, the drug should be administered again. If the patient still does not

Table 4–1
Anticholinergic Drugs

Generic Name	Brand Name	Tablet Size	Injectable	Usual Daily Oral Dose	Short-Term Intramuscular or Intravenous Dose
Benztropine mesylate	Cogentin, Tremin	0.5, 1.2 mg	1 mg per mL	1–4 mg one to three times	1–2 mg
Biperiden hydrochloride (tab) lactate (inj)	Akineton	2 mg	5 mg per mL	2 mg one to three times	2 mg
Ethopropazine hydrochloride	Parsidol	10, 50 mg	—	50–100 mg one to three times	—
Procyclidine hydrochloride	Kemadrin	5 mg	—	2.5–5 mg three times	—
Trihexyphenidyl hydrochloride	Artane, Trihexane, Trihexy-5	2, 5 mg elixir 2 mg per 5 mL	—	2–5 mg two to four times	—

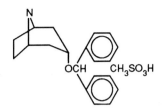

Benztropine mesylate

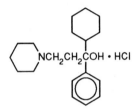

Trihexyphenidyl hydrochloride

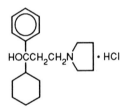

Procyclidine hydrochloride

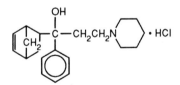

Biperiden hydrochloride

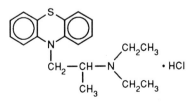

Ethopropazine hydrochloride

Figure 4–1. Molecular structures of selected anticholinergic drugs.

respond in another 20 to 30 minutes, a benzodiazepine (for example, lorazepam, 1 mg IM or IV) or an antihistamine (for example, diphenhydramine [Benadryl], 50 mg IM or IV) should be given.

For the treatment of chronic drug-induced extrapyramidal symptoms, the equivalent of 1 to 4 mg benztropine one to four times daily should be given. Patients usually respond to that dosage of benztropine in one to two days. The anticholinergic should be administered for four to eight weeks; then it should be discontinued to assess whether the patient still needs the drug. Anticholinergic drugs should be tapered over a one- to two-week period. If anticholinergics are not effective, diphenhydramine, amantadine, or a benzodiazepine can be tried.

Whether prophylaxis with anticholinergics is indicated when first giving a patient an antipsychotic has been debated. Clinicians in favor of prophylaxis argue that patient compliance is hindered if uncomfortable neurological adverse effects occur. Clinicians opposed to prophylactic treatment cite the increased risk of anticholinergic toxicity and possibly tardive dyskinesia. Studies have shown that prophylactic treatment with anticholinergic drugs does reduce the incidence of acute dystonic reactions. A reasonable compromise is to use prophylactic treatment in patients at high risk of acute dystonic reactions, primarily young male patients. Old adults and children are most sensitive to the effects of the drugs. At least one hour should elapse between the administration of antacids and the administration of anticholinergic drugs.

ADVERSE EFFECTS

The adverse effects of the anticholinergics are those resulting from the blockade of muscarinic acetylcholine receptors (Chapter 1 and Table 1–9). Anticholinergic drugs should be given cautiously, if at all, to patients with prostatic hypertrophy, urinary retention, narrow-arrow glaucoma, cardiovascular disease, or myasthenia gravis. The drugs should be used with caution in patients with hepatic or renal disease because the anticholinergic activity exacerbates those medical problems. The anticholinergics are occasionally used as drugs of abuse both on the street and by patients. Their abuse potential is related to their mild mood-elevating properties. The most serious adverse effect associated with anticholinergic toxicity is anticholinergic intoxication.

Those agents have not been studied in pregnancy. They have not been reported to cause problems in nursing babies; however, they may reduce the flow of breast milk in some patients.

Anticholinergic Intoxication

The symptoms of anticholinergic intoxication can include delirium, coma, seizures, extreme agitation, hallucinations, severe hypotension, supraventricular tachycardia, and the usual peripheral manifestations—flushing, mydriasis, dry skin, hyperthermia, and decreased bowel sounds. Treatment should begin with the immediate discontinuation of all anticholinergic drugs. The syndrome of anticholinergic intoxication can be diagnosed and treated with physostigmine (Antilirium, Eserine), an inhibitor of anticholinesterase, 1 to 2 mg IV (1 mg every two minutes) or IM every 30 or 60 minutes. Absorption of IM physostigmine can be erratic. The first dose should be repeated in 15 to 20 minutes if no response is seen. Benzodiazepines can be used to treat agitation. Treatment with physostigmine should be used only when emergency cardiac-monitoring and life-support services are available, because physostigmine can lead to serve hypotension and bronchial constriction. Those effects of physostigmine can be reversed with rapid IV administration of atropine, 0.5 mg per each milligram of physostigmine administered. Physostigmine is also contraindicated in patients with unstable vital signs, asthma, or a history of cardiac abnormalities. In general, physostigmine should be used only to confirm a diagnosis of anticholinergic activity or to treat the most serious symptoms of anticholinergic intoxication—seizures, severe hypotension, delirium.

DRUG-DRUG INTERACTIONS

The most common drug-drug interactions with the anticholinergic drugs occur when they are coadministered with psychotropics that also produce high anticholinergic activity, such as most antipsychotics, tricyclic and tetracyclic antidepressants, and monoamine oxidase inhibitors (MAOIs). Many over-the-counter cold preparations also produce significant anticholinergic activity. The coadministration of those drugs can result in a life-threatening anticholinergic intoxication syndrome. The drugs may have additive effects with central nervous system (CNS) depressants, including alcohol.

References

Arana G W, Goff D C, Baldessarini R J, Keepers G A: Efficacy of anticholinergic prophylaxis for neuroleptic-induced acute dystonia. Am J Psychiatry *145*: 993, 1988.

Davis J M, Dysken M W: The pharmacology of psychotropic drugs and drug-drug interactions. In *Comprehensive Textbook of Psychiatry*, ed 5, H I Kaplan, B J Sadock, editors, p 1662. Williams & Wilkins, Baltimore, 1989.

Dilsaver S C: Antimuscarinic agents as substances of abuse: A review. J Clin Psychopharmacol *8*: 14, 1988.

Goff D C, Arana G W, Greenblatt D J, Dupont R, Ornstein M, Harmatz J S, Shader R I: The effect of benztropine on haloperidol-induced dystonia, clinical efficacy, and pharmacokinetics: A prospective double-blind trial. J Clin Psychopharmacol *11* (2): 106, 1991.

Hidalgo H A, Mowers R M: Anticholinergic drug abuse. DICP *24*: 40, 1990.

Johnson A L, Hollister L E, Berger P A: The anticholinergic intoxication syndrome: Diagnosis and treatment. J Clin Psychiatry *42*: 313, 1981.

Keepers G A, Clappison V J, Casey D E: Initial anticholinergic prophylaxis for neuroleptic-induced extrapyramidal syndromes. Arch Gen Psychiatry *40*: 1113, 1983.

Modell J G, Tandon R, Beresford T P: Dopaminergic activity of the antimuscarinic antiparkinsonian agents. J Clin Psychopharmacol *9*: 347, 1989.

5

Antihistamines

Antihistamines are used in psychiatry primarily for the treatment of drug-induced extrapyramidal symptoms and as mild hypnotics and sedatives. Diphenhydramine (Benadryl) is used for the treatment of extrapyramidal symptoms and sometimes as a hypnotic; hydroxyzine hydrochloride (Atarax) and hydroxyzine pamoate (Vistaril) are used as sedatives. Cyproheptadine (Periactin) has been used for the treatment of inhibited male and female orgasm caused by tricyclic antidepressants, monoamine oxidase inhibitors, and fluoxetine (Prozac) (Figure 5–1).

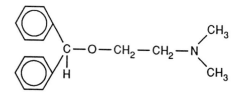

Diphenhydramine

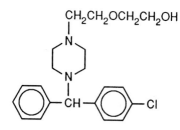

Hydroxyzine

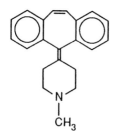

Cyproheptadine

Figure 5–1. Molecular structures of selected antihistamines.

PHARMACOLOGICAL ACTIONS

Both diphenhydramine and hydroxyzine are well absorbed from the gastrointestinal (GI) tract. Approximately 50 percent of diphenhydramine is metabolized in a first-pass effect by the liver, and the metabolites are excreted in the urine. The antiextrapyramidal effects of intramuscular (IM) diphenhydramine have their onset in 15 to 30 minutes; the sedative effects of diphenhydramine peak in one to three hours. Hydroxyzine is also metabolized by the liver, but its metabolites are excreted in feces. The sedative effects begin 30 to 60 minutes after administration and last four to six hours. Because both drugs are metabolized in the liver, patients with hepatic disease, such as cirrhosis, may attain high plasma concentrations with chronic administration. Both drugs have their primary therapeutic effects through antihistaminergic activity; however, both drugs also possess some antimuscarinic cholinergic activity. Cyproheptadine has potent antihistaminic and serotonin antagonist (5-hydroxytryptamine [$5-HT_2$]) properties. It is well absorbed after oral administration, and its metabolites are excreted in the urine.

INDICATIONS AND CLINICAL GUIDELINES

The use of antihistamines for drug-induced extrapyramidal disorders is a reasonable alternative to anticholinergics and amantadine (Symadine, Symmetrel), especially in patients who are particularly sensitive to anticholinergic effects but cannot tolerate amantadine. The antihistamines are relatively safe hypnotics, although they are not superior to benzodiazepines. The antihistamines have not been effective as chronic anxiolytic therapy for more than a few months. Either the benzodiazepines or buspirone (BuSpar) are preferable for such treatment. A listing of antihistamine preparations is given in Table 5–1.

Diphenhydramine is used in the acute and chronic treatment of drug-induced extrapyramidal symptoms and as a hypnotic. The drug is available in 25 and 50 mg tablets, 12.5 mg per 5 mL elixir, and 10 mg per mL and 50 mg per mL injectable forms. Injections given IM should be deep, since superficial injections can cause local irritation. Acute intravenous (IV) administration of 25 to 50 mg is an effective treatment for acute dystonic reactions. Treatment with 25 mg three times a day, up to 50 mg four times a day if necessary, can be used to treat drug-induced parkinsonism, akinesia, and rabbit syndrome (rapid, fine buccolingual movements). Diphenhydramine can be used as a hypnotic at a 50-mg dose. Doses of 100 mg have not been shown to be superior to doses of 50 mg.

Hydroxyzine is most commonly used as a sedative or short-term anxiolytic. Hydroxyzine is available in 10, 25, 50, and 100 mg tablets; 12.5 mg per 5 mL solution; and 10 mg per mL and 50 mg per mL injectable forms. Hydroxyzine should not be given IV, since it is irritating to the blood vessels. Doses of 50 to 100 mg orally (PO) four times a day for chronic treatment or 50 to 100 mg IM every four to six hours for acute treatment are usually effective.

The ability to achieve orgasm can be restored with 4 to 16 mg a day of cyproheptadine taken by mouth one or two hours before anticipated sexual activity. It is available in 4 mg tablets and 2 mg per 5 mL solution. Children and elderly patients are more sensitive to the effects of antihistamines than are young adults.

Table 5–1
Antihistamine Preparations

	Tablets (mg)	Capsules (mg)	Elixir[1] (mg/5 mL)	Solution[2] (mg/mL)	Parenteral (mg/mL)	Suspension[3] (mg/5 mL)	Cream*	Lotion*	Solution*
Diphenhydramine	25, 50	25, 50	12.5	8, 12.5	10, 50	—	1%, 2%	1%	1%, 2%
Hydroxyzine	10, 25, 50, 100	25, 50, 100	—	10	25, 50	25	—	—	—
Cyproheptadine	4	—	—	2	—	—	—	—	—

1 = A sweetened hydroalcoholic liquid intended for oral use.
2 = A drug incorporated into an aqueous or alcoholic solution.
3 = Undissolved drug dispersed in a liquid for oral or parenteral use.
* = Topical.

ADVERSE EFFECTS

Antihistamines are commonly associated with sedation, dizziness, and hypotension, all of which can be severe in elderly patients. Poor motor coordination can result in accidents; therefore, patients should be warned about driving or operating dangerous machinery. Other common adverse effects include epigastric distress, nausea, vomiting, diarrhea, and constipation. Because of the drugs' mild anticholinergic activity, dry mouth, urinary retention, blurred vision, and constipation can occur in some patients. Symptoms of intoxication include severe drowsiness, seizures, troubled breathing, insomnia, hallucinations, flushing of face, and feeling faint. Cyproheptadine has been associated with weight gain and has been used in anorexia nervosa to take advantage of that side effect.

Antihistamines should be used with caution in patients with urinary problems, asthma, enlarged prostate, or glaucoma.

Diphenhydramine and cyproheptadine should be used in pregnancy only if clearly needed. Hydroxyzine is contraindicated in early pregnancy because of reports of fetal damage in animals. Antihistamines are contraindicated in nursing mothers.

DRUG-DRUG INTERACTIONS

The sedative property of antihistamines can be additive with central nervous system (CNS) depressants, including alcohol, other sedative-hypnotic drugs, and many psychotropic drugs. The anticholinergic activity of diphenhydramine and hydroxyzine can be additive with other drugs, producing anticholinergic activity, sometimes resulting in severe anticholinergic symptoms or intoxication. Antihistamines should not be taken within two weeks of taking a monoamine oxidase inhibitor; their coadministration causes the side effects of antihistamines to become severe. Coadministration of antihistamines with opioids can increase the rush experienced by addicts; therefore, some abuse potential is associated with the compounds. In particular, hydroxyzine may potentiate the effects of meperidine (Demerol), so its use in preanesthetic adjunctive therapy should be modified on an individual basis. Cyproheptadine has been anecdotally reported to reverse the antidepressant effects of fluoxetine. Finally, it has been reported that hydroxyzine can falsely elevate the values of urinary 17-hydroxycorticosteroids when assayed with either the Porter-Silber or the Glenn-Nelson method.

References

Carruthers S G, Shoeman D W, Hignite C E, Azarnoff D L: Correlation between plasma diphenhydramine level and sedative and antihistamine effects. Clin Pharmacol Ther *23*: 375, 1978.

Gengo F M, Gabos C, Mechtler L: Quantitative effects of diphenhydramine on mental performance measured using an automobile driving simulator. Ann Allergy *64*: 520, 1990.

Goldbloom D S, Kennedy S H: Adverse interaction of fluoxetine and cyproheptadine in two patients with bulimia nervosa. J Clin Psychiatry *52*: 261, 1991.

Gorman J M, Davis J M: Antianxiety drugs. In *Comprehensive Textbook of Psychiatry*, ed 5, H I Kaplan, B J Sadock, editors, p 1579. Williams & Wilkins, Baltimore, 1989.

6

Barbiturates and Other Similarly Acting Drugs

The clinical use of barbiturates in psychiatry as sedative-hypnotics has been essentially eclipsed by the benzodiazepines. That change in clinical practice is based on the higher abuse potential and lower therapeutic index for barbiturates, compared with those for the benzodiazepines and buspirone (BuSpar).

PHARMACOLOGICAL ACTIONS

The barbiturates (Figure 6–1) are well absorbed after oral administration. The binding of barbiturates to plasma proteins is high, but lipid solubility varies. The individual barbiturates are differentially metabolized by the liver and are excreted by the kidneys. The half-lives of specific barbiturates range from 1 hour to 120 hours. Barbiturates may also induce hepatic enzymes, thereby reducing the levels of both the barbiturate and any other concurrently administered drugs metabolized by the liver. The mechanism of action for the barbiturates involves the γ-amino-butyric acid (GABA) receptor-benzodiazepine receptor-chloride ion channel complex.

INDICATIONS

There are currently six indications for barbiturate administration. First, amobarbital (Amytal) (50 to 250 mg intramuscular [IM]) may be used in emergency settings to control agitation. The use of IM lorazepam (Ativan) or diazepam (Valium), however, seems to be replacing that application of amobarbital. Second, amobarbital interviews are sometimes used for diagnostic purposes. Several studies report that other sedative drugs, including the benzodiazepines, are as effective in that application. Third, there are several reports that barbiturates can activate some catatonic patients, although benzodiazepines may also have that effect. Fourth, barbiturates may be indicated for use in patients who have serious adverse effects from benzodiazepines or buspirone. Fifth, some patients who do not respond adequately to benzodiazepines or buspirone may respond to barbiturates. Sixth, some patients, particularly elderly persons, who have received barbiturates in the past may insist on taking barbiturates, rather than trying a benzodiazepine or buspirone.

CLINICAL GUIDELINES

The dosages for barbiturates vary (Table 6–1), and treatment should begin with low dosages that are increased to achieve a clinical effect. Barbiturates with half-

General Formula:

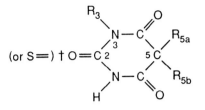

Barbiturate	R_{5a}	R_{5b}
Amobarbital	Ethyl	Isopentyl
Aprobarbital	Allyl	Isopropyl
Butabarbital	Ethyl	Sec-Butyl
Butalbital	Allyl	Isobutyl
Mephobarbital *	Ethyl	Phenyl
Metharbital *	Ethyl	Ethyl
Methohexital *	Allyl	1-Methyl-2-Pentynyl
Pentobarbital	Ethyl	1-Methylbutyl
Phenobarbital	Ethyl	Phenyl
Secobarbital	Allyl	1-Methylbutyl
Taibutal	Allyl	Sec-Butyl
Thiamyial †	Allyl	1-Methylbutyl
Thiopental †	Ethyl	1-Methylbutyl

* R_3 = H, except in mephobarbital, metharbital, and methohexital, where it is replaced by CH_3.
† O, except in thiamyial and thiopental, where it is replaced by S.

Figure from T W Rall: Hypnotics and sedatives: Ethanol. In Goodman and Gilman's The Pharmacological Basis of Therapeutics, ed 8, A Goodman Gilman, T W Rall, A S Nies, P Taylor, editors, p 358. Pergamon Press, New York, 1990. Used with permission.

Figure 6–1. Barbiturates currently available in the United States: names and structures.

lives in the 15- to 40-hour range are preferable, because longer-acting drugs build up in the body. The patient should be clearly instructed about the adverse effects and the potential for dependence associated with barbiturate treatment. Children and the elderly are more sensitive than are young adults to the effects of the drugs. Patients must be withdrawn from barbiturates gradually. The pentobarbital (Nembutal) challenge test can be used to estimate the dosage needed to prevent an abstinence syndrome. That approach is particularly useful when the patient's history regarding the daily dose of sedative-hypnotics consumed is unreliable (Table 6–2). Available preparations of selected barbiturates are given in Table 6–3.

ADVERSE EFFECTS

The adverse effects of barbiturates are similar to those for benzodiazepines, including paradoxical dysphoria, hyperactivity, and cognitive disorganization. The barbiturates differ from the benzodiazepines in their high abuse potential, marked development of tolerance, dependence, and low therapeutic index. Additional side effects include drowsiness, central nervous system (CNS) depression, irritability,

Table 6–1
Selected Barbiturates

Generic Name	DEA Control Level	Trade Name	Half-Life (hrs)	Sedative Adult Dose Range (mg per day)	Sedative Adult Single Dose Range (mg)	Hypnotic Dose Range (mg)
Amobarbital	II	Amytal	8–42	65–400	65–100	100–200
Butabarbital	III	Butisol	34–42	15–120	15–30	50–100
Mephobarbital	IV	Mebaral	11–67	32–400	32–100	—
Pentobarbital	II	Nembutal	15–48	30–120	30–40	100–200
Phenobarbital	IV	Luminal	80–120	15–600	15–60	100–200
Secobarbital	II	Seconal	15–40	—	—	100–300

Table 6–2
Pentobarbital Challenge Test

1. Give pentobarbital 200 mg orally.
2. Observe for intoxication after one hour (e.g., sleepiness, slurred speech, or nystagmus).
3. If patient is not intoxicated, give another 100 mg of pentobarbital every two hours (maximum 500 mg over six hours).
4. Total dose given to produce mild intoxication is equivalent to daily abuse level of barbiturates.
5. Substitute phenobarbital 30 mg (longer half-life) for each 100 mg of pentobarbital.
6. Decrease by about 10 percent a day.
7. Adjust rate if signs of intoxication or withdrawal are present.

and impairment of fine motor skills. The symptoms of barbiturate withdrawal are similar to but more marked than those for benzodiazepine withdrawal. Barbiturates are often lethal in overdoses because of respiratory depression, especially if the drugs are combined with alcohol intake, as is often seen clinically. Barbiturates affect the metabolism of the following drugs: anticoagulants, anticonvulsants, corticosteroids, adrenocorticotropic hormone (ACTH), estrogens, and progesterone. Barbiturates can decrease the effectiveness of oral contraceptives; therefore, an alternative method of birth control is recommended.

Barbiturates should not be used by pregnant or nursing women. Barbiturates should be used with caution in patients with a history of substance abuse, depression, diabetes, renal disease, severe anemia, pain, hyperthyroidism, or hypoadrenalism. Those agents can cause paradoxical excitation in both adults and children.

Intoxication is manifested by confusion or drowsiness, irritability, hyporeflexia or areflexia, ataxia, and nystagmus.

DRUG-DRUG INTERACTIONS

Barbiturates interact with many other drugs, and the clinician should consult a reference text for the interactions when prescribing barbiturates. The two most important interactions are the additive effects of other sedatives and the increased metabolism of many cardiac-related drugs and heterocyclic antidepressants.

Because of respiratory suppression, barbiturates should be used cautiously in patients with respiratory illness. Barbiturates are absolutely contraindicated in patients with acute intermittent porphyria, because barbiturates cause the production of porphyrins. Patients with hepatic cirrhosis may have very high plasma barbiturate concentrations because of their impaired ability to metabolize the drug.

OTHER SIMILARLY ACTING DRUGS

Four other classes of drugs—carbamates, piperidinediones, cyclic ethers, and tertiary carbinols—are still available for use as sedatives and hypnotics; however, those drugs are even more rarely used than the barbiturates because of their high abuse potential and potential toxic effects. Chloral hydrate is discussed in Chapter 13. The molecular structures of those drugs are given in Figure 6–2.

Table 6–3
Barbiturate Preparations

	Tablets	Capsules	Elixir	Parenteral	Rectal Suppositories
Amobarbital	30 mg	200 mg	—	250, 500 mg	—
Butabarbital	15, 30, 50, 100 mg	—	30 mg/5 mL, 33.3 mg/5 mL	—	—
Mephobarbital	32, 50, 100 mg	—	—	—	—
Pentobarbital	—	50, 100 mg	18.2 mg/5 mL	50 mg/mL	30, 60, 120, 200 mg
Phenobarbital	15, 16, 30, 32, 60, 65, 100 mg	16 mg	15 mg/5 mL, 20 mg/5 mL	30 mg/mL, 60 mg/mL, 65 mg/mL, 130 mg/mL	—
Secobarbital	—	50, 100 mg	—	50 mg/mL	—

Carbamates

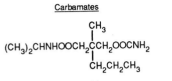

$(CH_3)_2CHNHOOCH_2CCH_2OOCNH_2$

Carisoprodol

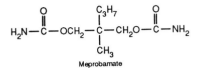

Meprobamate

Piperidinediones

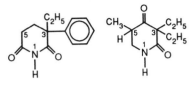

Glutethimide   Methyprylon

Cyclic Ethers

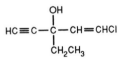

Paraldehyde

Tertiary Carbinols

$HC{\equiv}C-\underset{\underset{CH_2CH_3}{|}}{\overset{\overset{OH}{|}}{C}}-CH{=}CHCl$

Ethchlorvynol

Figure 6–2.   Molecular structures of other similarly acting drugs.

Carbamates

Meprobamate (Miltown, Equanil) and carisoprodol (Soma) are carbamates that are effective as anxiolytics, sedatives, hypnotics, and muscle relaxants. The drugs have a lower therapeutic index and a higher abuse potential than benzodiazepines, and their use is indicated only if the previously described drugs are not an option. The carbamates may have even more abuse potential and may be more dependence-inducing than the barbiturates.

The usual dosage of meprobamate is 400 mg three or four times daily. Drowsiness is a common adverse effect, and patients should be warned of the additive effects of sedative drugs. Sudden withdrawal may cause anxiety, restlessness, weakness, delirium, and convulsions. Adverse effects can include urticarial or erythematous rashes, anaphylactoid and other allergic reactions, angioneurotic edema, dermatitis, blood dyscrasias, gastrointestinal upsets, and extraocular muscular paralysis. Fatal overdoses can occur with meprobamate in doses as low as 12 g (thirty 400 mg tablets) without the ingestion of any other sedatives. Meprobamate is available in 200, 400, and 600 mg tablets and 200 and 400 mg extended-release capsules. Carisoprodol is available in 350 mg tablets.

Piperidinediones

Glutethimide (Doriden) and methyprylon (Noludar) are piperidinediones that are effective as hypnotics, sedatives, and anxiolytics but are even more subject to abuse and more lethal in overdoses than the barbiturates and carbamates. Glutethimide has a slow and unpredictable absorption after oral administration. Seizures, shock, and anticholinergic toxicity are more common in glutethimide overdoses than in barbiturate overdoses. It is a very rare patient for whom treatment with piperidinediones is indicated. Glutethimide is available in 500 mg tablets. Methyprylon is available in 200 mg tablets and 300 mg capsules.

Cyclic Ethers

Paraldehyde was introduced in 1882 as a hypnotic. When 5 mL is given IM or 5 to 10 mL administered orally, it is an effective, albeit old-fashioned, treatment for alcohol withdrawal symptoms, anxiety, and insomnia. Paraldehyde is almost completely metabolized, but its excretion in unmetabolized form by the lungs limits its usefulness because of its offensive taste and ubiquitous odor.

Tertiary Carbinols

Ethchlorvynol (Placidyl) is a tertiary carbinol, another nonbarbiturate sedative-hypnotic. It was marketed for use as a short-term treatment for insomnia. The drug is rapidly absorbed, with a fast onset of action. Its rapid distribution limits its duration of action. Most of the drug is metabolized by the liver. Ethchlorvynol has sedative-hypnotic, muscle relaxant, and anticonvulsant properties. The usual hypnotic dose is 500 mg at bedtime. It is available in 200, 500, and 750 mg capsules.

The drug has a significant potential for abuse, physical dependence, and tolerance. It is particularly dangerous in overdose. The lethal dose range is 10 to 25 grams, although death has been reported at 2.5 to 6 grams. There is little to recommend the drug, especially in view of the safe alternatives available. It is cross-tolerant with other sedative-hypnotics, and detoxification can be achieved with barbiturates by using the pentobarbital challenge.

References

Ator N A, Griffiths R R: Self-administration of barbiturates and benzodiazepines: A review. Pharmacol Biochem Behav 27: 391, 1987.

DeWit H, Griffiths R R: Testing the abuse liability of anxiolytic and hypnotic drugs in humans. Drug Alcohol Depend 28: 83, 1991.

Goodman R A, Mercy J A, Rosenberg M L: Drug use and interpersonal violence: Barbiturates detected in homicide victims. Am J Epidemiol 124: 851, 1986.

Gorman J M, Davis J M: Antianxiety drugs. In Comprehensive Textbook of Psychiatry, ed 5, H I Kaplan, B J Sadock, editors, p 1579. Williams & Wilkins, Baltimore, 1989.

Harris R A: Distinct actions of alcohols, barbiturates and benzodiazepines on GABA-activated chloride channels. Alcohol 7: 273, 1990.

Jensen C F, Cowley D S, Walker R D: Drug preferences of alcoholic polydrug abusers with and without panic. J Clin Psychiatry 51: 189, 1990.

McCall W V, Shelp F E, McDonald W M: Controlled investigation of the amobarbital interview for catatonic mutism. Am J Psychiatry 149: 202, 1992.

Sullivan J T, Sellers E M: Treatment of the barbiturate abstinence syndrome. Med J Aust 145: 456, 1986.

Taberber P V: The GABA system in functional tolerance and dependence following barbiturates, benzodiazepines, or ethanol: Correlation or causality? Comp Biochem Physiol 93: 241, 1989.

Yu S, Ho I K: Effects of acute barbiturate administration, tolerance and dependence on brain GAMA system: Comparison to alcohol and benzodiazepines. Alcohol 7: 261, 1990.

7

Benzodiazepines

Benzodiazepines are variously referred to as antianxiety agents, anxiolytics, and minor tranquilizers. The term "minor tranquilizer" is misleading, because using it may cause confusion between this class of drug and the major tranquilizers, a faulty but commonly used term for the antipsychotic drugs. Benzodiazepines are also classified as sedative-hypnotics. A sedative drug reduces daytime activity, tempers excitement, and generally quiets the patient. An anxiolytic drug reduces pathological anxiety. A hypnotic drug produces drowsiness and facilitates the onset and maintenance of sleep. In general, benzodiazepines act as hypnotics in high doses, as anxiolytics in moderate doses, and as sedatives in low doses. Recent indications for the benzodiazepines include panic disorder, phobias, and bipolar disorder. In addition, the benzodiazepines are used as anesthetics, anticonvulsants, and muscle relaxants.

The benzodiazepines have become the sedative-hypnotic drugs of first choice because they have a higher therapeutic index and significantly less abuse potential than many of the other sedative-hypnotics (for example, barbiturates), with the exception of buspirone (BuSpar). The term "benzodiazepine" is used to mean benzodiazepine agonist. However, a benzodiazepine antagonist, flumazenil (Mazicon), is available for the treatment of benzodiazepine overdose and is discussed in Chapter 21.

CLASSIFICATION

The benzodiazepine nucleus consists of a benzene ring fused to the seven-sided diazepine ring. All clinically important benzodiazepines also have a second benzene ring attached to the carbon at position 5 on the diazepine ring (Figure 7–1). The benzodiazepines can be classified according to the substitutions on the diazepine ring (Table 7–1). The 2-keto benzodiazepines have a keto group off the carbon atom in position 2 on the diazepine ring. Although chlordiazepoxide (Librium) has a different substitution ($-NHCH_1$) at that position, it is useful to classify it along with the 2-keto derivatives. Also, quazepam (Doral) substitutes a sulfur atom for the oxygen atom in the keto moiety. The 3-hydroxy benzodiazepines have a hydroxy group on the carbon atom at position 3 of the diazepine ring. The triazolo benzodiazepines have a triazolo ring fused to the nitrogen atom at position 1 and to the carbon atom at position 2 of the diazepine ring.

PHARMACOLOGICAL ACTIONS

Pharmacokinetics

With the exception of clorazepate (Tranxene), all the benzodizepines are completely absorbed unchanged from the gastrointestinal (GI) tract. Clorazepate is

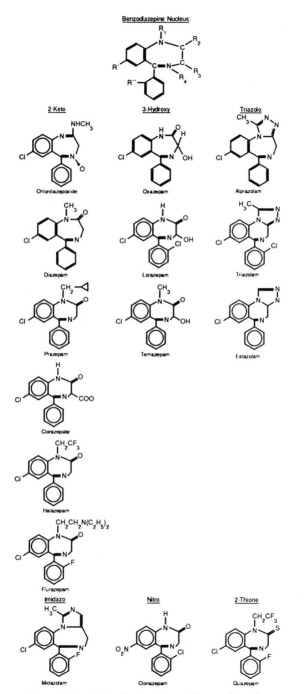

Figure 7–1. Molecular structures of benzodiazepines.

Table 7–1
Classification of Benzodiazepines

2-Keto	3-Hydroxy	Triazolo	Imidazo	Nitro	2-Thione
Chlordiazepoxide	Oxazepam	Alprazolam	Midazolam	Clonazepam	Quazepam
Diazepam	Lorazepam	Triazolam			
Prazepam	Temazepam	Estazolam			
Clorazepate					
Halazepam					
Flurazepam					

converted to desmethyldiazepam in the GI tract and is absorbed in that form. Absorption, attainment of peak levels, and onset of action are quickest for diazepam (Valium), lorazepam (Ativan), alprazolam (Xanax), triazolam (Halcion), and estazolam (ProSom). The rapid onset of effects is important to patients who take a single dose of benzodiazepines to calm an episodic burst of anxiety. The rapid onset of effects for those drugs can be partly attributed to their high lipid solubility, a characteristic that varies fivefold among the different benzodiazepines. The range of time to peak plasma level is one to three hours, although prazepam (Centrax) may take up to six hours. There may also be a secondary peak plasma level 6 to 12 hours after enterohepatic recirculation. Although several benzodiazepines are available in parenteral forms for intramuscular (IM) administration, only lorazepam has rapid and reliable absorption from that route. The use of IM lorazepam is beginning to replace the use of intravenous (IV) diazepam in psychiatric emergency settings.

The metabolism of benzodiazepines differs for the three classes. Chlordiazepoxide is metabolized to diazepam, then to desmethyldiazepam (nordiazepam), then to oxazepam, and finally to a glucuronide form. Diazepam, clorazepate, prazepam, and halazepam (Paxipam) are metabolized first to desmethyldiazepam and then follow the same route as chlordiazepoxide does. The metabolism of flurazepam (Dalmane) and quazepam follows similar biochemical steps. As a result of the slow metabolism of desmethyldiazepam, all the 2-keto benzodiazepines have plasma half-lives of 30 to more than 100 hours and are, therefore, the longest-acting benzodiazepines. The plasma half-life can be as high as 200 hours in persons who are genetically slow metabolizers of those compounds. Quazepam, a 2-thione benzodiazepine, also follows the same metabolic pathway as 2-keto benzodiazepines and, thus, has long half-life metabolites. Because the attainment of steady plasma levels of the drugs can take up to two weeks, patients may experience toxicity after 7 to 10 days of treatment with a dosage that may have seemed therapeutic to the clinician. Patients with hepatic disease and elderly patients are particularly likely to have toxic effects from benzodiazepines that are administered in repeated or high doses.

The 3-hydroxy benzodiazepines have short half-lives (10 to 30 hours), because they are directly metabolized by glucuronidation and, thus, have no active metabolites. The triazolo benzodiazepines are hydroxylated before they undergo glucuronidation. Alprazolam has a half-life of 10 to 15 hours, and triazolam has the shortest half-life (two to three hours) of all the orally administered benzodiazepines. Estazolam has a half-life of 10 to 24 hours.

Midazolam (Versed), an imidazobenzodiazepine, is available only in an injectable form. It is used for conscious sedation during medical procedures. It has no clinical use in psychiatry. It produces significant amnestic effects and can suppress respiration. Midazolam differs from other currently available benzodiazepines in that it is available only in a parenteral form and is used only by anesthesiologists. It forms a stable, water-soluble salt that permits its use in IV solutions.

Pharmacodynamics

The benzodiazepines bind to specific receptor sites that are associated with γ-aminobutyric acid (GABA) binding sites and chloride channels. Benzodiazepine binding increases the affinity of the GABA receptor for GABA, thereby increasing the flow of chloride ions into the neurons.

Recently, basic neuroscience research has found evidence for two subtypes of central nervous system (CNS) benzodiazepine receptors (also called omega receptors)—BZ_1 (also called omega$_1$) and BZ_2 (also called omega$_2$). BZ_1 receptors are believed to be involved in the mediation of sleep. BZ_2 receptors are believed to be involved in cognition, memory, and motor control. Theoretically, a benzodiazepine hypnotic that affects only BZ_1 receptors may have fewer adverse cognitive effects. Both quazepam and halazepam are more specific for the BZ_1 receptor than the BZ_2 receptor and, therefore, may be expected to be associated with less amnesia and other cognitive impairments.

Tolerance, Dependence, and Withdrawal

When benzodiazepines are used for short periods of time (one to two weeks) in moderate doses, there is usually no evidence of tolerance, dependence, or withdrawal. The very short-acting benzodiazepines (for example, triazolam) may be a slight exception to that rule, as some patients have reported increased anxiety the day after taking the drug. Some patients also report a tolerance to the anxiolytic effects of benzodiazepines and require increased doses to maintain clinical remission. There is also a cross-tolerance among most of the classes of antianxiety drugs, with the notable exception of buspirone.

The appearance of a withdrawal syndrome (also called a discontinuation syndrome) (Table 7–2) from benzodiazepines depends on the length of time a patient has taken the drug, the dosage the patient has been taking, the rate at which the drug is tapered, and the half-life of the particular compound. Abrupt discontinuation of benzodiazepines, particularly those with short half-lives, is associated with severe withdrawal symptoms. Serious symptoms may include depression, paranoia, delirium, and seizures. The incidence of the syndrome is controversial; however, some features of the syndrome may occur in as many as 50 percent of the patients treated with the drugs. The development of a severe withdrawal syndrome is seen only in patients who have taken high dosages for long periods. The appearance of the syndrome may be delayed for one to two weeks in patients who had been taking 2-keto benzodiazepines with very long half-lives. Alprazolam seems to be particularly associated with an immediate and severe withdrawal syndrome and should be tapered gradually.

Table 7–2
Commonly Observed Withdrawal Symptoms
(Benzodiazepine Withdrawal Syndrome)

Anxiety
Irritability
Insomnia
Fatigue
Headache
Muscle twitching or aching
Tremor, shakiness
Sweating
Dizziness
Concentration difficulties

*Nausea, loss of appetite
*Observable depression
*Depersonalization, derealization
*Increased sensory perception (smell, light, taste, touch)
*Abnormal perception or sensation of movement

Table from P P Roy-Byrne, D Hommer: Benzodiazepine withdrawal: Overview and implications for the treatment of anxiety. Am J Med *84*: 1041, 1988. Used with permission.
*Symptoms likely to represent true withdrawal, rather than an exacerbation or return of original anxiety.

INDICATIONS

Anxiety

The major clinical application for benzodiazepines in psychiatry is the treatment of anxiety—both idiopathic generalized anxiety disorder and anxiety associated with specific life events (for example, adjustment disorder with anxious mood). Most patients should be treated for a specific and relatively brief period. Some patients, however, may have a disorder that requires maintenance on the drugs.

Insomnia

Flurazepam, temazepam (Restoril), quazepam, estazolam, and triazolam are the benzodiazepines approved for use as hypnotics. They differ principally in their half-lives; flurazepam has the longest half-life, and triazolam has the shortest half-life. Flurazepam may be associated with minor cognitive impairment on the day after its administration, and triazolam may be associated with mild rebound anxiety. Temazepam may represent a reasonable compromise between those two adverse effects for the usual adult patient. Because of its higher specificity for BZ_1 receptors, quazepam may be associated with fewer adverse cognitive effects; however, quazepam shares the same final metabolite as flurazepam—desalkylflurazepam (half-life of about 100 hours)—and, therefore, may be associated with daytime impairment when used chronically. Estazolam produces a rapid onset of sleep and a hypnotic effect for six to eight hours.

Depression

In some outpatient studies, alprazolam has been shown to have antidepressant effects equal to those of the tricyclic antidepressants. The starting dosage for this indication should be 1 to 1.5 mg a day and should be raised 0.5 mg a day every three to four days. The maximal dosage is usually 4 to 5 mg a day, although some investigators and clinicians have used dosages as high as 10 mg a day. There is some controversy about the use of high dosages because of the possibility of withdrawal symptoms. It is particularly important to taper, rather than abruptly stop, alprazolam, usually at the rate of 0.5 mg a day every three to four days.

Bipolar Disorder

Clonazepam (Klonopin) has been shown to be effective in the management of acute mania and also as an adjuvant to lithium (Eskalith) therapy in lieu of antipsychotics. As an adjuvant to lithium, clonazepam may result in a longer time between cycles and fewer depressive episodes.

Panic Disorder and Social Phobia

In a number of studies, both alprazolam and clonazepam have been useful in treating panic disorder with and without agoraphobia and social phobia.

Akathisia

Standard anticholinergic drugs (for example, benztropine [Cogentin, Tremin]) are often ineffective in treating drug-induced akathisia. The first-line drug for akathisia is most commonly a β-adrenergic antagonist (for example, propranolol [Inderal]); however, several studies have found that benzodiazepines are also effective in treating some cases of akathisia.

Other Psychiatric Indications

Chlordiazepoxide (Librium) is used to manage the symptoms of alcohol withdrawal. The benzodiazepines (especially IM lorazepam) are used to manage both drug-induced (except amphetamine) and psychotic agitation in the emergency room. There are a few reports of the use of high dosages of benzodiazepines in patients with schizophrenia who had not responded to antipsychotics or who were unable to take the traditional drugs because of adverse effects. It is reported that benzodiazepines may be of help in some patients with tardive dyskinesia. There are reports of the successful use of intramuscular lorazepam for the treatment of catatonia.

Medical Indications

Benzodiazepines are used as anticonvulsants, muscle relaxants, and adjuvants in anesthesia. They are also used in some patients with tension headaches, tremors, or nausea and vomiting caused by chemotherapy.

CLINICAL GUIDELINES

The clinical decision to treat a patient for anxiety with a benzodiazepine should be carefully considered. Organic causes for anxiety—such as thyroid dysfunction, caffeinism, and medications—should be ruled out. The benzodiazepine should be started at a very low dosage, and the patient should be instructed regarding the sedative properties and abuse potential of the drug. An estimated length of therapy should be decided at the beginning of therapy, and the need for continued therapy should be reevaluated at least monthly because of the problems associated with long-term use. When the medication is to be discontinued, the drug must be tapered slowly (25 percent a week); otherwise, recurrence or rebound of symptoms is likely to occur. Monitoring of any withdrawal symptoms (possibly with a standardized rating scale) and support of the patient are helpful in the successful accomplishment of benzodiazepine discontinuation. Concurrent use of carbamazepine (Tegretol) during benzodiazepine discontinuation has been reported in a few studies to permit a more rapid and better-tolerated withdrawal than does a gradual taper alone. The dose range of carbamazepine used to facilitate withdrawal is 400 to 500 mg a day.

Some clinicians report particular difficulty in tapering and discontinuing alprazolam, particularly in patients who have been receiving high dosages for long periods of time. There have been reports of successful discontinuation of alprazolam by switching to clonazepam, which is then gradually withdrawn.

Children and the elderly are more susceptible than are young adults to the side effects of benzodiazepines.

Benzodiazepine withdrawal syndrome occurs when patients discontinue benzodiazepines abruptly. Ninety percent of patients after long-term use experience the syndrome on withdrawal of the drug, even if tapered slowly (although only to a mild to moderate degree). Benzodiazepine withdrawal syndrome consists of anxiety, nervousness, diaphoresis, restlessness, irritability, fatigue, light-headedness, tremor, insomnia, and weakness. The higher the dose and the shorter the half-life, the worse the withdrawal syndrome is.

Duration of Treatment

Benzodiazepines can be used to treat illnesses other than anxiety disorders. In such cases the duration of treatment should generally be similar to that for the standard drugs used to treat those disorders. The use of benzodiazepines over a long period of time for the chronically anxious patient is often valuable although controversial. In his 1980 textbook on drug treatment in psychiatry, Donald Klein, M.D., stated: "There are many reports of patients maintained on benzodiazepines for years with apparent benefit and without the development of tolerance. Nonetheless, it is dubious practice to prescribe such medications indefinitely without accompanying psychotherapy.''

Choice of Drug and Potency

Clinicians need to choose among the array of benzodiazepines available (Table 7–3). The drugs primarily differ in their half-lives. Another difference is in the rate of onset of their anxiolytic effects and potency. Potency is a general term used to express the pharmacological activity of a drug. Some benzodiazepines are more potent than others in that one compound requires a relatively smaller dose than another compound to achieve the same effect. Table 7–3 lists the approximate dose equivalents of various benzodiazepines. Clonazepam requires 0.25 mg to achieve the same effect as 5 mg of diazepam and is a high-potency benzodiazepine. Conversely, oxazepam has an approximate dose equivalent of 15 and is a low-potency drug. The four high-potency benzodiazepines—alprazolam, triazolam, estazolam, and clonazepam—are the drugs indicated for the new applications, such as depression, bipolar disorder, panic disorder, and phobias.

The advantages of the long half-life drugs include less frequent dosing, less variation in plasma concentration, and less severe withdrawal phenomena; the disadvantages include drug accumulation, increased risk of daytime psychomotor impairment, and more daytime sedation. The advantages of short half-life drugs include no drug accumulation and less daytime sedation; the disadvantages include more frequent dosing and earlier and more severe withdrawal syndromes. Rebound insomnia and anterograde amnesia (particularly with triazolam) are also more of a problem with short half-life drugs.

DRUG COMBINATIONS

The most common drug combination is the use of benzodiazepines as hypnotics in patients who are also being treated with other drugs for schizophrenia or mood disorders (Table 7–4). The combination of a benzodiazepine and an antidepressant may be indicated in the treatment of markedly anxious depressed patients or patients with panic disorder. There are several reports that the combined use of alprazolam with antipsychotics may further reduce psychotic symptoms in patients who had not responded adequately to the antipsychotic alone. The combined use of benzodiazepines with tricyclic antidepressants may improve compliance by reducing subjective side effects and producing an immediate reduction of anxiety and insomnia. However, the combination may also cause excessive sedation and cognitive impairment, and it significantly adds to the risk of overdose.

ADVERSE EFFECTS

The most common adverse effect of benzodiazepines is drowsiness, occurring in approximately 10 percent of patients, and patients should be advised not to drive or use dangerous machinery while taking the drugs. Some patients also experience dizziness (less than 1 percent) and ataxia (less than 2 percent). The most serious

Table 7–3
Benzodiazepines

Drug	Approximate Dose Equivalents[1]	Dosage Forms	Benzodiazepines Rate of Absorption	Major Active Metabolites	Average Half-Life of Metabolites (hrs)	Short-Acting/ Long-Acting[3]	Usual Adult Dosage Range (mg per day)
Alprazolam (Xanax)	0.5	0.25, 0.5, 1, 2 mg tablets	Medium	α-Hydroxyalprazolam, 4-hydroxyalprazolam	12	Short	0.5–6
Chlordiazepoxide (Librium)	10	5, 10, 25 mg tablets; 5, 10, 25 mg capsules; 100 mg parenteral	Medium	Desmethylchlordiazepoxide, demoxepam, desmethyldiazepam, oxazepam	100	Long	15–100
Clonazepam (Klonopin)	0.25	0.5, 1, 2 mg tablets	Rapid	None	34	Long	0.5–10
Clorazepate (Tranxene)	7.5	3.75, 7.5, 11.25, 15, 22.5 mg tablets; 3.75, 7.5, 15 mg capsules	Rapid	Desmethyldiazepam, oxazepam	100	Long	7.5–60
Diazepam (Valium)	5	2, 5, 10 mg tablets; 15 mg capsules (extended release); 5 mg/ mL parenteral; 5 mg/5 mL, 5 mg/ mL solution	Rapid	Desmethyldiazepam, oxazepam	100	Long	2–60
Estazolam (ProSom)	0.33	1, 2 mg tablets	Rapid	4-Hydroxy estazolam, 1-oxo-estazolam	17	Short	1–2

Flurazepam (Dalmane)	5	15, 30 mg tablets	Rapid	Desalkylflurazepam, N-1-hydroxyethylflurazepam	100	Long	15–30
Halazepam (Paxipam)	20	20, 40 mg tablets	Medium	Desmethyldiazepam, oxazepam	100	Long	60–160
Lorazepam (Ativan)	1	0.5, 1, 2 mg tablets; 2 mg/mL, 4 mg/mL parenteral	Medium	None	15	Short	2–6
Midazolam (Versed)[2]	1.25–1.7	1 mg/mL, 5 mg/mL parenteral	N/A	1-Hydroxymethylmidazolam	2.5	Short	Parenteral form only: 7.5–45
Oxazepam (Serax)	15	15 mg tablets; 10, 15, 30 mg capsules	Slow	None	8	Short	30–120
Prazepam (Centrax)	10	10 mg tablets; 5, 10, 20 mg capsules	Slow	Desmethyldiazepam, oxazepam	100	Long	20–60
Quazepam (Doral)	5	7.5, 15 mg tablets	Rapid	2 oxoquazepam, N-desalkyl-2-oxoquazepam, and 3-hydroxy-2-oxoquazepam glucuronide	100	Long	7.5–30
Temazepam (Restoril)	5	15, 30 mg tablets	Medium	None	11	Short	15–30
Triazolam (Halcion)	0.1–0.03	0.125, 0.25 mg tablets	Rapid	None	2	Short	0.125–0.25

[1] High-potency drugs have an approximate dose equivalent of under 1.0; 1.0–10–medium potency; over 10–low potency.
[2] Used only by anesthesiologists.
[3] Short-acting benzodiazepines have a half-life of under 25 hrs.

Table 7–4
Interactions of Benzodiazepines with Other Drugs

Decrease absorption
  Antacids

Increase central nervous system depression
  Antihistamines
  Barbiturates and similarly acting drugs
  Cyclic antidepressants
  Ethanol

Increase benzodiazepine levels (compete for microsomal enzymes; probably little or no effect on lorazepam, oxazepam, temazepam)
  Cimetidine
  Disulfiram
  Erythromycin
  Estrogens
  Fluoxetine
  Isoniazid

Decrease benzodiazepine levels
  Carbamazepine (possibly other anticonvulsants)

Table from G W Arana, S E Hyman: *Handbook of Psychiatric Drug Therapy*, ed 2, p 159. Little, Brown, Boston, 1991. Used with permission.

adverse effects of benzodiazepines occur when other sedative drugs, such as alcohol, are taken concurrently. The combinations can result in marked drowsiness, disinhibition, or even respiratory depression. Other relatively rare adverse effects include weakness, nausea, vomiting, blurred vision, and epigastric distress. There have been several reports of mild cognitive deficits that could impair job performance in patients who are taking benzodiazepines. Anterograde amnesia has also been associated with benzodiazepines, particularly high-potency drugs. A rare, paradoxical increase in aggression has been reported in patients given a benzodiazepine. Allergic reactions to the drugs are also rare, but there are a few reports of maculopapular rashes and generalized itching. Benzodiazepines can produce clinically significant impairment of respiration in patients with chronic obstructive pulmonary disease or sleep apnea. Benzodiazepines should be used with caution in patients with a history of substance abuse, organic brain disease, renal disease, hepatic disease, porphyria, CNS depression, or myasthenia gravis.

Triazolam (Halcion) has received significant attention in the media because of an alleged association with serious, aggressive behavioral manifestations. Although little evidence supports the association, the Upjohn Company, which manufactures triazolam, has issued a statement emphasizing that the drug is best used as a short-term (less than 10 days) treatment for insomnia and that physicians should carefully evaluate the emergence of any abnormal thinking or behavioral changes in patients treated with triazolam, giving appropriate consideration to all potential causes.

Some data suggest that benzodiazepines are teratogenic; therefore, their use during pregnancy is not advised. The use of benzodiazepines in the third trimester, moreover, can precipitate a withdrawal syndrome in the newborn. Benzodiazepines are secreted in the breast milk in sufficient concentrations to affect the newborn. Benzodiazepines may cause dyspnea, bradycardia, and drowsiness in nursing babies. Symptoms of intoxication include confusion, slurred speech, ataxia, drowsiness, dyspnea, and hyporeflexia.

Abuse and Dependence

Some persons may take single doses of benzodiazepines for recreational purposes. Patients who take prescribed benzodiazepines may have both a physical dependence and a psychological dependence on the drugs and insist on taking them against the clinician's advice. As previously mentioned, withdrawal syndromes do occur, although much less often than with many other drugs in this class, such as barbiturates and carbamates.

Overdoses

Overdoses with benzodiazepines have a predictably favorable outcome unless other drugs—such as alcohol, antipsychotics, and antidepressants—have also been ingested. In those cases, respiratory depression, coma, seizures, and death are much more likely.

DRUG-DRUG INTERACTIONS

Cimetidine (Tagamet), disulfiram (Antabuse), isoniazid (Nydrazid), and estrogens increase the plasma levels of 2-keto benzodiazepines. Antacids and food may decrease the absorption of benzodiazepines, and smoking may increase the metabolism of benzodiazepines. The benzodiazepines may increase the plasma levels of phenytoin (Dilantin) and digoxin (Lanoxin). All benzodiazepines have additive central nervous system (CNS) depressant effects with other sedative drugs. Ataxia and dysarthria may occur when relatively high doses of lithium, antipsychotics, and clonazepam are combined.

ZOLPIDEM

Zolpidem (Ambien) is a new hypnotic medication that appears to bind to the GABA-benzodiazepine receptor complex. It is not a member of the benzodiazepine class, however, but is an imidazopyridine. It is available in 5, 10, 15, and 20 mg tablets, and a single 10 mg tablet is the usual bedtime dose. It has a half-life of about two to three hours and is metabolized primarily by conjugation. Emesis and dysphoric reactions have been reported as adverse effects.

References

American Psychiatric Association: *A Task Force Report: Benzodiazepine Dependence, Toxicity, and Abuse.* American Psychiatric Association, Washington, 1990.
Ankier S I, Goa K L: Quazepam: A preliminary review of its pharmacodynamic and pharmacokinetic properties, and therapeutic efficacy in insomnia. Drugs *35*: 42, 1988.
Busto U E, Sykora K, Sellers E M: A clinical scale to assess benzodiazepine withdrawal. J Clin Psychopharmacol *9*: 412, 1989.
Cohn J B, Wilcox C S, Bremner J, Ettinger M: Hypnotic efficacy of estazolam compared with flurazepam in outpatients with insomnia. J Clin Pharmacol *31*: 747, 1991.
Dement W C, Greenblatt D J (editors): Pharmacokinetic and clinical considerations in selecting appropriate benzodiazepine hypnotic therapy. J Clin Psychiatry *52* (9, Suppl): 2, 1991.

Dubin W R: Rapid tranquilization: Antipsychotics or benzodiazepines? J Clin Psychiatry 49 (12, Suppl): 5, 1988.

Estazolam: A new benzodiazepine hypnotic. Med Lett Drugs Ther 33: 91, 1991.

Ghadirian A-M, Annable L, Bélanger M-C: Lithium, benzodiazepines, and sexual function in bipolar patients. Am J Psychiatry 149: 801, 1992.

Gillin J C, Spinweber C L, Johnson L C: Rebound insomnia: A critical review. J Clin Psychopharmacol 9: 161, 1989.

Noyes R, Garvey M J, Cook B L, Perry P J: Benzodiazepine withdrawal: A review of the evidence. J Clin Psychiatry 49: 382, 1988.

Rickels K, Case W G, Schweizer E, Garcia-España F, Fridman R: Long-term benzodiazepine users 3 years after participation in a discontinuation program. Am J Psychiatry 148: 757, 1991.

Rickels K, Schweizer G, Case G, Greenblatt D J: Long-term therapeutic use of benzodiazepines. Arch Gen Psychiatry 47: 899, 1990.

Rosenbaum J, editor: High-potency benzodiazepines: Emerging uses in psychiatry. J Clin Psychiatry 51 (5, Suppl): 2, 1990.

Roth M: Anxiety disorders and the use and abuse of drugs. J Clin Psychiatry 50 (11, Suppl): 30, 1989.

Sachs G S, Rosenbaum J F, Jones L: Adjunctive clonazepam for maintenance treatment of bipolar affective disorder. J Clin Psychopharmacol 10: 42, 1990.

Uhlenhuth E H, deWit H, Balter M B, Johanson C E, Mellinger G D: Risks and benefits of long-term benzodiazepine use. J Clin Psychopharmacol 8: 161, 1988.

Walsh J K, Mahowald M W: Avoiding the blanket approach to insomnia: Targeted therapy for specific causes. Postgrad Med 90: 211, 1991.

Zorumski C F, Isenberg K E: Insights into the structure and function of GABA-benzodiazepine receptors: Ion channels and psychiatry. Am J Psychiatry 148: 162, 1991.

8

Bromocriptine

Bromocriptine (Parlodel) is a mixed dopamine agonist-antagonist that is used primarily for the treatment of Parkinson's disease (Figure 8–1). Some data indicate that bromocriptine may be useful in the treatment of neuroleptic malignant syndrome. The data are less robust in support of the use of bromocriptine for the treatment of cocaine withdrawal and depressive disorder. Any clinician who uses bromocriptine for those psychiatric indications should conduct a review of the recent literature about those novel applications, which remain controversial. Bromocriptine is available in 2.5 mg tablets and 5 mg capsules.

PHARMACOLOGICAL ACTIONS

Bromocriptine is rapidly but only partially (about 30 percent) absorbed from the gastrointestinal (GI) tract. Peak concentrations are achieved 1½ to 3 hours after oral administration. No active metabolites have been identified. Bromocriptine is metabolized in the liver and is excreted in the bile.

Depending on dosage, bromocriptine has two effects on dopamine function. At low dosages, bromocriptine primarily affects presynaptic dopamine type 2 (D_2) receptors as an agonist, thus inhibiting the release of dopamine. At higher dosages, bromocriptine acts directly on postsynaptic dopamine receptors, thus acting as a direct dopamine agonist. That differential activity is due to the increased sensitivity of presynaptic dopamine D_2 receptors to dopamine agonist compounds.

INDICATIONS

The three indications for bromocriptine in psychiatry that have the best data for support are neuroleptic malignant syndrome, cocaine withdrawal, and depression. Much less well-supported indications include tardive dyskinesia, mania, and

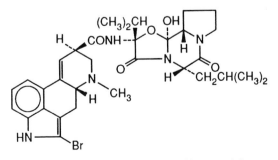

Figure 8–1. Molecular structure of bromocriptine.

schizophrenia. In rare cases, bromocriptine may be implemented as a treatment for antipsychotic-induced galactorrhea and extrapyramidal symptoms.

CLINICAL GUIDELINES

Neuroleptic Malignant Syndrome

Bromocriptine may be effective in neuroleptic malignant syndrome for two possible reasons: First, dopamine antagonists may interfere with hypothalamic thermoregulatory functions. Second, dopamine antagonists may prolong muscle contraction in the periphery. The dopaminergic agonist activity of bromocriptine theoretically reverses those effects.

Of primary importance in the treatment of neuroleptic malignant syndrome is the recognition of the syndrome. The first steps in management are the discontinuation of the antipsychotic drug and the initiation of supportive care. If bromocriptine or other drugs are used to treat neuroleptic malignant syndrome, the earlier they are begun, the greater benefit they are to the patient. Amantadine (Symmetrel), another dopamine agonist, and dantrolene (Dantrium), a direct-acting skeletal muscle relaxant, have also been reported to be of benefit in the treatment of neuroleptic malignant syndrome.

Treatment usually begins with 2.5 to 5.0 mg orally three times daily. The dosage can then be increased gradually to 60 mg a day in divided doses to control fever, rigidity, and autonomic instability. The length of treatment is from 2 to 56 days.

Cocaine Withdrawal

Bromocriptine has been used to treat both the withdrawal symptoms of cocaine and the long-term craving for cocaine. The clinical trials for those uses have not been especially well controlled, and the uses, therefore, should be considered of unknown efficacy. Dosages for the treatment of cocaine-related disorders range from 0.625 to 12.5 mg a day.

Depression

Although theories of depression have emphasized the roles of serotonin and norepinephrine, data support the role of dopamine in the mood disorders; depression is associated with too little dopamine, and mania is associated with too much dopamine. In the studies of bromocriptine in depression, the daily dosages have ranged from 2.5 to 200 mg, and treatment response has taken from four days to four weeks. The use of bromocriptine in the treatment of depression should be considered an experimental treatment that is used only after many other treatments have failed.

Anxiety

Bromocriptine may have anxiolytic properties at dosages of 10 mg a day, particularly in obsessive-compulsive disorder.

ADVERSE EFFECTS

Nausea and various GI disturbances are common dose-related side effects of bromocriptine. Some patients have headache, dizziness, and sedation. Paradoxical side effects in some patients are abnormal involuntary movements and psychotic symptoms. The drug may affect the cardiovascular system; for example, it may cause an exacerbation of angina.

Bromocriptine should be used with caution in a patient with hypertension or hepatic disease. It is not recommended for pregnant or breast-feeding patients.

DRUG-DRUG INTERACTIONS

The concurrent use of bromocriptine and drugs that have dopamine antagonist activity (for example, phenothiazines, butyrophenones) may decrease the therapeutic effects of each drug. The use of bromocriptine in conjunction with antihypertensive agents may produce additive hypotensive effects. Ergot alkaloids and bromocriptine should not be used concurrently, as they may cause hypertension and myocardial infarction. Progestins, estrogens, and oral contraceptives may interfere with the effects of bromocriptine.

References

Fayen M, Goldman M B, Moulthrop M A, Luchins D J: Differential memory function with dopaminergic versus anticholinergic treatment of drug-induced extrapyramidal symptoms. Am J Psychiatry *145*: 483, 1988.

Kranzler H R, Bauer L O: Effects of bromocriptine on subjective and autonomic responses to cocaine-associated stimuli. NIDA Res Monogr *105*: 505, 1991.

Mueller P S: Neuroleptic malignant syndrome. Psychosomatics *26*: 654, 1985.

Mueller P S: Neuroleptic malignant syndrome: Comment. Am J Psychiatry *143*: 674, 1986.

Perovich R M, Lieberman J A, Fleischhacker W W, Alvir J: The behavioral toxicity of bromocriptine in patients with psychiatric illness. J Clin Psychopharmacol *9*: 417, 1989.

Pope H G, Keck P E, McElroy S L: Frequency and presentation of neuroleptic malignant syndrome in a large psychiatric hospital. Am J Psychiatry *143*: 1227, 1986.

Preston K L, Sullivan J T, Strain E C, Bigelow G E: Effects of cocaine alone and in combination with bromocriptine in human cocaine abusers. NIDA Res Monogr *105*: 507, 1991.

Ross R G, Ward N G: Bromocriptine abuse. Biol Psychiatry *31*: 404, 1992.

Sakkas P, Davis J M, Hua J, Wang Z: Pharmacotherapy of neuroleptic malignant syndrome. Psychiatric Ann *21*: 157, 1991.

Sitland-Marken P A, Wells B G, Froemming J H, Chu C-C, Brown C S: Psychiatric applications of bromocriptine therapy. J Clin Psychiatry *51*: 68, 1990.

9

Bupropion

Bupropion (Wellbutrin) is a unicyclic antidepressant that is unrelated either to the tricyclic and tetracyclic antidepressants or to the monoamine oxidase inhibitors (Figure 9–1). The drug was introduced in the United States and then withdrawn because of the occurrence of seizures in some patients taking the drug. The drug has now been reintroduced with specific recommendations regarding dose ranges to limit the occurrence of seizures.

PHARMACOLOGICAL ACTIONS

Bupropion is well absorbed from the gastrointestinal (GI) tract and is metabolized by the liver, with its metabolites excreted by the kidneys. The mean half-life is 12 hours. Two metabolites of the drug, hydroxybupropion and threohydrobupropion, may be related to its clinical and adverse effects. One study found that plasma hydroxybupropion concentrations above 1,250 μg per mL were associated with a lack of clinical response. The mechanism of action for the antidepressant effects of bupropion is unknown. Although it was initially thought that bupropion may act through the blockade of dopamine reuptake, one study found an increase in homovanillic acid (a metabolite of dopamine) to be associated with a lack of clinical response. It is possible that bupropion has some as yet unidentified effect on noradrenergic neural transmission.

INDICATIONS

The primary indication for bupropion is the treatment of major depression. As an antidepressant, bupropion is as effective as standard antidepressant therapies and is associated with significantly fewer adverse effects, thus making bupropion a reasonable first-line drug for the treatment of depression.

CLINICAL GUIDELINES

Bupropion is available in 75 and 100 mg tablets. Initiation of treatment in the average adult patient should be at 100 mg orally (PO) twice a day (bid). On the fourth day of treatment, the dosage can be raised to 100 mg PO three times a day (tid). Because 300 mg is the recommended dosage, it seems reasonable to maintain the patient on that dosage for several weeks before further increasing the dosage. Because of the risk of seizures, increases in dosage should never exceed 100 mg in a three-day period; a single dose of bupropion should never exceed 150 mg, and the total daily dose should not exceed 450 mg.

Bupropion should be given cautiously to patients with hepatic and renal diseases

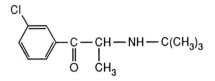

Figure 9–1. Molecular structure of bupropion.

because of the potential accumulation of the drug in the body. Although bupropion is associated with minimal effects on cardiac conduction, the limited clinical experience makes it advisable to use the drug cautiously in patients with cardiac disease. Because of the increased incidence of seizures in patients with anorexia nervosa, bulimia nervosa, or a history of such disorders, bupropion should not be used in such patients. Bupropion is also contraindicated in patients with the following: seizure disorder; history of head trauma, central nervous system (CNS) tumor, or other organic brain disease; electroencephalogram (EEG) abnormalities; recent withdrawal from benzodiazepines or alcohol; and ingestion of other psychotropics that may affect seizure level, such as antipsychotics and lithium. Bupropion can be used in the elderly; however, it has not been studied in children.

ADVERSE EFFECTS

Most notable about bupropion is the absence of significant drug-induced orthostatic hypotension, weight gain, daytime drowsiness, and anticholinergic effects; however, some patients may experience dry mouth or constipation. In fact, weight loss may occur in approximately 25 percent of patients. Bupropion may be a drug to consider early in the treatment of depressed patients with preexisting cardiovascular disease. The most common adverse effects are headache, insomnia, upper respiratory complaints, and nausea. Restlessness, agitation, and irritability may also occur. Bupropion may cause menstrual irregularities in some patients. Although clinical experience is limited to fewer than 20 cases, overdoses of bupropion up to 4,200 mg when taken alone have not been fatal, thus suggesting that bupropion is significantly safer than conventional antidepressant drugs. At dosages less than 450 mg a day, the incidence of seizures is approximately 0.4 percent, which is fourfold that of standard antidepressants. The risk of seizures increases dramatically to about 4 percent in dosages from 450 to 600 mg a day. Bupropion may be less likely than tricyclics to cause a switch into mania or rapid cycling in bipolar disorder patients; however, the drug can cause mania in some patients. The use of bupropion in pregnant women has not been studied. Bupropion is not recommended during breast feeding, because it does pass into breast milk.

DRUG-DRUG INTERACTIONS

Bupropion should not be coadministered with monoamine oxidase inhibitors (MAOIs); if bupropion treatment is indicated, MAOIs should be discontinued at least two weeks before giving bupropion. Although clinical experience is limited, care should be exercised when coadministering bupropion with other drugs metabolized by the liver, such as carbamazepine (Tegretol), cimetidine (Tagamet), barbiturates, and phenytoin (Dilantin). Coadministration with other antidepressants, lithium, or alcohol may increase the risk of seizures.

References

Ames D, Wirshing W C, Szuba M P: Organic mental disorders associated with bupropion in three patients. J Clin Psychiatry *53*: 53, 1992.

Calabrese J R, Markovitz P J: Treatment of depression: New pharmacologic approaches. Prim Care *18*: 421, 1991.

Davidson J: Seizures and bupropion: A review. J Clin Psychiatry *50*: 256, 1989.

Davis J M, Dysken M W: The pharmacology of psychotropic drugs and drug-drug interactions. In *Comprehensive Textbook of Psychiatry*, ed 5, H I Kaplan, B J Sadock, editors, p 1662. Williams & Wilkins, Baltimore, 1989.

Feighner J P, Gardner E A, Johnston J A, Batey S R, Khayrallah M A, Ascher J A, Lineberry C G: Double-blind comparison of bupropion and fluoxetine in depressed outpatients. J Clin Psychiatry *52*: 329, 1991.

Golden R N, Rudorfer M V, Sherer M A, Linnoila M, Potter W Z: Bupropion in depression: I. Biochemical effects and clinical response. II. The role of metabolites in clinical outcome. Arch Gen Psychiatry *45*: 139, 145, 1988.

Goodnick P J: Blood levels and acute response to bupropion. Am J Psychiatry *149*: 399, 1992.

James W A, Lippman S: Bupropion: Overview and prescribing guidelines in depression. South Med J *84*: 222, 1991.

Johnston J A, Lineberry C G, Ascher J A, Davidson J, Khayrallah M A, Feighner J P, Stark P: A 102-center prospective study of seizure in association with bupropion. J Clin Psychiatry *52*: 450, 1991.

Journal of Clinical Psychiatry: New directions in the treatment of depression: Bupropion. J Clin Psychiatry *44* (5, Sec 2): 2, 1983.

Roose S P, Dalack G W, Glassman A H, Woodring S, Walsh B T, Giardina E G V: Cardiovascular effects of bupropion in depressed patients with heart disease. Am J Psychiatry *148*: 512, 1991.

10

Buspirone

Buspirone (BuSpar) is a novel azaspirone anxiolytic drug that offers a distinct and important alternative to treatment with benzodiazepines for anxiety. Buspirone is an exception to the general rule that anxiolytic drugs are also sedatives and hypnotics. In contrast to the benzodiazepines, buspirone carries a low potential for abuse and is not associated with withdrawal phenomena or sedation and cognitive impairment.

PHARMACOLOGICAL ACTIONS

Buspirone is well absorbed from the gastrointestinal (GI) tract and unaffected by food intake, and its metabolism involves both the liver and the kidneys. The drug reaches peak plasma levels 60 to 90 minutes after administration. The short half-life (2 to 11 hours) and the absence of active metabolites necessitate three-times-daily dosing.

In contrast to benzodiazepines and barbiturates, which act on the γ-aminobutyric acid (GABA)-associated chloride ion channel, buspirone has no effect on that receptor mechanism. Rather, buspirone acts as an agonist or partial agonist on serotonin type 1_A receptors. Some reports have noted the influence of buspirone on dopaminergic neurons; however, it has not been shown that this is of any clinical significance in the production of anxiolytic or adverse effects. Figure 10–1 shows the molecular structure of buspirone.

INDICATIONS

The primary indication for buspirone treatment is anxiety, particularly generalized anxiety disorder. Although further research is required, several reports have suggested that buspirone is effective in controlling anxiety and aggression in developmentally disabled persons. Buspirone may be useful in treating emotional and behavioral problems in brain-injured and elderly patients. Buspirone augmentation may lead to symptomatic improvement in fluoxetine (Prozac)-treated patients with depression or obsessive-compulsive disorder. Most available data suggest that buspirone should not be used for the treatment of panic disorder. Because it does not act on the GABA-chloride channel complex, buspirone is not recommended for the treatment of withdrawal from benzodiazepines, alcohol, or other sedative drugs. Available data indicate that the use of buspirone in the elderly, in the same dosages as for nonelderly adults, is safe and effective.

There are advantages and disadvantages to both benzodiazepines and buspirone. The beneficial effects of benzodiazepines are felt the same day they are started, and the full clinical response takes only days, whereas buspirone has no immediate

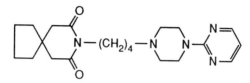

Figure 10–1. Molecular structure of buspirone.

effect, and the full clinical response may take two to four weeks. Sometimes the sedative effects of benzodiazepines, which are not found with buspirone, are desirable; however, those sedative effects are also associated with impaired motor performance and cognitive deficits, such as impaired memory. The major disadvantage of benzodiazepine treatment is its addictive potential and the development of withdrawal phenomena on discontinuation. Buspirone is not associated with any abuse potential, even in groups of patients who are at high risk for addictive behavior.

CLINICAL GUIDELINES

Buspirone is available in 5 and 10 mg tablets, and treatment is usually initiated with 5 mg orally (PO) three times a day. The dosage can be raised 5 mg every two to three days to the usual dosage range of 15 to 30 mg a day. The maximum dosage is 60 mg a day.

Buspirone is as useful as the benzodiazepines in the treatment of anxiety in patients who have not received benzodiazepines in the past. Buspirone does not achieve the same response, however, in patients who have received benzodiazepines in the past. The reason is probably the absence of the immediate mildly euphoric and sedative effects of the benzodiazepines. The most common clinical problem, therefore, is how to start giving buspirone to a patient who is currently taking benzodiazepines. There are two alternatives. First, it is possible to start buspirone treatment gradually while the benzodiazepine is being withdrawn. Second, it is possible to start buspirone treatment and bring the patient up to a therapeutic dosage for two to three weeks while the patient is still receiving the regular dosage of benzodiazepine, at which point the benzodiazepine can be tapered. A few initial reports indicate that the coadministration of buspirone and benzodiazepines may be effective in the treatment of anxiety that has not responded to treatment with either drug alone. Buspirone can be used in the elderly; however, no specific information is available about its use in children.

ADVERSE EFFECTS

The most common adverse effects are headache, nausea, dizziness, and, rarely, insomnia. No sedation is associated with buspirone; some patients report a minor feeling of restlessness, although that symptom may reflect incompletely treated anxiety. No deaths have been reported from overdoses of buspirone, and the median lethal dose (LD_{50}) is estimated to be 160 to 550 times the recommended daily dose. Buspirone should be used with caution in patients with hepatic or renal disease, in pregnant women, and in nursing mothers, although it is not known whether the drug passes into breast milk.

DRUG-DRUG INTERACTIONS

One study reports that the coadministration of buspirone and haloperidol (Haldol) resulted in increased blood concentrations of haloperidol. Buspirone should not be used with monoamine oxidase inhibitors (MAOIs) unless a two-week washout period of the MAOI has occurred.

References

Godd D C, Midha K K, Brotman A W, McCormick S, Waites M, Amico E T: An open trial of buspirone added to neuroleptics in schizophrenic patients. J Clin Psychopharmacol *11*: 193, 1991.

Gorman J M, Davis J M: Antianxiety drugs. In *Comprehensive Textbook of Psychiatry*, ed 5, H I Kaplan, B J Sadock, editors, p 1579. Williams & Wilkins, Baltimore, 1989.

Hart R P, Colenda C C, Hamer R M: Effects of buspirone and alprazolam on the cognitive performance of normal elderly subjects. Am J Psychiatry *148*: 73, 1991.

Jacobsen F M: Possible augmentation of antidepressant response by buspirone. J Clin Psychiatry *52*: 217, 1991.

Manfredi R L, Kales A, Vgontzas A N, Bixler E O, Isaac M A, Falcone C M: Buspirone: Sedative or stimulant effect? Am J Psychiatry *148*: 1213, 1991.

Rickels K: Buspirone in clinical practice. J Clin Psychiatry *51* (9, Suppl): 51, 1990.

Rickels K, Amsterdam J, Clary C, Hassman J, London J, Puzzuoli G, Schweizer E: Buspirone in depressed outpatients: A controlled study. Psychopharmacol Bull *26*: 163, 1990.

Rickels K, Amsterdam J D, Clary C, Puzzuoli G, Schweizer E: Buspirone in major depression: A controlled study. J Clin Psychiatry *52*: 34, 1991.

Robinson D, Napoliello M J, Schenk J: The safety and usefulness of buspirone as an anxiolytic drug in elderly versus young patients. Clin Ther *10*: 740, 1988.

Sussman N: Treatment of anxiety with buspirone. Psychiatr Ann *17*: 114, 1987.

Taylor D P: Buspirone: A new approach to the treatment of anxiety. FASEB J *2*: 2445, 1988.

Tollefson G D, Montague-Clouse J, Tollefson S L: Treatment of comorbid generalized anxiety in a recently detoxified alcoholic population with a selective serotonergic drug (buspirone). J Clin Psychopharmacol *12*: 19, 1992.

11

Calcium Channel Inhibitors

Three calcium channel inhibitors (also called calcium channel blockers) have been used for neuropsychiatric disorders and are available in the United States: verapamil (Calan, Isoptin), diltiazem (Cardizem), and nifedipine (Adalat, Procardia) (Figure 11–1). The major medical indications for the drugs are angina and specific types of cardiac arrhythmias; the major psychiatric indication is bipolar disorder.

PHARMACOLOGICAL ACTIONS

The calcium ion is a major intracellular second messenger. Intraneuronal calcium has many functions, including the activation of calcium-dependent protein kinases. The calcium channel inhibitors inhibit the influx of calcium into neurons through one type of voltage-dependent calcium channel called the L-type calcium channel. The calcium channel inhibitors bind to the channel and inhibit its opening. Nifedipine (a dihydropyridine) binds to a different part of the channel from verapamil and diltiazem (both nondihydropyridines).

The calcium channel inhibitors are well absorbed from the gastrointestinal (GI) tract, but all three are substantially metabolized by the liver in a first-pass effect. There are considerable intraindividual and interindividual variations in the plasma concentrations of the drugs after a single dose. Verapamil is the most commonly used calcium channel inhibitor in psychiatry. The half-life of verapamil after the first dose is two to eight hours; the half-life increases to 5 to 12 hours after the first few days of therapy. According to some studies, verapamil does pass the blood-brain barrier and reaches the cerebrospinal fluid (CSF) in concentrations approximately 0.05 percent that of plasma.

INDICATIONS

Hypertensive Crisis Associated with Monoamine Oxidase Inhibitors

Nifedipine—which, among other effects, rapidly reduces arterial blood pressure—can be used to treat the hypertensive crisis associated with the use of monoamine oxidase inhibitors (MAOIs). Patients should be instructed to bite into a 20-mg capsule of nifedipine, to swallow its contents with water, to contact their physician, and to go to an emergency room. Some controversy surrounds the efficacy of its indication and use.

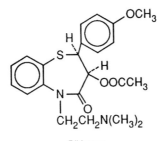

Diltiazem

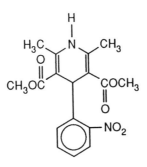

Nifedipine

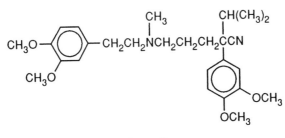

Verapamil

Figure 11–1. Molecular structures of calcium channel inhibitors.

Bipolar Disorder

The major indication for calcium channel inhibitors is in the acute and maintenance treatment of bipolar disorder, especially in patients who have not responded to or cannot tolerate lithium or carbamazepine (Tegretol). Verapamil is the calcium channel inhibitor that has been most studied in those cases, and a number of double-blind, placebo-controlled studies have shown it to be effective. Because of potential drug-drug interactions with lithium and carbamazepine, however, the drug should be coadministered with lithium and carbamazepine with caution. Some patients who are treated simultaneously with lithium and calcium channel inhibitors may experience neurotoxicity.

Movement Disorders

Many reports have described improvement with calcium channel inhibitors in various movement disorders; however, those reports require verification by controlled studies. The movement disorders include tardive dyskinesia, Tourette's disorder, and Huntington's chorea.

Other Disorders

Most studies have not found a beneficial clinical effect of calcium channel inhibitors in the treatment of schizophrenia, although some data suggest that verapamil may reduce depressive or negative symptoms slightly. Calcium channel inhibitors have generally not been effective in the treatment of major depression. Other possible applications include premenstrual syndrome, primary degenerative dementia of the Alzheimer's type, panic disorder, pain control, stuttering, and violent behavior.

CLINICAL GUIDELINES

Verapamil is available in 40, 80, and 120 mg tablets; 180 and 240 mg extended-release tablets; and 120 and 240 mg capsules. It is also available in a 2.5 mg/mL parenteral form. The starting dosage is 40 mg orally (PO) three times a day and can be raised in increments every four to five days up to 80 to 120 mg three times a day. The patient's blood pressure, pulse, and electrocardiogram (ECG) (in patients over 40 years old or with a history of cardiac illness) should be followed routinely. Diltiazem is available in 30, 60, 90, and 120 mg tablets and 60, 90, and 120 mg capsules. It should be started at 30 mg PO four times a day and can be increased up to a maximum of 360 mg a day. Nifedipine is available in 10 and 20 mg capsules and 30, 60, and 90 mg tablets. It should be started at 10 mg PO three or four times a day and can be increased up to a maximum dosage of 180 mg a day.

The elderly are more sensitive to the drugs than are younger adults. No specific information is available regarding the use of the agents in children.

ADVERSE EFFECTS

The most common adverse effects associated with calcium channel inhibitors are hypotension and bradycardia, which sometimes necessitate discontinuing the drug. The calcium channel inhibitors interfere with atrioventricular (AV) conduction and can lead to AV heart block, especially in elderly patients. In all patients with heart disease, especially conduction defects, the drugs should be used with extreme caution. Common GI symptoms include constipation, nausea, and occasionally dry mouth, GI distress, or diarrhea. Adverse effects in the central nervous system (CNS) include dizziness, headache, and fatigue. Rare adverse effects that have been reported include, with diltiazem, hyperactivity, akathisia, parkinsonism; with nifedipine, depression; and with verapamil, delirium, hyperprolactinemia, and galactorrhea. The drugs have not been evaluated in pregnant women, but they do pass into breast milk.

DRUG-DRUG INTERACTIONS

Calcium channel inhibitors should not be prescribed for patients taking β-adrenergic antagonists, hypotensives (for example, diuretics, vasodilators, angiotensin-converting enzyme inhibitors), or antiarrhythmic drugs (for example, quinidine, digoxin [Lanoxin]) without consultation with the patient's internist or cardiologist. Verapamil and diltiazem but not nifedipine have been reported to precipitate carbamazepine-induced neurotoxicity. Cimetidine (Tagamet) has been reported to increase plasma concentrations of nifedipine and diltiazem.

References

Freeman T W, Clothier J L, Pazzaglia P, Lesem M S, Swann A C: A double-blind comparison of valproate and lithium in the treatment of acute mania. Am J Psychiatry *149*: 108, 1992.

Garza-Tervino E D, Overall J E, Hollister L E: Verapamil versus lithium in acute mania. Am J Psychiatry *149*: 121, 1992.

Grebb J A, Shelton R C, Taylor E H, Bigelow L B: A negative, double-blind, placebo-controlled, clinical trial of verapamil in chronic schizophrenia. Biol Psychiatry *21*: 691, 1986.

Höschl C, Koźený J: Verapamil in affective disorders: A controlled, double-blind study. Biol Psychiatry *25*: 128, 1989.

Kaplan P M, Boggiano W E: Anticonvulsants, noradrenergic drugs, and other organic therapies. In *Comprehensive Textbook of Psychiatry*, ed 5, H I Kaplan, B J Sadock, editors, p 1681. Williams & Wilkins, Baltimore, 1989.

Klein E, Uhde T W: Controlled study of verapamil for treatment of panic disorder. Am J Psychiatry *145*: 431, 1988.

Kushnir S L, Ratner J T: Calcium channel blockers for tardive dyskinesia in geriatric psychiatric patients. Am J Psychiatry *146*: 1218, 1989.

Pollack M H, Rosenbaum J F, Hyman S E: Calcium channel blockers in psychiatry. Psychosomatics *28*: 356, 1987.

Thulin T: Calcium antagonists: Assessment of side affects. Scand J Prim Health Care Suppl *1*: 81, 1990.

Tollefson G D: Short-term effects of the calcium channel blocker nimodipine (Bay-e-9736) in the management of primary degenerative dementia. Biol Psychiatry *27*: 1133, 1990.

12

Carbamazepine

Carbamazepine (Tegretol) is an iminodibenzyl drug, structurally similar to imipramine (Tofranil), and approved for use in the United States for the treatment of temporal lobe epilepsy and trigeminal neuralgia (Figure 12–1). A large body of data supports the use of carbamazepine for the treatment of acute mania and for the prophylactic treatment of bipolar disorder.

PHARMACOLOGICAL ACTIONS

Pharmacokinetics

Carbamazepine is absorbed slowly and erratically from the gastrointestinal (GI) tract, although absorption is enhanced when it is taken with meals. Peak plasma levels are reached two to eight hours after a single dose; steady-state levels are reached after two to four days on a steady dosage. The half-life of carbamazepine at the initiation of treatment has a wide range; during chronic administration the half-life ranges from 12 to 17 hours. Carbamazepine is metabolized in the liver and is excreted by the kidneys. The 10-, 11-epoxide metabolite is active as an anticonvulsant, although its activity in the treatment of bipolar disorder is unknown. Recent reports have indicated that carbamazepine can lose one third of its potency when stored in a humid environment. Manufacturers are now advising consumers not to store the drug in such environments as bathrooms.

Pharmacodynamics

The anticonvulsant effects of carbamazepine may be mediated through peripheral benzodiazepine receptors located in the brain, potentiation of α_2-adrenergic receptors, or stabilization of sodium channels on neurons. Central benzodiazepine receptors are more or less the same as the γ-aminobutyric acid (GABA) type A receptor and are acted on by benzodiazepines. Those receptors are associated with the GABA binding site and chloride ion channel. Peripheral benzodiazepine receptors, which exist in both the periphery and the central nervous system (CNS), are thought to be regulators of calcium channel function. That potential effect of carbamazepine is interesting theoretically in the light of the increasing use of calcium channel inhibitors (Chapter 11) for the treatment of bipolar disorder.

Theoretically, another basis for the antimanic effect of carbamazepine involves the concept of kindling. Kindling is the electrophysiological process in which repeated subthreshold stimulations of a neuron eventually generate an action potential. It has been hypothesized that bipolar disorder represents a covert form of limbic epilepsy, which is responsive to carbamazepine; however, electroenceph-

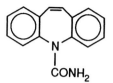

Figure 12–1. Molecular structure of carbamazepine.

alograms (EEGs) are normal in the majority of bipolar disorder patients who respond to carbamazepine.

INDICATIONS

Manic Episodes

Carbamazepine may be as effective as lithium (Eskalith) in the control of manic episodes. Nevertheless, lithium is still the drug of choice because of the absence of significant advantages of carbamazepine over lithium and the rare association of carbamazepine with severe adverse effects. Current clinical and research experience suggests, however, that carbamazepine may be more effective in the treatment of rapidly cycling bipolar disorder patients or patients with dysphoric manic episodes. Carbamazepine can be used alone or with an antipsychotic drug for the treatment of manic episodes, although carbamazepine-induced CNS adverse effects (drowsiness, dizziness, ataxia) with that combination are increasingly emerging. Patients who do not respond to lithium alone may respond when carbamazepine is added to the lithium treatment. If patients then respond, an attempt should be made to withdraw the lithium to see if the patient can be treated with carbamazepine alone. When lithium and carbamazepine are used together, the clinician should minimize or discontinue any antipsychotics, sedatives, or anticholinergic drugs the patient may be taking to reduce the increased risks of adverse effects associated with taking multiple drugs. The lithium and the carbamazepine should both be used at standard therapeutic plasma concentrations before a trial of combined therapy is considered to have been a therapeutic failure. Carbamazepine plasma concentrations from 8 to 12 μg per mL should be achieved for the treatment of manic episodes. A three-week trial of carbamazepine at therapeutic plasma concentrations is usually sufficient to determine whether the drug is effective.

Bipolar Disorder

Carbamazepine alone or in combination with lithium is an effective prophylactic treatment for bipolar disorder. It reduces the frequency of both manic and depressive episodes in 50 to 70 percent of patients.

Schizoaffective Disorder

Patients with schizoaffective disorder, as defined by the revised third edition of *Diagnostic and Statistical Manual of Mental Disorders* (DSM-III-R), probably constitute a particularly heterogeneous group of patients, some of whom may have a form of bipolar disorder. Both lithium and carbamazepine are usually effective treatments for those patients, although as yet there is no method for predicting the response of schizoaffective patients to those drugs.

Depression

The available data suggest that carbamazepine is an effective treatment for depression in some patients. Approximately 25 to 33 percent of depressed patients respond to carbamazepine; that percentage is significantly smaller than the 60 to 70 percent for standard antidepressants. Carbamazepine is an alternative for depressed patients who have not responded to conventional treatments, including electroconvulsive therapy (ECT).

Impulse Control Disorders

Several studies have reported carbamazepine to be effective in controlling impulsive, aggressive behavior in nonpsychotic patients. Other drugs for impulse control disorders, particularly episodic dyscontrol, include lithium, propranolol (Inderal), and antipsychotics. Because of the risk of serious adverse effects with carbamazepine, clinical trials with those other agents are warranted before a trial with carbamazepine.

Other Disorders

According to several studies, carbamazepine is as effective as the benzodiazepines in the control of symptoms associated with alcohol withdrawal. However, the lack of any advantage of carbamazepine over the benzodiazepines and the potential risk of adverse effects with carbamazepine limit the clinical usefulness of that application. Carbamazepine is also effective in controlling nonacute agitation and aggressive behavior in schizophrenic patients. Diagnoses to be ruled out before treatment with carbamazepine is begun include schizophrenic agitation, akathisia, and neuroleptic malignant syndrome. Lorazepam (Ativan) (1 to 2 mg every two to four hours) is more effective than carbamazepine for the control of acute agitation.

CLINICAL GUIDELINES

Pretreatment Medical Evaluation

The patient's medical history should include information about preexisting hematological, hepatic, and cardiac diseases, because all three can be relative contraindications to carbamazepine treatment. Patients with hepatic disease require only one third to one half the usual dose; the clinician should be cautious about raising the dose in such patients and should only do so slowly and gradually. Laboratory examination should include a complete blood count with platelet count, liver function tests, serum electrolytes, and an electrocardiogram (ECG) in patients over 40 years of age or with preexisting cardiac disease. An electroencephalogram (EEG) is not necessary before the initiation of treatment, but it may be helpful in documenting objective changes correlated with clinical improvement.

Initiation of Treatment and Plasma Levels

Carbamazepine is available in 100 and 200 mg tablets and as a 100 mg per 5 mL suspension. The usual starting dosage is 200 mg orally (PO) two times a day. Carbamazepine should be taken with meals, and the drug should be stored in a cool, dry place; carbamazepine stored in a bathroom medicine cabinet can lose up to one third of its activity. In an inpatient setting with seriously ill patients, the dosage can be raised by not more than 200 mg a day until a dosage of 600 to 1,000 mg a day is reached. Otherwise, in less ill patients and in outpatients, the dosage should be raised more slowly (200 mg every two to four days) to reduce the occurrence of minor adverse effects, such as nausea, vomiting, drowsiness, and dizziness. Plasma concentrations should be obtained when a patient has been receiving a steady dosage for at least five days. Blood for the determination of plasma levels is drawn in the morning before the first dose of carbamazepine is given. Although therapeutic concentrations for the treatment of epilepsy are 6 to 10 μg per mL, the therapeutic range for psychiatric indications is slightly higher, 8 to 12 μg per mL. Dosages required to achieve that level usually range from 400 to 1,600 mg a day in divided doses, with a mean around 1,000 mg a day. Some patients require doses as high as 2,200 mg a day to obtain therapeutic blood concentrations of carbamazepine.

Routine Laboratory Monitoring

The most serious potential adverse effects of carbamazepine are agranulocytosis and aplastic anemia. Patients should inform the physician immediately if fever, sore throat, infections, mouth ulcers, easy bruising, pallor, weakness, petechiae, or bleeding develops. The complete blood count (CBC), platelet count, electrolytes, and carbamazepine plasma concentration should be determined every two weeks for the first two months of treatment and quarterly thereafter. Liver and renal function tests should be conducted after the first month, then every three months for the first year, then annually. Transient leukopenias occur in approximately 10 percent of patients during the first few months and do not require discontinuation of treatment. Carbamazepine should be discontinued if laboratory values are lower than any of the following: total white blood cell count, 3,000 mm^3; neutrophils, 1,500 per mm^3; erythrocytes, 4.0 $\times$ 10^6 per mm^3; hematocrit, 32 percent; hemoglobin, 11 gm per 100 mL; platelet count, 100,000 per mm^3; reticulocyte count, 0.3 percent; serum iron level, 150 mg per 100 mL. A hematological consultation should be obtained if any such situation arises. Elderly patients are more likely to

TABLE 12–1
Comparative and Differential Side Effects Profile of Lithium Carbonate and Carbamazepine

Side effects	Lithium Carbonate	Carbamazepine	Lithium and Carbamazepine Combination
White blood count	↑	↓	↑, —, Li*
Diabetes insipidus	↑	↓	↑, Li*
Thyroid hormones T₃, T₄	↓	↓	↓ ↓
TSH	↑	(—)	↑, Li*
Serum calcium	(↑)	↓	(↑), (Li*)
Weight gain	(↑)	(—)	
Tremor	(↑)	(—)	
Memory disturbances	(↑)	?	
Diarrhea	(↑)	—	
Teratogenic effects	(↑)	—	
Psoriasis	(↑)	(—)	
Pruritic rash (allergy)	—	↑	
Agranulocytosis	—	(↑)	
Hepatitis	—	(↑)	
Hyponatremia, water intoxication	—	(↑)	
Dizziness, ataxia, diplopia	—	↑	
Hypercortisolism, escape from dexamethasone suppression	—	↑	

Table adapted from Robert M. Post, M.D. Used with permission.
Side effects:
   ↑ : Increase
   ↓ : Decrease
   ( ): Inconsistent or rare
   —: Absent
↓ ↓ : Potentiation
   Li*: Effect of lithium predominates

have side effects than are younger adults. Children are more likely to experience behavior changes than are adults.

ADVERSE EFFECTS

Although the benign hematological effects are not dose-related, most of the adverse effects of carbamazepine are correlated with plasma concentrations above 9 μg per mL. A comparison of the adverse effects for lithium and carbamazepine is given in Table 12–1. The most serious but rare adverse effects of carbamazepine are blood dyscrasias, hepatitis, and exfoliative dermatitis. Otherwise, carbamazepine is relatively well tolerated by patients except for mild GI and CNS effects that can be significantly reduced if the drug dosage is increased slowly and minimal effective plasma concentrations are maintained.

Blood Dyscrasias

Severe blood dyscrasias (aplastic anemia, agranulocytosis) occur in approximately 1 in 20,000 patients treated with carbamazepine. The early identification of those disorders through patient education about symptoms and with routine laboratory testing can reduce the likelihood of a serious outcome.

Hepatitis

Within the first few weeks of therapy, carbamazepine can cause both a hypersensitivity hepatitis associated with increases in liver enzymes and a cholestasis associated with elevated bilirubin and alkaline phosphatase. Hepatitis will recur if the drug is introduced and can be fatal.

Exfoliative Dermatitis

Stevens-Johnson syndrome of exfoliative dermatitis is a rare complication of carbamazepine requiring discontinuation of the drug. More common are urticaria and pruritic and erythematous rashes.

Gastrointestinal Adverse Effects

The most common adverse effects of carbamazepine are nausea, vomiting, gastric distress, constipation, diarrhea, and anorexia. The severity of the adverse effects is reduced if the dosage of carbamazepine is increased slowly.

Central Nervous System Adverse Effects

Acute confusional states can occur with carbamazepine alone but occur more often in combination with lithium or antipsychotic drugs. The symptoms include drowsiness, confusion, ataxia, hyperreflexia, clonus, and tremor. Elderly patients and patients with organic brain disease are at increased risk. The much more common CNS effects of dizziness, ataxia, clumsiness, and sedation are commonly associated with carbamazepine treatment, although they are reduced by a slower upward titration of the dosage.

Thyroid Adverse Effects

A decrease in L-triiodothyronine (T_3), thyroxine (T_4), and the free T_4 index can occur with carbamazepine treatment, although the development of hypothyroidism is rare. Patients who are taking both carbamazepine and lithium are at a greater risk of developing hypothyroidism than are patients who are taking either drug alone.

Overdoses

No fatalities have been reported from overdoses of carbamazepine when taken alone. The symptoms of overdose include sinus tachycardia, atrioventricular (AV) conduction defects, seizures, coma, nystagmus, hyporeflexia or hyperreflexia, rigidity, orofacial dyskinesias, and mild respiratory depression.

TABLE 12–2
Clinically Important Interactions Between Carbamazepine and Other Drugs

Influences of Other Drugs on Carbamazepine

Increased carbamazepine levels and toxicity produced by 　Danazol 　Diltiazem (not nifedipine) 　Erythromycin (and analogs) 　Influenza vaccine 　Isoniazid (not tranylcypromine) 　Nafimidone 　Triacetyloleandomycin 　Verapamil 　Viloxazine Decreased carbamazepine levels produced by 　Phenobarbital 　Phenytoin 　Primidone 　Theophylline 　Tricyclic antidepressants	Increased carbamazepine levels not associated with marked toxicity 　Cimetidine (mild acute increases; none after 　　one week) 　Josamycin 　Nicotinamide 　Propoxyphene 　Valproic acid (increases epoxide only)

Influences of Carbamazepine on Other Drugs

Carbamazepine decreases levels or effects of 　Clonazepam 　Cyclosporine 　Dexamethasone 　Dicoumarol 　Doxycycline 　Ethosuximide 　Haloperidol 　Pregnancy tests 　Theophylline 　Valproic acid 　Warfarin	Carbamazepine increases 　Clomipramine 　Desmethylclomipramine 　Escape from dexamethasone suppression 　Phenytoin 　Tricyclic antidepressants

Table by Robert M. Post, M.D. Modified by Eugene Rubin, M.D.

Other Adverse Effects

Although the teratogenicity of carbamazepine is unknown, its use in pregnancy should be undertaken only if absolutely necessary. Carbamazepine is secreted in breast milk; therefore, women taking carbamazepine should not breast-feed their babies. Carbamazepine decreases cardiac conduction (although less than the tricyclic antidepressants do) and can, thus, exacerbate preexisting cardiac disease. Photosensitivity has been reported. Carbamazepine has been associated with the development of hyponatremia; therefore, if signs of neurotoxicity emerge, that condition should be considered. Carbamazepine should be used with caution in patients with glaucoma, prostatic hypertrophy, diabetes, or a history of alcohol abuse.

DRUG-DRUG INTERACTIONS

Potential drug-drug interactions of carbamazepine are listed in Table 12–2. Coadministration with lithium, antipsychotic drugs, verapamil (Calan, Isoptin), or nifedipine (Adalat, Procardia) can precipitate carbamazepine-induced CNS adverse effects. Carbamazepine can decrease the blood concentrations of oral contraceptives, resulting in breakthrough bleeding and uncertain prophylaxis against pregnancy. Carbamazepine should not be administered with monoamine oxidase inhibitors (MAOIs), which should be discontinued for two weeks before starting to give carbamazepine.

References

Adamee R E: Does kindling model anything clinically relevant? Biol Psychiatry *27*: 249, 1990.

Carpenter W T, Kurz R, Kirkpatrick B, Hanlon T E, Summerfelt A T, Buchanan R W, Waltrip R W, Breier A: Carbamazepine maintenance treatment in outpatient schizophrenics. Arch Gen Psychiatry *48*: 69, 1991.

Cullen M, Mitchell P, Brodaty H, Boyce P, Parker G, Hickie I, Wilhelm K: Carbamazepine for treatment-resistant melancholia. J Clin Psychiatry *52*: 472, 1991.

Gleason R P, Schenider L S: Carbamazepine treatment of agitation in Alzheimer's outpatients refractory to neuroleptics. J Clin Psychiatry *51*: 115, 1990.

Kaplan P M, Boggiano W E: Anticonvulsants, noradrenergic drugs, and other organic therapies. In *Comprehensive Textbook of Psychiatry*, ed 5, H I Kaplan, B J Sadock, editors, p 1681. Williams & Wilkins, Baltimore, 1989.

Kessler A J, Barklage N E, Jefferson J W: Mood disorders in the psychoneurologic borderland: Three cases of responsiveness to carbamazepine. Am J Psychiatry *146*: 81, 1989.

Ketter T A, Post R M, Worthington K: Principles of clinically important drug interactions with carbamazepine: Part I. J Clin Psychopharmacol *11*: 198, 1991.

Ketter T A, Post R M, Worthington K: Principles of clinically important drug interactions with carbamazepine: Part II. J Clin Psychopharmacol *11*: 306, 1991.

Kramlinger K G, Post R M: Addition of lithium carbonate to carbamazepine: Hematological and thyroid effects. Am J Psychiatry *147*: 615, 1990.

Kramlinger K G, Post R M: The addition of lithium to carbamazepine: Antidepressant efficacy in treatment-resistant depression. Arch Gen Psychiatry *46*: 794, 1989.

Leinonen E, Lillsunde P, Laukkanen V, Ylitalo P: Effects of carbamazepine on serum antidepressant concentrations in psychiatric patients. J Clin Psychopharmacol *11*: 313, 1991.

Lerer B, Moore N, Meyendorff E, Cho S-R, Gershorn S: Carbamazepine versus lithium in mania: A double-blind study. J Clin Psychiatry *48*: 89, 1987.

Lusznat R M, Murphy D P, Nunn C M: Carbamazepine vs lithium in the treatment and prophylaxis of mania. Br J Psychiatry *153*: 198, 1988.

Malcolm R, Ballenger J C, Sturgis E T, Anton R: Double-blind controlled trial comparing carbamazepine to oxazepam treatment of alcohol withdrawal. Am J Psychiatry *146*: 617, 1989.

Neppe W M, editor: Carbamazepine use in neuropsychiatry. J Clin Psychiatry *49*(4, Suppl): 2, 1988.

Post R M, Leverich G S, Rosoff A S, Altshuler L L: Carbamazepine prophylaxis in refractory affective disorders: A focus on long-term follow-up. J Clin Psychopharmacol *10*: 318, 1990.

Post R M, Weiss S R B, Chuang D-M: Mechanisms of action of anticonvulsants in affective disorders: Comparisons with lithium. J Clin Psychopharmacol *12*: 23S, 1992.

Schweizer E, Rickels K, Case W G, Greenblatt D J: Carbamazepine treatment in patients discontinuing long-term benzodiazepine therapy: Effects on withdrawal severity and outcome. Arch Gen Psychiatry *48*: 448, 1991.

Stuppaeck C, Barnas C, Miller C, Schwitzer J, Fleischhacker W W: Carbamazepine in the prophylaxis of mood disorders. J Clin Psychopharmacol *10*: 39, 1990.

Tohen M, Castillo J, Cole J O, Miller M G, de los Heros R, Farrer R J: Thrombocytopenia associated with carbamazepine: A case series. J Clin Psychiatry *52*: 496, 1991.

13

Chloral Hydrate

Chloral hydrate (Noctec) is one of the oldest sedative-hypnotic drugs still in use, having been used since 1869. Because of the introduction of many compounds since that time, chloral hydrate is now used only as a very short-term (two- to three-day) hypnotic. Its chemical formula is $CCl_3CH(OH)_2$. A discussion of other sedative-hypnotic drugs similar to chloral hydrate appears in Chapter 6.

PHARMACOLOGICAL ACTIONS

Chloral hydrate is well absorbed from the gastrointestinal (GI) tract. The parent compound is metabolized within minutes by the kidneys, the liver, and the red blood cells. An active metabolite, trichloroethanol, has a half-life of approximately 8 to 11 hours. A dose of chloral hydrate induces sleep in 30 to 60 minutes and maintains sleep for four to eight hours. The pharmacodynamic basis for the hypnotic effect of chloral hydrate is not known.

INDICATIONS

The major indication for chloral hydrate is insomnia. Whether chloral hydrate affects rapid eye movement (REM) sleep is controversial; however, there is no REM rebound after discontinuation of chloral hydrate therapy. Chronic treatment with chloral hydrate is associated with an increased incidence and severity of adverse effects. Tolerance develops to the hypnotic effects of chloral hydrate after two weeks of treatment. Chloral hydrate is available in 250 and 500 mg capsules, 250 and 500 mg per 5 mL solutions, and 325, 500, and 650 mg rectal suppositories. The standard dose of chloral hydrate is 500 to 2,000 mg at bedtime. The drug is an irritant that can be administered with milk or antacids to decrease gastric irritation.

In addition to the development of tolerance, dependence on chloral hydrate can occur, with symptoms similar to those of alcohol dependence. The lethal dose of chloral hydrate is between 5,000 and 10,000 g, thus making chloral hydrate a particularly poor choice for potentially suicidal patients. The lethality of chloral hydrate is potentiated by other central nervous system (CNS) depressants, including alcohol. Chloral hydrate is not expected to cause particular difficulties in children or the elderly; however, no specific information is available.

ADVERSE EFFECTS

The most common GI adverse effects are nausea, vomiting, and diarrhea; however, those effects can be somewhat reduced by taking the drug with extra water. Patients should be warned that there may be residual daytime sedation and impaired motor coordination. With long-term use and with overdose, gastritis and gastric ulceration can develop. Hepatic and renal damage can follow overdose attempts, resulting in jaundice and albuminuria. Chloral hydrate should be avoided in patients with severe renal, cardiac, or hepatic disease or with porphyria. Chloral hydrate may aggravate gastrointestinal (GI) inflammatory conditions. It should not be used during pregnancy. It passes into the breast milk. Symptoms of intoxication include confusion, ataxia, dysarthria, bradycardia, arrhythmia, and severe drowsiness.

DRUG-DRUG INTERACTIONS

Patients who have received chloral hydrate less than 24 hours before receiving intravenous furosemide (Lasix) can have diaphoresis, flushes, and an unsteady blood pressure. Reports are somewhat controversial concerning the potentiation of warfarin (Coumadin) when coadministered with chloral hydrate.

References

Gorman J M, Davis J M: Antianxiety drugs. In *Comprehensive Textbook of Psychiatry*, ed 5, H I Kaplan, B J Sadock, editors, p 1579. Williams & Wilkins, Baltimore, 1989.

Graham S R, Day R O, Lee R, Fulde G W: Overdose with chloral hydrate: A pharmacological and therapeutic review. Med J Aust *149*: 686, 1988.

Keeter S, Benator R M, Weinberg S M, Hartenburg M A: Sedation in pediatric CT: National survey of current practice. Radiology *175*: 745, 1990.

Schuler M E: Augmentation of chloral hydrate induced sleep by centrally acting hypertensive agents. Proc West Pharmacol Soc *25*: 347, 1982.

14

Clonidine

Clonidine (Catapres) is an α_2-adrenergic receptor agonist used primarily as a hypotensive agent (Figure 14–1). Its major indications in psychiatry are the control of the withdrawal symptoms from opioids and the treatment of Tourette's disorder.

PHARMACOLOGICAL ACTIONS

Clonidine is well absorbed from the gastrointestinal (GI) tract and reaches peak plasma levels in one to three hours. Approximately 35 percent of the drug is metabolized by the liver, and 65 percent is excreted in both unchanged and metabolized forms by the kidneys. The half-life of the parent compound is 6 to 20 hours, and there are no active metabolites. The agonist effects on presynaptic α_2-adrenergic receptors result in a decrease in the amount of neurotransmitter released from the nerve terminal.

CLINICAL GUIDELINES AND INDICATIONS

Clonidine is available in 0.1, 0.2, and 0.3 mg tablets. The usual starting dosage is 0.1 mg orally (PO) twice a day and can be raised by 0.1 mg a day to an appropriate level. Clonidine must always be tapered when it is discontinued to avoid rebound hypertension, which occurs approximately 20 hours after the last clonidine dose. The elderly are more sensitive to the drug than are younger adults. Children are susceptible to the same side effects as are adults.

Opioid Withdrawal

Clonidine is effective in reducing the autonomic symptoms of opiate withdrawal (hypertension, tachycardia, dilated pupils, sweating, lacrimation, rhinorrhea) but not the associated subjective sensations. Clonidine can be used as a method of withdrawing a patient from methadone. Usually, dosages of 0.15 mg twice a day are sufficient for that purpose. For clonidine to be effective for that indication, it

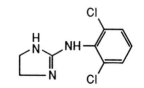

Figure 14–1. Molecular structure of clonidine.

88

is presumably affecting the activity of the locus ceruleus neurons. Clonidine should be withheld if patients become hypotensive (blood pressure less than 90/60).

Tourette's Disorder

Some clinicians now use clonidine as a first-line drug for the treatment of Tourette's disorder instead of the standard drugs, haloperidol (Haldol) and pimozide (Orap), because of the serious adverse effects associated with those antipsychotics. The starting pediatric or child dosage is 0.05 mg a day, although it can be raised to 0.3 mg a day in divided doses. It takes up to three months to observe the beneficial effects of clonidine in the disorder.

Other Disorders

Other potential indications include the anxiety disorders (panic disorder, phobias, obsessive-compulsive disorder, posttraumatic stress disorder, generalized anxiety disorder), mania (possibly synergistic with lithium or carbamazepine [Tegretol]), and schizophrenia (in which it may help reduce tardive dyskinetic movements).

ADVERSE EFFECTS

The most common adverse effects associated with clonidine are dry mouth and eyes, fatigue, sedation, dizziness, nausea, hypotension, and constipation, which result in approximately 10 percent of patients choosing to discontinue the drug. Some patients may experience sexual dysfunction. Uncommon central nervous system (CNS) adverse effects include insomnia, anxiety, and depression; rare CNS adverse effects include vivid dreams, nightmares, and hallucinations. Fluid retention associated with clonidine treatment can be treated with diuretics. Patients who overdose on clonidine can present with coma and constricted pupils, symptoms similar to an opioid overdose. Other symptoms of overdose are decreased blood pressure, pulse, and respiratory rates. Clonidine should be used with caution in patients with heart disease, renal disease, Raynaud's syndrome, or a history of depression. Clonidine should be avoided during pregnancy. It is excreted in breast milk.

DRUG-DRUG INTERACTIONS

The most relevant drug-drug interaction is that the coadministration of clonidine with tricyclic antidepressants can inhibit the hypotensive effects of clonidine. The drug may enhance the CNS depressive effects of barbiturates, alcohol, or other sedatives. Concomitant use of β-blockers can increase the severity of rebound phenomena when clonidine is discontinued.

References

Charney D C, Heninger G R, Kleber H D: The combined use of clonidine and naltrexone as a rapid, safe, and effective treatment of abrupt withdrawal from methadone. Am J Psychiatry *143*: 831, 1986.

Cuthill J D, Baroniada V, Salvatori V A, Viguie F: Evaluation of clonidine suppression of opiate withdrawal reactions: A multidisciplinary approach. Can J Psychiatry *35*: 377, 1990.

Fankhauser M P, Karumanchi V C, German M L, Yates A, Karumanchi S D: A double-blind, placebo-controlled study of the efficacy of transdermal clonidine in autism. J Clin Psychiatry *53*: 77, 1992.

Giannini A J, Pascarzi G A, Loiselle R H, Price W A, Giannini M C: Comparison of clonidine and lithium in the treatment of mania. Am J Psychiatry *143*: 1608, 1986.

Hardy M-C, Lecrubier Y, Widlöcher D: Efficacy of clonidine in 24 patients with acute mania. Am J Psychiatry *143*: 1450, 1986.

Heidemann S M, Sarnaik A P: Clonidine poisoning in children. Crit Care Med *18*: 618, 1990.

Kaplan P M, Boggiano W E: Anticonvulsants, noradrenergic drugs, and other organic therapies. In *Comprehensive Textbook of Psychiatry*, ed 5, H I Kaplan, B J Sadock, editors, p 1681. Williams & Wilkins, Baltimore, 1989.

Leckman J F, Hardin M T, Riddle M A, Stevenson J, Ort S I, Cohen D J: Clonidine treatment of Gilles de la Tourette's syndrome. Arch Gen Psychiatry *48*: 324, 1991.

Leckman J F, Ort S, Caruso K A, Anderson G M, Riddle M A, Cohen D J: Rebound phenomena in Tourette's syndrome after abrupt withdrawal of clonidine. Arch Gen Psychiatry *43*: 1168, 1986.

Ornish S A, Zisook S, McAdams L A: Effects of transdermal clonidine treatment on withdrawal symptoms associated with smoking cessation: A randomized, controlled trial. Arch Intern Med *148*: 2027, 1988.

15

Clozapine: Antipsychotic

Clozapine (Clozaril) is a newly available alternative drug for the treatment of psychotic disorders, particularly schizophrenia (Figure 15–1). It is a dibenzodiazepine, not to be confused with the drug clonazepam (Klonopin), which is a benzodiazepine. Clozapine is unique among the antipsychotics in that its use is not associated with extrapyramidal adverse effects or with tardive dyskinesia. The major disadvantage of clozapine is a 1 to 2 percent incidence of agranulocytosis in patients who take the drug.

PHARMACOLOGICAL ACTIONS

Clozapine is rapidly absorbed from the gastrointestinal (GI) tract, and peak plasma levels are reached in one to four hours. The drug is completely metabolized, with a half-life of approximately 16 hours. It is not known whether the metabolites are active. Clozapine differs from all other available antipsychotic drugs, which have their major effects as antagonists of dopamine receptors, particularly D_2 receptors. The antiserotonergic (5-hydroxytryptamine [5-HT$_2$]), antiadrenergic (α_1 and α_2), anticholinergic (muscarinic), and antihistaminergic (H_1) activities are significantly more potent than the antidopaminergic activity of clozapine. Moreover, its D_1 antagonist activity is much greater than its D_2 antagonist activity. Clozapine is more effective in blocking dopaminergic activity in the cortical and limbic dopamine neurons than in the dopamine neurons in the basal ganglia; that observation may explain the lack of extrapyramidal adverse effects with clozapine. Some researchers have hypothesized that the combined antagonist activity of clozapine on multiple neurotransmitters results in its antipsychotic activity.

INDICATIONS

The major indication for clozapine at this time is the treatment of psychotic patients, usually affected with schizophrenia, who have not responded to traditional antipsychotic drugs (Chapter 19) or who cannot tolerate the adverse effects asso-

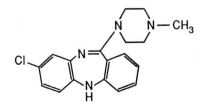

Figure 15–1. Molecular structure of clozapine.

ciated with those drugs. Clozapine has been shown to be as effective as standard antipsychotics in both the short-term and the long-term management of psychosis. Lorazepam (Ativan) can be used when adjunctive drugs are necessary to control agitation. However, caution is advised when prescribing clozapine with benzodiazepines in view of reports of increased side effects in that combination. Clozapine has been reported to be more effective than standard drugs in reducing the negative symptoms of schizophrenia. Approximately 30 percent of patients who have not responded to standard antipsychotic treatments do respond to clozapine treatment. Low-dose clozapine (25 to 125 mg a day) has recently been used in the treatment of parkinsonism.

CLINICAL GUIDELINES

The clinical guidelines are not standardized as to which patients warrant a trial of clozapine. A patient who has been unsuccessfully treated with two or three different antipsychotic drugs from different classes in sufficient doses (1,000 mg chlorpromazine [Thorazine] equivalents), each for at least two months, is probably a candidate for treatment with clozapine. In such situations the clinician must confirm that the patient has been compliant with drug therapy and that no unusual pharmacokinetic factors have been operative. Some patients treated with standard antipsychotic drugs have intolerable adverse effects—such as parkinsonism, akathisia, and tardive dyskinesia—that cannot be controlled by other drugs. Those patients are also candidates for treatment with clozapine. Clozapine may be of particular use in patients with coexisting Parkinson's disease and psychosis. Clozapine may be likely to cause side effects in the elderly. Its use in elderly adults and in children has not been specifically studied.

The clinician must explain the risks and the benefits of clozapine treatment to prospective patients and their families. The informed consent procedure should be documented in the patient's chart.

The patient's preadministration history should include information on blood disorders, epilepsy, and any hepatic or renal diseases. Blood disorders and epilepsy are contraindications to clozapine therapy. Hepatic and renal diseases make it imperative that clozapine be administered at low dosages. Preadministration laboratory examination should include an electrocardiogram (ECG), several complete blood counts (CBCs) with white blood cell counts (WBCs), which can then be averaged, and liver and renal function tests. Clozapine is available in 25 and 100 mg tablets; 1 mg of clozapine is equivalent to approximately 2 mg of chlorpromazine. The initial dosage is usually 25 mg one or two times daily, which can be raised gradually to 300 mg a day divided into two or three daily doses. The gradual increase in dosage is necessitated by the development of hypotension, syncope, and sedation, adverse effects to which patients have tolerance with continued treatment. The usual effective treatment range is 400 to 500 mg a day, although dosages up to 600 mg a day are not unusual. After the decision to terminate the drug, clozapine treatment should be tapered whenever possible to avoid cholinergic rebound symptoms of diaphoresis, flushing, diarrhea, and hyperactivity.

Laboratory Monitoring

Weekly WBCs are indicated to monitor the patient for the development of agranulocytosis. Although careful monitoring is quite expensive, early identification of agranulocytosis can prevent a fatal outcome. If the WBC is less than 3,000 cells per mm^3 or the granulocyte count is less than 1,500 per mm^3, clozapine should be discontinued, and a hematological consultation should be obtained. If the WBC is less than 2,000 cells per mm^3, a bone marrow aspiration should be conducted to evaluate hematopoietic activity. Patients with agranulocytosis from clozapine should not be reexposed to the drug. Physicians can monitor the WBC through any laboratory. Proof of monitoring must be presented to the pharmacist weekly in order to obtain medication.

Blood levels of clozapine indicate that therapeutic effects occur when levels are above 350 ng per mL.

ADVERSE EFFECTS

The feature of clozapine that distinguishes it from standard antipsychotics is the absence of extrapyramidal adverse effects. Clozapine does not cause acute dystonia, parkinsonism, akathisia, rabbit syndrome, or akinesia. It also appears that clozapine does not cause tardive dyskinesia. Because of its weak effects on D_2 receptors, clozapine does not affect prolactin secretion; thus, clozapine does not cause sexual or reproductive adverse effects or galactorrhea. Its use in pregnancy has not been studied. Clozapine may pass into breast milk.

The two most serious adverse effects associated with clozapine use are agranulocytosis and seizures. Agranulocytosis is defined as a decrease in the number of white blood cells, with a specific decrease in the number of polymorphonuclear leukocytes, and a relative lymphopenia. The erythrocyte and platelet concentrations are unaffected. Agranulocytosis occurs in 1 to 2 percent of patients treated with clozapine; that percentage contrasts with an incidence of 0.04 to 0.5 percent of patients treated with standard antipsychotics. Early studies showed that one third of patients who developed agranulocytosis from clozapine died; careful clinical monitoring in the United States in recent years has prevented fatalities. The vast majority of patients recover from agranulocytosis if the condition is recognized early and clozapine is discontinued. Agranulocytosis can appear precipitously or gradually; it most often develops in the first six months of treatment, although it can appear much later. Clozapine is also associated with the development of benign cases of leukocytosis, leukopenia, eosinophilia, and elevated erythrocyte sedimentation rates.

Clozapine is also associated with the development of seizures. Approximately 14 percent of patients taking more than 600 mg a day of clozapine, 1.8 percent of patients taking 300 to 600 mg a day, and 0.6 percent of patients taking less than 300 mg a day have seizures. Those percentages are higher than those of standard antipsychotics. If seizures develop in a patient, clozapine should be temporarily stopped. Phenobarbital treatment can be initiated, and clozapine can be restarted at approximately 50 percent of the previous dosage, then very gradually raised again. Carbamazepine (Tegretol) should not be used in combination with clozapine because of its association with agranulocytosis.

The most common adverse effects associated with clozapine treatment are sedation, tachycardia, constipation, dizziness, hypotension, hyperthermia, and sialorrhea. Weight gain, fainting spells, myoclonus, periodic catalepsy, gastrointestinal upset, and anticholinergic side effects have also been reported. The tachycardia is due to vagal inhibition and can be treated with peripherally acting β-adrenergic antagonists, such as atenolol (Tenormin, Tenoretic), although that treatment may aggravate the hypotensive effects of the clozapine. Hyperthermia of 1 to 2°F may develop, causing concern regarding the development of an infection because of agranulocytosis. Clozapine should be withheld, and, if the WBC is normal, clozapine can be reinstituted more slowly and at a lower dosage.

DRUG-DRUG INTERACTIONS

Clozapine should not be used with any other drug that is also associated with the development of agranulocytosis. Such drugs include carbamazepine, propylthiouracil, sulfonamides, and captopril (Capoten). Central nervous system (CNS) depressants, alcohol, or tricyclic antidepressants coadministered with clozapine may increase the risk of seizures, sedation, or cardiac effects. Lithium combined with clozapine may increase the risk of seizures, confusion, and movement disorders. An adverse interaction may occur when clozapine and cimetidine (Tagamet) are combined. Concomitant use of clozapine and benzodiazepines has been associated with a significant percentage of the reported cases of orthostasis and syncope associated with clozapine.

References

Baldessarini R, Frankenburg F: Clozapine: A novel antipsychotic agent. N Engl J Med *324*: 746, 1991.
Buch D L: Clozapine: A novel antipsychotic. Am Fam Physician *45*: 795, 1992.
Cheng Y F, Lundberg T, Bondesson U, Lindström L, Gabrielsson J: Clinical pharmacokinetics of clozapine in chronic schizophrenic patients. Eur J Clin Pharmacol *34*: 445, 1988.
Davies M A, Conley R R, Schulz S C, Bell-Delaney J: One-year follow-up of 24 patients in a clinical trial of clozapine. Hosp Community Psychiatry *42*: 628, 1991.
Davis J M, Barter J T, Kane J M: Antipsychotic drugs. In *Comprehensive Textbook of Psychiatry*, ed 5, H I Kaplan, B J Sadock, editors, p 1591. Williams & Wilkins, Baltimore, 1989.
Green A I, Salzman C: Clozapine benefits and risks. Hosp Community Psychiatry *41*: 379, 1990.
Jann M W: Clozapine. Pharmacotherapy *11*: 179, 1991.
Kane J, Honigfeld G, Singer J, Meltzer H: Clozaril Collaborative Study Group: Clozapine for the treatment-resistant schizophrenic. Arch Gen Psychiatry *45*: 789, 1988.
Leadbetter R, Shutty M, Pavalonis D, Viewig V, Higgins P, Downs M: Clozapine-induced weight gain: Prevalence and clinical relevance. Am J Psychiatry *149*: 68, 1992.
Lieberman J A, Johns C A, Kane J M, Rai K, Pisciotta A V, Saltz B L, Howard A: Clozapine-induced agranulocytosis: Non-cross-reactivity with other psychotropic drugs. J Clin Psychiatry *49*: 271, 1988.
Lieberman J A, Kane J M, Johns C A: Clozapine: Guidelines for clinical management. J Clin Psychiatry *50*: 329, 1989.
Marder S R, Van Putten T: Who should receive clozapine? Arch Gen Psychiatry *45*: 865, 1988.
Meltzer H Y, Bastani B, Kwon K Y, Ramirez L F, Burnett S, Sharpe J: A prospective study of clozapine

in treatment-resistant schizophrenic patients: I. Preliminary report. Psychopharmacology *99*(Suppl): S68, 1989.

Small J G, Milstein V, Marhenke J D, Hall D D, Kellams J J: Treatment outcome with clozapine in tardive dyskinesia, neuroleptic sensitivity, and treatment-resistant psychosis. J Clin Psychiatry *48*: 263, 1987.

Wolters E C, Hurwitz T A, Mak E, Teal P, Peppard F R, Remick R, Caine S, Caine D B: Clozapine in the treatment of parkinsonian patients with dopaminomimetic psychosis. Neurology *40*: 832, 1990.

16

Dantrolene

Dantrolene (Dantrium) is a direct-acting skeletal-muscle relaxant. Derived from hydantoin, it is unrelated structurally or pharmacologically to other skeletal-muscle relaxants. Its molecular structure is given in Figure 16–1.

PHARMACOLOGICAL ACTIONS

Pharmacodynamics

Dantrolene produces skeletal-muscle relaxation by directly affecting the contractile response of the muscle at a site beyond the myoneural junction. Dantrolene dissociates excitation-contraction coupling by interfering with the release of calcium from the sarcoplasmic reticulum.

Pharmacokinetics

Approximately one third of orally administered dantrolene is slowly absorbed from the gastrointestinal (GI) tract. Nevertheless, at sufficient dosages, consistent plasma levels can be maintained. The average absorption half-life in adults is just over one hour. Peak blood concentrations occur about five hours after oral administration (PO). The elimination half-life of dantrolene is about nine hours after a 100 mg dose. Dantrolene is metabolized by the liver and is excreted in the urine.

Dantrolene is largely bound to plasma proteins. It crosses the placenta.

INDICATIONS

The primary psychiatric indication for intravenous (IV) dantrolene is spasticity in neuroleptic malignant syndrome. Dantrolene is almost always used in conjunction with appropriate supportive measures and a dopamine receptor agonist (Chapter 8). Because of its potential for severe side effects, dantrolene should not be used in psychiatry for long-term treatment.

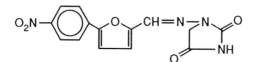

Figure 16–1. Molecular structure of dantrolene.

CLINICAL GUIDELINES

In addition to immediate discontinuation of antipsychotic drugs, medical support to cool the patient, and the monitoring of vital signs and renal output, dantrolene in doses of 1 mg per kg PO four times a day or 1 to 5 mg per kg IV may reduce the muscle spasms in neuroleptic malignant syndrome. Dantrolene is supplied as 25 mg, 50 mg, and 100 mg capsules, in addition to a 20 mg parenteral preparation. Dantrolene has not been tested in the elderly. Testing in children has not revealed any problems unique to them.

ADVERSE EFFECTS

Many of the serious side effects of dantrolene are associated with long-term treatment. The side effects include hepatitis, seizures, and pleural effusion with pericarditis. The effects have not been shown to be associated with short-term IV use. Muscle weakness, drowsiness, dizziness, light-headedness, nausea, diarrhea, malaise, and fatigue are the most common adverse effects of dantrolene. Those effects are generally transient. The central nervous system (CNS) effects of dantrolene may include speech disturbances, headache, visual disturbances, alteration of taste, mental depression, confusion, hallucinations, nervousness, insomnia, and the exacerbation or precipitation of seizures. Dantrolene should be used with caution in patients with hepatic, renal, or chronic lung disease. Dantrolene has not been shown to cause problems during pregnancy or while a woman is breast-feeding.

DRUG-DRUG INTERACTIONS

The risk of liver toxicity may be increased in patients taking estrogens. Dantrolene should be used with caution in patients who are using other drugs that produce drowsiness, most notably benzodiazepines. IV dantrolene should not be used with calcium channel blockers.

References

Burch E A, Montoya J: Neuroleptic malignant syndrome in an AIDS patient. J Clin Psychopharmacol 9: 228, 1989.

Mueller P S: Neuroleptic malignant syndrome. Psychosomatics 26: 654, 1985.

Pennati A, Sacchetti E, Calzeroni A: Dantrolene in lethal catatonia. Am J Psychiatry 148: 268, 1991.

Sakkas P, Davis J M, Hua J, Wang Z: Pharmacotherapy of neuroleptic malignant syndrome. Psychiatric Ann 21: 157, 1991.

Sewell D D, Jasta D U: Neuroleptic malignant syndrome: A review. Yakubutsu Seishin Kada 9: 319, 1989.

Shalav A, Hermash H, Munitz H: Mortality from neuroleptic malignant syndrome. J Clin Psychiatry 50: 18, 1989.

17

Disulfiram

Disulfiram (Antabuse) is used in the treatment of alcoholism. Its main effect is to produce an extremely unpleasant reaction in a person who ingests even a small amount of alcohol while disulfiram is in the system. The molecular formula is given in Figure 17–1.

PHARMACOLOGICAL ACTIONS

Disulfiram is an aldehyde dehydrogenase inhibitor that interferes with the metabolism of alcohol by producing a marked increase in blood acetaldehyde levels. The accumulation of acetaldehyde (to a level up to 10 times higher than normally occurs in the normal metabolism of alcohol) produces a vast array of unpleasant reactions called the disulfiram-alcohol (DA) reaction, characterized by the following signs and symptoms: nausea, throbbing headache, vomiting, hypertension, flushing, sweating, thirst, dyspnea, tachycardia, chest pain, vertigo, and blurred vision. The reaction occurs almost immediately after the ingestion of one drink and may last up to 30 minutes.

Disulfiram is almost completely absorbed from the gastrointestinal tract after oral administration. It is metabolized in the liver and excreted in the urine. It is lipid-soluble and has a half-life estimated at 60 to 120 hours. One to two weeks may be needed before disulfiram is totally eliminated from the body after the last dose has been taken.

CLINICAL GUIDELINES

Disulfiram is supplied in tablets of 250 mg and 500 mg. The usual initial dosage is 500 mg a day taken by mouth for the first one to two weeks, followed by a maintenance dose of 250 mg a day. The dosage should not exceed 500 mg a day. The maintenance dosage range is 125 to 500 mg a day.

The patient should be instructed that the ingestion of even the smallest amount of alcohol will bring on the DA reaction, with all its unpleasant effects. In addition, the patient should be warned against ingesting any alcohol-containing preparations, such as cough drops, tonics of any kind, and alcohol-containing

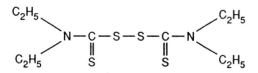

Figure 17–1. Molecular formula of disulfiram.

foods and sauces. Some reactions have occurred in men who used alcohol-based after-shave lotion and inhaled the fumes; therefore, precautions should be extremely explicit and should include any topically applied preparation containing alcohol, such as perfume.

Disulfiram should not be administered until the patient has abstained from alcohol for at least 12 hours. Patients should be warned that the DA reaction may occur as long as one to two weeks after the last dose of disulfiram. Patients should carry identification cards describing the DA reaction and the name and telephone number of the physician to be called.

Baseline and follow-up blood counts and transaminase levels are recommended by the manufacturer because of reports of blood dyscrasias, hepatitis, and hypersensitivity to disulfiram. Disulfiram is not indicated for children, adolescents, or pregnant women and should be used with extreme caution in patients over 50 years of age.

Because of the risk of severe and fatal reactions, disulfiram therapy is used less often today than previously.

Trial with Alcohol

Some clinicians stimulate a DA reaction in patients to convince them of the drug's unpleasant effects. However, because of the risk of cardiovascular collapse and death in some patients, that procedure is no longer advisable. Most patients are convinced of the DA reaction when the physician graphically describes it.

Combination Therapies

Disulfiram is rarely effective as the sole treatment approach in alcoholism, even in highly motivated patients. It should be combined with psychotherapy and group techniques, such as Alcoholics Anonymous (AA). Careful follow-up is always indicated to monitor compliance.

ADVERSE EFFECTS

The intensity of the DA reaction varies with each patient. In extreme cases it is marked by respiratory depression, cardiovascular collapse, myocardial infarction, convulsions, and death. Therefore, disulfiram is contraindicated in a patient with significant pulmonary or cardiovascular disease. In addition, disulfiram should be used with caution, if at all, in a patient with nephritis, brain damage, hypothyroidism, diabetes, hepatic disease, seizures, polydrug dependence, or an abnormal electroencephalogram (EEG). Most fatal reactions occur in patients who are taking more than 500 mg a day of disulfiram and who consume more than three ounces of alcohol. Treatment of severe DA reaction is supportive to prevent shock.

The adverse effects of disulfiram in the absence of alcohol include fatigue, dermatitis, impotence, optic neuritis, mental changes, and liver damage. A metabolite of disulfiram inhibits dopamine hydroxylase; disulfiram can cause or exacerbate psychosis and should not be used in patients with psychotic disorders.

DRUG-DRUG INTERACTIONS

Disulfiram increases the blood concentration of diazepam (Valium), paraldehyde, phenytoin (Dilantin), caffeine, tetrahydrocannabinol, barbiturates, anticoagulants, isoniazid (Cotinazin), and tricyclic antidepressants.

References

Banys P: The clinical use of disulfiram (Antabuse): A review. Special Issue: Pharmacological adjuncts and nutritional supplements in the treatment of drug dependence. J Psychoactive Drugs *20*: 243, 1988.

Elder I R, Voris J C, Sebastian P S, Acevedo A G: Disulfiram compliance as a function of patient motivation, program philosophy and side effects. J Alcohol Drug Educ *34*: 23, 1988.

Friedman T C, Fulop G: Disulfiram use at hospital-based and free-standing alcoholism treatment centers. J Subst Abuse Treat *5*: 139, 1988.

Fuller R K: Current status of alcoholism treatment outcome research: 51st Annual Meeting of the Committee on Problems of Drug Dependence (Keystone, Colorado). NIDA Res Monogr *95*: 85, 1989.

Kingsbury S J, Salzman C: Disulfiram in the treatment of alcoholic patients with schizophrenia. Hosp Community Psychiatry *41*: 133, 1990.

Kranzler H R, Dolinsky Z, Kaplan R F: Giving ethanol to alcoholics in a research setting: Its effect on compliance with disulfiram treatment. Br Addict *85*: 119, 1990.

Larson E W, Olincy A, Rummans T A, Morse R M: Disulfiram treatment of patients with both alcohol dependence and other psychiatric disorders: A review. Alcoholism *16*: 125, 1992.

Liskow B, Nickel E, Tunley N, Powell B J: Alcoholics' attitudes toward and experiences with disulfiram. Am J Drug Alcohol Abuse *16*: 147, 1990.

18

L-Dopa

L-Dopa, also known as levodopa (Larodopa), is a dopamine agonist used primarily for the treatment of drug-induced extrapyramidal disorders, such as parkinsonism. The molecular structure of L-dopa is given in Figure 18–1.

PHARMACOLOGICAL ACTIONS

Pharmacokinetics

L-Dopa is rapidly absorbed after oral administration, with peak plasma levels reached after 30 minutes to two hours. The half-life of L-dopa is one to three hours. Absorption of levodopa can be significantly reduced by changes in gastric pH and by ingestion with meals. L-Dopa is almost entirely decarboxylated in the periphery by L-amino acid decarboxylase. Dopamine, the decarboxylated form of levodopa, is pharmacologically active. But dopamine does not cross the blood-brain barrier. The strategy of combining L-dopa with a peripheral inhibitor of L-dopa decarboxylase, such as carbidopa, results in more efficient delivery of dopa to the central nervous system (CNS). An available combination of L-dopa and carbidopa is Sinemet. Dopamine is rapidly and completely metabolized mainly to DOPAC and homovanillic acid and is excreted in the urine.

Pharmacodynamics

L-Dopa, once converted to dopamine, replenishes depleted stores of endogenous dopamine.

INDICATIONS

Although there is no primary psychiatric indication for L-dopa, the drug may be useful in the treatment of extrapyramidal signs and symptoms—such as parkinsonism, akinesia, and rabbit syndrome (focal perioral tremor of the choreoath-

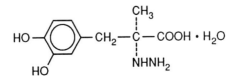

Figure 18–1. Molecular structure of L-dopa.

etoid type)—caused by the administration of antipsychotic drugs. L-Dopa may also relieve the symptoms of restless legs syndrome.

CLINICAL GUIDELINES

L-Dopa combined with a peripheral decarboxylase inhibitor, carbidopa, is the therapy of choice for idiopathic parkinsonism. Starting dosages of 100 mg three times a day may be increased until the patient is functionally improved. Hyperkinesias, in the form of chorea or dystonia, are dose-related side effects. Particularly after prolonged therapy, periods of profound bradykinesia may alternate with periods when the patient can move well or is hyperkinetic (on-off phenomenon or end-of-dose deterioration). Careful titration of L-dopa, avoidance of protein intake during the day hours, or the addition of a direct dopamine receptor agonist, bromocriptine (Parlodel), may ameliorate the syndrome. Parkinsonism resistant to L-dopa may respond to small doses of bromocriptine (between 2.5 and 30 mg). L-Dopa is available in 100 mg, 250 mg, and 500 mg tablets and capsules. The elderly are particularly sensitive to L-dopa's effects. The drug has not been studied in children.

ADVERSE EFFECTS

Side effects commonly occur with L-dopa therapy. Most side effects are dose-related or associated with withdrawal. The side effects seen early in treatment include nausea, vomiting, and cardiac arrythmias. After long-term use, patients may experience abnormal involuntary movements and psychiatric disturbances. L-Dopa may exacerbate or precipitate psychotic symptoms. Up to 12 percent of patients treated with L-dopa experience mania. L-Dopa may induce orthostatic hypotension. Abrupt discontinuation of L-dopa has been reported to cause symptoms similar to neuroleptic malignant syndrome. The risk may be high if the patient is taking a dopamine receptor antagonist, such as a phenothiazine or haloperidol (Haldol). L-Dopa should not be administered during pregnancy. It inhibits lactation and may be secreted in breast milk.

DRUG-DRUG INTERACTIONS

Drugs that block dopamine type 2 (D_2) receptors—most notably phenothiazines, haloperiodol, and other drugs used to treat psychosis—reverse the therapeutic effects of L-dopa. Concurrent use of tricyclic antidepressant drugs and L-dopa can result in rigidity, agitation, and tremor. L-Dopa may potentiate the hypotensive effects of diuretics and antihypertensive medications. L-Dopa should not be used in conjunction with monoamine oxidase inhibitors (MAOIs). MAOIs should be discontinued at least two weeks before the initiation of L-dopa therapy. Benzodiazepines, phenytoin (Dilantin), and pyridoxine may interfere with the therapeutic effects of L-dopa. Selegiline (Eldepryl) may increase the effects of L-dopa.

References

Fayen M, Goldman M B, Moulthrop M A, Luchins D J: Differential memory function with dopaminergic versus anticholinergic treatment of drug-induced extrapyramidal symptoms. Am J Psychiatry *145*: 483, 1988.

Geminiani G, Cesana B M, Scigliano G, Soliveri P: Variation of therapeutic response in Parkinson's disease: A retrospective study. Acta Neurol Scand *81*: 397, 1990.

Kaplan B, Mason N A: Levodopa in restless legs syndrome. Ann Pharmacother *26*: 214, 1992.

Ludatscher J I: Stable remission of tardive dyskinesia by L-dopa. J Clin Psychopharmacol *9*: 39, 1989.

Ray S R, Opler L A: L-Dopa in the treatment of negative schizophrenic symptoms: A single-subject experimental study. Int J Psychiatry Med *15*: 293, 1986.

19

Dopamine Receptor Antagonists: Antipsychotics

Dopamine receptor antagonists make up the largest group of drugs known as *antipsychotics*. The antipsychotics are a seemingly diverse group of drugs that have the single common pharmacodynamic property of antagonizing dopamine receptors (except for clozapine [Clozaril], which is discussed in Chapter 15). The drugs have also been referred to as *neuroleptics* and *major tranquilizers*. The term "neuroleptic" refers more to the neurological or motor effects of the drugs. The term "major tranquilizer" inaccurately implies that the primary effect of the drugs is merely to sedate patients; it also confounds the drugs with the so-called minor tranquilizers, such as the benzodiazepines. A common mistake is to use the term "phenothiazine" as synonymous with the term "antipsychotic"; the phenothiazine antipsychotics are only one class of antipsychotic drugs.

The major use of antipsychotics is to treat schizophrenia, although the drugs are also used to treat agitation and psychosis associated with other psychiatric and organic disorders. Antipsychotics have little or no abuse potential.

CLASSIFICATION

Seven classes of drugs can be grouped together as antipsychotic dopamine receptor antagonists (Figure 19–1).

Phenothiazines

All the phenothiazines have the same three-ring phenothiazine nucleus but differ in the side chains joined to the nitrogen atom of the middle ring. The phenothiazines are typed according to the aliphatic (for example, chlorpromazine [Thorazine]), piperazine (for example, fluphenazine [Prolixin, Permitil]), or piperidine (for example, thioridazine [Mellaril]) nature of the side chain.

Thioxanthenes

The thioxanthene three-ring nucleus differs from the phenothiazine nucleus by the substitution of a carbon atom for the nitrogen atom in the middle ring. The two available thioxanthenes have either an aliphatic (chlorprothixene [Taractan]) or a piperazine (thiothixene [Navane]) side chain.

Dibenzoxazepines

The dibenzoxazepines are based on another modification of the three-ring phenothiazine nucleus. The only dibenzoxazepine available in the United States is loxapine (Loxitane), which has a piperazine side chain.

Dihydroindoles

The only dihydroindole available in the United States, molindone (Moban, Lidone), has somewhat unusual properties, such as not inducing weight gain and perhaps being less epileptogenic than the phenothiazines.

Butyrophenones

Only two butyrophenones are available in the United States—haloperidol (Haldol) and droperidol (Inapsine). Haloperidol is perhaps the most widely used antipsychotic, and droperidol is used as an adjuvant in anesthesia. Some research groups, however, have been using droperidol as an intravenous (IV) antipsychotic drug in emergency settings. Spiroperidol is a butyrophenone compound widely used in research studies to label dopamine receptors.

Diphenylbutylpiperidines

Diphenylbutylpiperidines are somewhat similar structurally to the butyrophenones. Only one diphenylbutylpiperidine, pimozide (Orap), is available in the United States and is approved for treating Tourette's disorder. In Europe, however, pimozide has been shown to be an effective antipsychotic agent. A controversial clinical and research observation about pimozide is that it may be more effective than the other antipsychotics in reducing the deficit or negative symptoms of schizophrenia.

Benzamides

No benzamide derivatives are available in the United States; however, there is considerable evidence that sulpiride (Dogmatil) is an effective antipsychotic associated with fewer neurological side effects than are the other antipsychotics.

PHARMACOLOGICAL ACTIONS

Pharmacokinetics

Although the pharmacokinetic details for the antipsychotics vary widely (for example, half-lives ranging from 10 to 20 hours), the most important clinical generalization is that all the antipsychotics currently available in the United States can be given in one daily dose once the patient is in a stable condition and has

Phenothiazines

Aliphatic

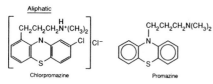

Chlorpromazine

Promazine

Triflupromazine

Piperazine

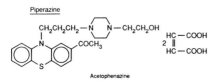

Acetophenazine

Fluphenazine

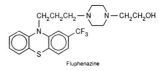

Perphenazine

Prochlorperazine

Trifluoperazine

Piperidine

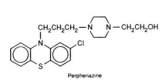

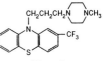

Mesoridazine

Thoridazine

Thioxanthenes

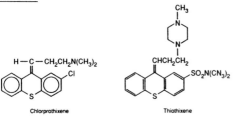

Chlorprothixene

Thiothixene

Figure 19–1. Molecular structures of dopamine receptor antagonists and reserpine.

Dibenzoxazepine

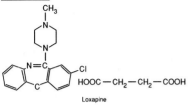

Loxapine

Dihydroindole

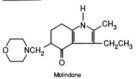

Molindone

Butyrophenones

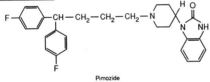

Droperidol

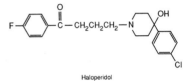

Haloperidol

Diphenylbutylpiperidine

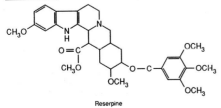

Pimozide

Benzamide

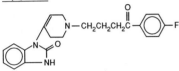

Sulpiride (not available in U.S.)

Rauwolfia Alkaloid

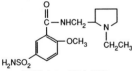

Reserpine

Figure 19–1. Molecular structures of dopamine receptor antagonists and reserpine (continued).

adjusted to any adverse effects. Most antipsychotics are incompletely absorbed after oral administration. In addition, most have high binding to plasma proteins, volumes of distribution, and lipid solubilities. Antipsychotic drugs are metabolized in the liver and reach steady-state plasma levels in 5 to 10 days. There is some evidence that, after a few weeks of administration, chlorpromazine, thiothixene, and thioridazine induce metabolic enzymes, thereby decreasing the plasma concentrations. Chlorpromazine is notorious among psychopharmacologists for having more than 150 metabolites, some of which are active. The nonaliphatic phenothiazines and the butyrophenones have few metabolites, but the activity of those metabolites is still controversial. The potential presence of active metabolites complicates the interpretation of plasma drug levels that report the presence of only the parent compound.

Pharmacodynamics

The potency of antipsychotic drugs to reduce psychotic symptoms is most closely correlated with the affinity of those drugs with the dopamine type 2 (D_2) receptor. The mechanism of therapeutic action for antipsychotic drugs is thought to be as D_2 receptor antagonists, preventing the binding of endogenous dopamine to that type of dopaminergic receptor. There are two caveats to that hypothesis. First, although the dopamine receptor blocking effect occurs immediately, the full antipsychotic effects may take weeks to develop. That observation suggests that some more slowly developing homeostatic change in the brain is the actual mechanism of action for the antipsychotic effects of the drugs. Second, although the correlation of dopamine blocking effects with the clinical potency has led to the dopamine hypothesis of schizophrenia, it is also true that the drugs reduce psychotic symptoms regardless of the diagnosis. The therapeutic effects of dopamine receptor blockade, therefore, are not unique to the pathophysiology of schizophrenia.

Most of the neurological and endocrinological adverse effects of antipsychotics can also be explained by the blockade of dopamine receptors. Various antipsychotics, however, also block noradrenergic, cholinergic, and histaminergic receptors, thus accounting for the variation in adverse effects profiles seen among the drugs.

Although the potency of the antipsychotics varies widely (Table 19–1), all available antipsychotics are equally efficacious in the treatment of schizophrenia. No type of schizophrenia or set of symptoms has been demonstrated conclusively to be more effectively treated by any single class of antipsychotics (with the possible exception of clozapine and pimozide for negative symptoms). The therapeutic index for antipsychotics is very favorable and has contributed to the unfortunate practice of routinely using high doses of the drugs. Recent investigations of the dose-response curve for antipsychotics indicate that the equivalent of 10 to 20 mg of haloperidol is usually efficacious for either the short-term or the long-term treatment of schizophrenia. Antipsychotics may have a bell-shaped dose-response curve. Overly high doses of antipsychotics may lead to neurological side effects, such as akinesia and akathisia, which are difficult to distinguish from an exacerbation of psychosis. Moreover, excessively high doses of some antipsychotics become less effective in reducing psychotic symptoms.

Although patients can build up a tolerance to most of the adverse effects caused by antipsychotics, patients do not build up a tolerance to the antipsychotic effect. It is wise, nevertheless, to taper the dosage when the drugs are being discontinued, as there may be rebound effects from the other neurotransmitter systems that the drug blocked. Cholinergic rebound, for example, can produce a flulike syndrome in patients.

INDICATIONS

Idiopathic Psychoses

Idiopathic psychoses include schizophrenia, schizophreniform disorder, schizoaffective disorder, delusional disorder, brief reactive psychosis, manic episode, and major depressive episode with psychotic features. Antipsychotics are effective in both the short-term and the long-term management of those conditions; that is, antipsychotics both reduce acute symptoms and prevent future exacerbations. Antipsychotics are often used in combination with antimanic drugs to treat bipolar disorder and in combination with antidepressants to treat major depression with psychotic features. Because of the potential adverse effects of repeatedly administering antipsychotics, maintenance treatment with the drugs is indicated primarily for schizophrenia and in some cases of schizoaffective disorder.

Antipsychotics are superior to placebos in the treatment of acute and chronic schizophrenia and in the control of other agitated and psychotic behavior. Approximately 70 percent of patients improve significantly with antipsychotic treatment. The onset of sedation is rapid, often within one hour after intramuscular (IM) administration of the drugs. Antipsychotic activity has a slower onset, but most therapeutic gain occurs in the first six weeks of therapy. Patients may continue to improve, however, for up to six months. Antipsychotics are most effective against the positive symptoms of psychosis, such as agitation and hallucinations. Although the negative symptoms are less affected by antipsychotic treatment, with continued treatment many patients become less socially withdrawn.

Secondary Psychoses

Secondary psychoses are associated with an identified organic cause, such as a brain tumor or drug intoxication. The high-potency antipsychotics are usually safer to use in such patients because of their lower cardiotoxic and epileptogenic potential. Antipsychotic drugs should not be used to treat drug intoxications or withdrawals when there is an increased risk of seizures. The drug of choice in such cases is usually a benzodiazepine. Psychosis secondary to amphetamine intoxication, however, is an indication for antipsychotic treatment if a pharmacological treatment is required.

TABLE 19–1
Dopamine Receptor Antagonist Drugs, Trade Names, Potencies, and Dosages

Generic Name	Trade Name	Potency* (mg of drug equivalent to 100 mg chlorpromazine)	Usual Adult Dosage Range (mg per day)	Usual Single IM Dosage (mg)
Phenothiazines				
Aliphatic				
Chlorpromazine	Thorazine	100—low	300–800	25–50
Triflupromazine	Vesprin	25–50—low	100–150	20–60
Promazine	Sparine	40—low	40–800	50–150
Piperazine				
Prochlorperazine	Compazine	15—medium	40–150	10–20
Perphenazine	Trilafon	10—medium	8–40	5–10
Trifluoperazine	Stelazine	3–5—high	6–20	1–2
Fluphenazine	Prolixin, Permitil	1.5–3—high	1–20	2–5
Acetophenazine	Tindal	25—medium	60–120	—
Butaperazine	Repoise (not sold in U.S.)	10—medium	—	—
Carphenazine	Proketazine (not sold in U.S.)	25—medium	—	—

Piperidine				
Thioridazine	Mellaril	100—low	200–700[1]	—
Mesoridazine	Serentil	50—low	75–300	25
Piperacetazine	Quide (not sold in U.S.)	10—medium	—	—
Thioxanthenes				
Chlorprothixene	Taractan	50—low	50–400	25–50
Thiothixene	Navane	2–5—high	6–30	2–4
Dibenzoxazepine				
Loxapine	Loxitane	10–15—medium	60–100	12.5–50
Dihydroindole				
Molindone	Moban, Lidone	6–10—medium	50–100	—
Butyrophenones				
Haloperidol	Haldol	2–5—high	6–20	2–5
Droperidol	Inapsine	10—medium	—	—
Diphenylbutylpiperidine				
Pimozide	Orap	1—high	1–10[2]	—

*Recommended adult dosages are 200 to 400 mg a day of chlorpromazine or an equivalent amount of another drug.
[1]Maximum 800 mg.
[2]Second-line drug because of cardiotoxicity.

Severe Agitation or Violent Behavior

The administration of antipsychotics calms most severely agitated or violent patients, although the use of a sedative drug (for example, benzodiazepine or barbiturate) may be preferable in some cases. The agitation associated with delirium and dementia, most common in elderly patients, is an indication for antipsychotics. Small dosages of high-potency drugs (for example, 0.5 to 1 mg a day of haloperidol) are usually the best choice. The repeated administration of antipsychotics to control disruptive behavior in mentally retarded children is a controversial indication.

Movement Disorders

Both the psychosis and the movement disorder of Huntington's chorea are often treated with antipsychotics. The drugs are also used to treat the motor and vocal tics of Tourette's disorder.

Other Psychiatric Indications

The use of thioridazine to treat depression with marked anxiety or agitation has been approved by the Food and Drug Administration (FDA). Some clinicians use small dosages of antipsychotics (0.5 mg of haloperidol or 25 mg of chlorpromazine two to three times a day) to treat severe anxiety. In addition, some investigators have reported using antipsychotics to control the behavioral turmoil in patients with borderline personality disorder. But because of the possible long-term adverse effects of antipsychotics, they should be used in those other psychiatric conditions only after more conventional drugs have been tried.

CLINICAL GUIDELINES

Antipsychotic drugs are remarkably safe in short-term use, and, if necessary, a clinician can administer the drugs without conducting a physical or laboratory examination of the patient. The major contraindications to antipsychotics are (1) a history of a serious allergic response; (2) the possibility that the patient has ingested a drug that will interact with the antipsychotic to induce central nervous system (CNS) depression (for example, alcohol, opioids, barbiturates, benzodiazepines) or anticholinergic delirium (for example, scopolamine [Donnatal], possibly phencyclidine [PCP]); (3) the presence of a severe cardiac abnormality; (4) a high risk of seizures from organic or idiopathic causes; (5) the presence of narrow-angle glaucoma or prostatic hypertrophy (or other conditions that cause urinary retention) if an anticholinergic antipsychotic is to be used; and (6) the presence of or a history of tardive dyskinesia. Antipsychotics should be administered with caution in patients with hepatic disease. In the usual assessment, however, it is best to obtain a complete blood count (CBC) with white blood cell indexes, liver function tests, and an electrocardiogram (ECG), especially in women over 40 and men over 30. The elderly and children are more sensitive to side effects than are young adults.

Choice of Drug

The general guidelines for choosing a particular psychotherapeutic drug should be followed (Chapter 1). If no other rationale prevails, the choice should be based on adverse effect profiles, as described below, and the psychiatrist's preference. Although high-potency antipsychotics are associated with more neurological adverse effects, current clinical practice greatly favors using them because of the higher incidence of other adverse effects (for example, cardiac, hypotensive, epileptogenic, sexual, and allergic) with the low-potency drugs. There is a myth in psychiatry that hyperexcitable patients respond best to chlorpromazine because it is more sedating, whereas withdrawn patients respond best to high-potency antipsychotics, such as fluphenazine. That hypothesis has never been proved; if sedation is a desired goal, either the antipsychotic can be given in divided doses or a sedative drug, such as a benzodiazepine, can also be administered.

A clinical observation supported by some research is that an unpleasant reaction by the patient to the first dose of an antipsychotic correlates highly with future poor response and noncompliance. Such experiences include a subjective negative feeling, oversedation, and acute dystonia. If a patient reports such a reaction, the clinician may be well advised to switch the patient to a different antipsychotic.

Dosage and Schedule

Various patients may respond to widely different dosages of antipsychotics; therefore, there is no set dosage for any given antipsychotic drug. It is reasonable clinical practice to start each patient at a low dosage and increase it as necessary. It is important to remember that the maximal effects of a particular dosage may not be evident for four to six weeks. Available preparations of dopamine receptor antagonists are given in Table 19–2.

Short-term treatment.   The equivalent of 5 mg of haloperidol is a reasonable dose for an adult patient in an acute state. A geriatric patient may benefit from as little as 1 mg of haloperidol. The administration of more than 50 mg of chlorpromazine in one injection, however, may result in serious hypotension. The administration of the antipsychotic IM results in peak plasma levels in approximately 30 minutes, versus 90 minutes with the oral route. The patient should be observed for one hour; after that time, most clinicians administer a second dose of the antipsychotic.

Rapid neuroleptization is the practice of administering hourly IM doses of antipsychotic medications until the desired clinical effect is achieved. Several research studies have shown, however, that merely waiting several more hours after one dose of an antipsychotic results in the same clinical improvement as that seen with repeated doses of antipsychotics. The clinician must be careful to prevent patients from becoming violent while they are psychotic. Psychiatrists can do so by temporarily using physical restraints until the patients can control their behavior.

Because the administration of very high doses of high-potency antipsychotics is not associated with a higher incidence of adverse effects, the practice of giving very large cumulative antipsychotic doses in the emergency setting has become common. Physicians, therefore, may be pressured by their staff members to use

TABLE 19–2
Dopamine Receptor Antagonist Preparations

	Tablets	Capsules	Solution	Parenteral	Rectal Suppositories
Acetophenazine	20 mg	—	—	—	—
Chlorpromazine	10, 25, 50, 100, 200 mg	30, 75, 150, 200, 300 mg	10 mg/5 mL, 30 mg/mL, 100 mg/mL	25 mg/mL	25, 100 mg
Chlorprothixene	10, 25, 50, 100 mg	—	100 mg/5 mL (suspension)	12.5 mg/mL	—
Droperidol	—	—	—	2.5 mg/mL	—
Fluphenazine	1, 2.5, 5, 10 mg	—	2.5 mg/5 mL, 5 mg/mL	2.5 mg/mL (IM only)	—
Fluphenazine decanoate	—	—	—	25 mg/mL	—
Fluphenazine enanthate	—	—	—	25 mg/mL	—
Haloperidol	0.5, 1, 2, 5, 10, 20 mg	—	2 mg/mL	5 mg/mL (IM only)	—
Haloperidol decanoate	—	—	—	50 mg/mL, 100 mg/mL (IM only)	—

Loxapine	—	5, 10, 25, 50 mg	25 mg/mL	50 mg/mL	—
Mesoridazine	10, 25, 50, 100 mg	—	25 mg/mL	25 mg/mL	—
Molindone	5, 10, 25, 50, 100 mg	—	20 mg/mL	—	—
Perphenazine	2, 4, 8, 16 mg	—	16 mg/5 mL	5 mg/mL	—
Pimozide	2 mg	—	—	—	—
Prochlorperazine	5, 10, 25 mg	10, 15, 30 mg	5 mg/5 mL	5 mg/mL	2.5, 5, 25 mg
Promazine	25, 50, 100 mg	—	—	25 mg/mL, 50 mg/mL	—
Thioridazine	10, 15, 25, 50, 100, 150, 200 mg	—	25 mg/5 mL, 100 mg/5 mL, 30 mg/mL, 100 mg/mL	—	—
Thiothixene	—	1, 2, 5, 10, 20 mg	5 mg/mL	10 mg (IM only), 2 mg/mL (IM only)	—
Trifluoperazine	1, 2, 5, 10 mg	—	—	—	—
Triflupromazine	—	—	—	10 mg/mL, 20 mg/mL	—

repeated administrations of antipsychotics. But hypotension can be a serious complication resulting from the repeated administration of low-potency antipsychotics.

Clinicians usually attempt to achieve sedation, in addition to the reduction of psychosis, with repeated administrations of antipsychotics. It may be reasonable, therefore, to use a sedative agent, rather than an antipsychotic, after one or two doses of the antipsychotic. Possible sedatives include lorazepam (Ativan) (2 mg IM) and amobarbital (Amytal) (50 to 250 mg IM).

Early treatment. The equivalent of 10 to 20 mg of haloperidol or 400 mg of chlorpromazine a day is adequate treatment for most patients with schizophrenia. Some research suggests that 5 mg of haloperidol or 200 mg of chlorpromazine may, in fact, be just as effective. It is wise to use divided doses when initiating the therapy. That practice reduces the incidence and the severity of adverse effects and may help sedate the patient. The sedative effects of antipsychotics last only a few hours, in contrast to the antipsychotic effects, which last for one to three days. After approximately one week of treatment, it is usually helpful to give the entire dose of the antipsychotic at bedtime. That practice usually helps the patient sleep and reduces the incidence of adverse effects. In elderly patients treated with low-potency antipsychotics, however, the practice may increase the risk of their falling if they get out of the bed during the night.

It is common clinical practice to order medications to be given as needed (PRN). Although that practice may be reasonable during the first few days that a patient is hospitalized, the time on antipsychotic drugs, rather than an increase in dosage, is what produces therapeutic improvement. Again, clinicians may feel pressured by their staff members to write PRN antipsychotic orders. The orders for PRN medications should include the specific symptoms, how often the drugs should be given, and how many doses can be given each day. Clinicians may choose to use small doses for the PRNs (for example, 2 mg of haloperidol) or may use a benzodiazepine (for example, 2 mg lorazepam IM).

Maintenance treatment. A patient with schizophrenia should continue to receive an effective dosage of antipsychotics for at least six months after improvement. For a patient who has had only one or two psychotic episodes and has been in a stable clinical state for six months, it is reasonable to attempt to reduce the dosage by 50 percent gradually over three to six months. After the patient has had another six months in a stable clinical state, another 50 percent dosage reduction may be indicated. Some research data suggest that many patients with schizophrenia can be maintained with the equivalent of 5 mg of haloperidol a day. It is wise for the clinician to know enough about the patient's life to try to predict upcoming stressors, during which times the patient's antipsychotic dosage should perhaps be increased.

Patients who have had three or more exacerbations of schizophrenic symptoms should probably continue to receive antipsychotics indefinitely, although attempts to reduce the dosage may be warranted every four to five years if the patient has been clinically stable. Although antipsychotic drugs are effective, patients may report that they prefer being off the drugs, because they feel better without them. Normal persons who have taken antipsychotic drugs report a sense of dysphoria. The clinician must discuss maintenance medication with the patients and take into account the patients' wishes, the severity of their illness, and the quality of their support systems.

TABLE 19–3
Use of Long-Acting Dopamine Receptor Antagonists

Dosage
  a. Stabilize patient on lowest effective dose of oral preparation.
  b. Usual dosage conversion:
    10 mg/day oral fluphenazine = 12.5–25 mg/2 weeks fluphenazine decanoate
    10 mg/day oral haloperidol = 100–200 mg/4 weeks haloperidol decanoate
  c. As with all other antipsychotic medications, the lowest effective dose should be used. Note that patients with chronic schizophrenia have been adequately maintained on doses of fluphenazine decanoate as low as 5 mg/2 weeks.
  d. Supplementation with oral medication may be necessary for the first several months until the optimum dosage regimen has been determined.

Techniques of Injection
  a. Using a 2-inch needle, inject no more than 3 cc of medication per injection into upper quadrant of buttock (to inject more than 3 cc, use alternate buttocks and vary injection sites).
  b. After drawing up medication, draw a small air bubble of 0.1 cc into syringe and change needle for injection.
  c. Wipe injection site with alcohol swab and allow to dry before giving injection, otherwise alcohol may infiltrate subcutaneous tissue and cause local irritation.
  d. Stretch the skin over the injection site to one side and hold firmly.
  e. Inject medication slowly, including air bubble, which forces last drop from needle into the muscle and prevents any medication from being deposited in subcutaneous tissue as needle is withdrawn.
  f. Wait about 10 seconds before withdrawing needle, then do so quickly and release skin.
  g. Do not massage injection site, as this may force medication to ooze from muscle and infiltrate subcutaneous tissue.
  h. Precautions should also be taken with glass ampules to avoid injection of glass particles.

Table from J M Silver, S C Yudofsky: Psychopharmacology and electroconvulsive therapy. In *The American Psychiatric Press Textbook of Psychiatry*, J A Talbott, R E Hales, S C Yudofsky, p 782. American Psychiatric Press, Washington, 1988.
Adapted from M C Belanger, G Chouinard: Technique for injecting long-acting neuroleptics. Br J Psychiatry *141*: 316, 1982. Used with permission.

Alternative maintenance regimens.   Alternative maintenance regimens have been designed to reduce both the risk of long-term adverse effects and any unpleasantness associated with taking antipsychotic medications. Intermittent medication is the use of antipsychotics only when patients require them. That arrangement requires that the patients or their caretakers be both willing and able to watch carefully for early signs of clinical exacerbations. At the earliest signs of such problems, antipsychotic medications should be reinstituted for a reasonable period, usually one to three months.

Drug holidays are regular two- to seven-day periods during which the patient is not given antipsychotic medications. Currently, no evidence indicates that drug holidays reduce the risk of long-term adverse effects from antipsychotics, and it is possible that drug holidays increase the incidence of noncompliance.

Long-acting depot antipsychotics.   Because some patients with schizophrenia do not reliably comply with oral antipsychotic regimens, it may be reasonable to treat them with long-acting depot preparations (Table 19–3). The preparations are usually administered IM once every one to four weeks by a clinician. The clinician, therefore, immediately knows if a patient has missed a dose of medication. Depot antipsychotics may be associated with more adverse effects, including tardive dyskinesia. Although that concern is controversial, clinicians should probably refrain from using depot forms unless the patient is unable to comply with oral medications.

Two depot preparations (a decanoate and an enanthate) of fluphenazine and a decanoate preparation of haloperidol are available in the United States. The preparations are injected IM into an area of large muscle tissue, from where they are absorbed slowly into the blood. Decanoate preparations can be given less frequently than are enanthate preparations because they are absorbed more slowly. Although it is not absolutely necessary to stabilize a patient on the oral (PO) preparation of the specific drug before initiating the depot form, it is good practice to give at least one PO dose of the drug to assess the possibility of any adverse effect, such as severe extrapyramidal symptoms or an allergic reaction.

It is difficult to predict the correct dosage or time interval for depot preparations. It is reasonable to begin with 12.5 mg (0.5 cc) of either fluphenazine preparations or 25 mg (0.5 cc) of haloperidol decanoate. If symptoms emerge in the next two to four weeks, the patient can be treated temporarily with additional oral medications or with additional small depot injections. After three to four weeks the depot injection can be increased to include the supplemental doses given during the initial period.

A good reason to initiate depot treatment with low doses is that the absorption of the preparations may be faster at the onset of treatment, resulting in frightening episodes of dystonia that eventually discourage compliance with the medication. Some clinicians keep patients drug-free for three to seven days before initiating depot treatment and give very small doses of the depot preparations (3.125 mg fluphenazine or 6.25 mg haloperidol) every few days to avoid those initial problems. Because the major indication for depot medication is poor compliance with oral forms, it may be wise to go slowly with what is practically the last method of achieving compliance.

ADVERSE EFFECTS

Nonneurological Adverse Effects

One generalization about the adverse effects of antipsychotics is that low-potency drugs cause most nonneurological adverse effects and that high-potency drugs cause most neurological adverse effects (Table 19–4).

Orthostatic (postural) hypotension. Orthostatic (postural) hypotension is mediated by adrenergic blockade and is most common with chlorpromazine and thioridazine (Table 19–4). It occurs most frequently during the first few days of treatment, and patients readily have a tolerance to it. It is most apt to occur when high doses of intramuscular, low-potency antipsychotics are given. The chief dangers of the adverse effect are that the patients may faint, fall, and injure themselves, although such occurrences are uncommon. When using IM low-potency antipsychotics, the clinician should measure the patients' blood pressure (lying and standing) before and after the first dose and during the first few days of treatment. When appropriate, patients should be warned of the adverse effects and given the usual instructions—to rise from bed gradually, sit at first with their legs dangling, wait for a minute, and sit or lie down if they feel faint. Support hose may help with

TABLE 19–4
Relative Adverse Effects of Dopamine Receptor Antagonists

	Sedation	Anticholinergic	Hypotension	Extrapyramidal
Acetophenazine	Low	Low	Low	Medium
Chlorpromazine	High	High	High	Low
Chlorprothixene	High	High	High	Low
Fluphenazine	Medium	Low	Low	High
Haloperidol	Low	Low	Low	High
Loxapine	Medium	Medium	Medium	High
Mesoridazine	Medium	High	Medium	Medium
Molindone	Medium	Medium	Low	High
Perphenazine	Low	Low	Low	High
Pimozide	Low	Low	Low	High
Thioridazine	High	High	High	Low
Thiothixene	Low	Low	Low	High
Trifluoperazine	Medium	Low	Low	High
Triflupromazine	High	Medium	High	Medium

the symptom. If low-potency antipsychotics are used by patients with cardiac problems, the dosage should be increased slowly.

If hypotension does occur in patients receiving the medications, the symptoms can usually be managed by having the patients lie down with the feet higher than the head. On rare occasions, volume expansion or vasopressor agents, such as norepinephrine, may be indicated. Because hypotension is produced by α-adrenergic blockade, the drugs also block the α-adrenergic stimulating properties of epinephrine, leaving the β-adrenergic stimulating effects untouched. Therefore, administering epinephrine results in a paradoxical worsening of hypotension and so is contraindicated in cases of antipsychotic-induced hypotension. Pure α-adrenergic pressors, such as metaraminol (Aramine) and norepinephrine (levarterenol [Levophed]), are the drugs of choice in the treatment of the disorder.

Peripheral anticholinergic effects. Peripheral anticholinergic effects are common and consist of dry mouth and nose, blurred vision, constipation, urinary retention, and mydriasis. Some patients also have nausea and vomiting. Chlorpromazine, thioridazine, mesoridazine (Serentil), and trifluoperazine (Stelazine) are potent anticholinergics (Table 19–4). Anticholinergic effects can be particularly severe if a low-potency antipsychotic is used with a tricyclic antidepressant and an anticholinergic drug; such a practice is seldom warranted.

Dry mouth can be a troubling symptom for patients. They should be advised to rinse out the mouth frequently with water and not to chew gum or candy containing sugar, as that can result in fungal infections of the mouth or an increased incidence of dental caries. Constipation should be treated with the usual laxative preparations, but the condition can progress to paralytic ileus. Pilocarpine may be used in such situations, although the relief is only transitory. A decrease in the antipsychotic or a change to another drug is warranted in such cases. Bethanechol (Urecholine) (20 to 40 mg a day) may be useful in some patients with urinary retention.

Endocrine effects. Blockade of the dopamine receptors in the tuberoinfundibular tract results in increased secretion of prolactin, which can result in breast enlargement, galactorrhea, impotence in men, and amenorrhea and inhibited orgasm in women. Both sexes may report decreased libido, and women may have a false pregnancy test result while taking some antipsychotics. Thioridazine is particularly associated with decreased libido and retrograde ejaculation in male patients. Psychiatrists may not find out about the disturbing sexual adverse effects of an antipsychotic if they do not ask about them specifically. Another adverse effect of antipsychotics is the inappropriate secretion of antidiuretic hormone. Some patients' glucose tolerance test results shift in a diabetic direction because of antipsychotic administration.

Skin effects.   Allergic dermatitis and photosensitivity occur in a small percentage of patients, most commonly those taking low-potency drugs, particularly chlorpromazine. A variety of skin eruptions—urticarial, maculopapular, petechial, and edematous eruptions—have been reported. The eruptions occur early in treatment, generally in the first few weeks, and remit spontaneously. A photosensitivity reaction that resembles a severe sunburn also occurs in some patients taking chlorpromazine. Patients should be warned of that adverse effect, should spend no more than 30 to 60 minutes in the sun, and should use sun screens. Chlorpromazine is also associated with some cases of blue-gray discoloration of the skin over areas exposed to sunlight. The skin changes often begin with a tan or golden brown color and progress to such colors as slate gray, metallic blue, and purple.

Ophthalmological effects.   Thioridazine is associated with irreversible pigmentation of the retina when given in dosages of more than 800 mg a day. The pigmentation is similar to that seen in retinitis pigmentosa, and it can progress even after the thioridazine is stopped and can result in blindness.

Chlorpromazine may induce whitish-brown granular deposits concentrated in the anterior lens and posterior cornea, visible only by slit-lens examination. They progress to opaque white and yellow-brown granules, often stellate in shape. Occasionally, the conjunctiva is discolored by a brown pigment. Retinal damage is not seen in the patients, and their vision is almost never impaired. The majority of patients who show the deposits are those who have ingested 1 to 3 kg of chlorpromazine throughout their lives.

Cardiac effects.   Low-potency antipsychotics are more cardiotoxic than are high-potency drugs. Chlorpromazine causes prolongation of the QT and PR intervals, blunting of T waves, and depression of the ST segment. Thioridazine, in particular, has marked effects on the T wave, and the unique cardiac effects may be why overdoses of the piperidine phenothiazines are the most lethal among the antipsychotics.

Sudden death.   The cardiac effects of antipsychotics have been hypothesized to be related to sudden death in patients treated with the drugs. Careful evaluation of the literature, however, suggests that it is premature to attribute the sudden deaths to the antipsychotic drugs. Supporting that view is the observation that the introduction of antipsychotics had no effect on the incidence of sudden death in schizophrenic patients. In addition, both low-potency and high-potency drugs were involved in the cases. Furthermore, many reports were of patients with other medical problems, treated with other drugs.

Weight gain.   A common adverse effect of treatment with antipsychotics is weight gain, which can be significant in some cases. Molindone and, perhaps, loxapine are not associated with the symptom and may be indicated in patients for whom weight gain is a serious health hazard or a reason for noncompliance.

Hematological effects. A leukopenia with a white blood count (WBC) around 3,500 is a common but not serious problem. A life-threatening hematological problem is agranulocytosis, occurring most often with chlorpromazine and thioridazine but seen with almost all antipsychotics. It occurs most frequently during the first three months and with an incidence of 1 in 500,000. Routine complete blood counts (CBCs) are not indicated; however, if a patient reports a sore throat and fever, a CBC should be done immediately to check for the possibility. If the blood indexes are low, the antipsychotic should be stopped, and the patient should be transferred to a medical facility. The mortality rate for the complication may be as high as 30 percent. Thrombocytopenic or nonthrombocytopenic purpura, hemolytic anemias, and pancytopenia may occur rarely in patients treated with antipsychotics.

Jaundice. In the early days of chlorpromazine treatment, jaundice was not unusual, occurring in about 1 out of every 100 patients treated. Recently, for unexplained reasons, the incidence of chlorpromazine-induced jaundice has dropped considerably. Although accurate data are lacking, the incidence is probably in the range of 1 out of every 1,000 patients treated.

The jaundice occurs most often in the first five weeks of treatment and is generally preceded by a flulike syndrome. It is generally wise to discontinue chlorpromazine if patients have jaundice, although the value of the practice has never been proved. Indeed, patients have continued to receive chlorpromazine throughout the illness without adverse effects. Chlorpromazine-associated jaundice has also recurred in patients as long as 10 years later.

Jaundice has also been reported to occur with promazine (Sparine), thioridazine, mepazine (Pacalal), and prochlorperazine (Compazine) and very rarely with fluphenazine and trifluoperazine. No convincing evidence indicates that haloperidol or many of the other nonphenothiazine antipsychotics can produce jaundice. The majority of the cases reported in the literature are still associated with the use of chlorpromazine.

Overdoses of antipsychotics. With the exception of overdoses from thioridazine and mesoridazine, the outcome of antipsychotic overdose is favorable unless the patient has also ingested other CNS depressants, such as alcohol and benzodiazepines. The symptoms of overdose include drowsiness, which may progress to delirium, coma, dystonias, and seizures. The pupils are mydriatic; deep tendon reflexes are decreased; tachycardia and hypotension are present; and the electroencephalogram (EEG) shows diffuse slowing and low voltage. The piperazine phenothiazines can lead to heart block and ventricular fibrillation, resulting in death.

The treatment should include gastric lavage and activated charcoal followed by catharsis. Convulsions can be treated with IV diazepam (Valium) or phenytoin (Dilantin). Hypotension should be treated with either norepinephrine or dopamine, not epinephrine.

Pregnancy and lactation. If possible, antipsychotics should be avoided during pregnancy, particularly in the first trimester, unless the benefit outweighs the risk. Antipsychotic use in the second and third trimesters is unlikely to cause fetal malformations. Behavioral disturbance in the neonate is possible. High-potency agents are preferable as first-time management in view of the potential hypotension caused by thioridazine and aliphatic phenothiazines and the possible increased risk of fetal malformation with chlorpromazine. Haloperidol and phenothiazines pass into breast milk. It is not known if loxapine, molindone, or pimozide pass into breast milk. There is no clear contraindication to breast feeding in mothers who are taking phenothiazines.

Neurological Adverse Effects

Epileptogenic effects. Antipsychotic administration is associated with a slowing and an increased synchronization of the EEG. That effect may be the mechanism by which some antipsychotics decrease the seizure threshold. Chlorpromazine, loxapine, and other low-potency antipsychotics are thought to be more epileptogenic than are high-potency drugs, especially molindone. The risk of inducing a seizure by drug administration warrants consideration when the patient already has a seizure disorder or an organic brain lesion.

Sedation. Sedation is primarily a result of the blockade of histamine type 1 receptors. Chlorpromazine is the most sedating antipsychotic; thioridazine, chlorprothixene, and loxapine are also very sedating; and the high-potency antipsychotics are much less sedating (Table 19–4). Patients should be warned about driving or operating machinery when first treated with antipsychotics. Giving the entire antipsychotic dose at bedtime usually eliminates any problems from sedation, and tolerance to the adverse effect often develops.

Central anticholinergic effects. The symptoms of central anticholinergic activity include severe agitation; disorientation to time, person, or place; hallucinations; seizures; high fever; and dilated pupils. Stupor and coma may ensue. The treatment consists of discontinuing the causal agent, close medical supervision, and physostigmine (Antilirium, Eserine((2 mg by slow IV infusion, repeated within one hour as necessary). Too much physostigmine is dangerous, and symptoms of physostigmine toxicity include hypersalivation and sweating. Atropine sulfate (0.5 mg) can reverse the effects.

Dystonias. Approximately 10 percent of all patients experience dystonias as an adverse effect of antipsychotics, usually in the first few hours or days of treatment. Dystonic movements result from a slow, sustained muscular contraction or spasm that can result in an involuntary movement. Dystonias can involve the neck (spasmodic torticollis or retrocollis), jaw (forced opening resulting in a dislocation or trismus), tongue (protrusions, twisting), or the entire body (opisthotonos). Involvement of the eyes can result in an oculogyric crisis, characterized by their upward lateral movement. Unlike other dystonias, an oculogyric crisis may also occur late in treatment. Other dystonias include blepharospasm and glossopharyngeal dystonias, resulting in dysarthria, dysphagia, and even cyanosis. Children are particularly likely to evidence opisthotonos, scoliosis, lordosis, and writhing movements. Dystonias can be painful and frightening and often result in later noncompliance.

Dystonias are most common in young men (less than 40 years old) but can occur at any age in either sex. Although they are most common with IM doses of high-potency antipsychotics, dystonias can occur with any antipsychotic but are rare with thioridazine. The mechanism of action is thought to be the dopaminergic hyperactivity in the basal ganglia that occurs when the CNS levels of the anti-

TABLE 19–5
Drug Treatment of Extrapyramidal Disorders

Generic Name	Trade Name	Usual Daily Dosage	Indications
Anticholinergic			
Benztropine	Cogentin, Tenormin	PO 0.5–2 mg tid; IM or IV 1–2 mg	Acute dystonic reaction, parkinsonism, akinesia, akathisia, rabbit syndrome
Biperiden	Akineton	PO 2–6 mg tid; IM or IV 2 mg	
Procyclidine	Kemadrin	PO 2.5–5 mg bid-qid	
Trihexyphenidyl	Artane, Pipanol	PO 2–5 mg tid	
Ethopropazine	Parsidol	PO 50–100 mg bid-qid	
Orphenadrine	Norflex, Dispal	PO 50–100 mg bid-qid; IV 60 mg	
Antihistaminergic			
Diphenhydramine	Benadryl	PO 25 mg qid; IM or IV 25 mg	Acute dystonic reaction, parkinsonism, akinesia, rabbit syndrome
Dopamine agonists			
Amantadine	Symmetrel	PO 100–200 mg bid	Parkinsonism, akinesia, rabbit syndrome
β-Adrenergic antagonists			
Propranolol	Inderal	PO 20–40 mg tid	Akathisia
α-Adrenergic antagonists			
Clonidine	Catapres	PO 0.1 mg tid	Akathisia
Benzodiazepines			
Clonazepam	Klonopin	PO 1 mg bid	Akathisia, acute dystonic reactions
Lorazepam	Ativan	PO 1 mg tid	

psychotic begin to fall. Dystonias can fluctuate spontaneously, responding to reassurance and resulting in the clinician's false impression that the movement is hysterical. The differential diagnosis should include seizures and tardive dyskinesia. Prophylaxis with anticholinergics or related drugs (Table 19-5) usually prevents the development of dystonias. Treatment with IM anticholinergics or IV or IM diphenhydramine (Benadryl) (50 mg) almost always relieves the symptoms. Diazepam (10 mg IV), amobarbital, caffeine sodium benzoate, and hypnosis have also been reported to be effective. Although tolerance to the adverse effect usually develops, it is sometimes prudent to change the antipsychotic if the patient is particularly concerned about the reaction's recurrence.

Parkinsonian effects. Parkinsonian adverse effects occur in approximately 15 percent of patients, usually within 5 to 90 days of the treatment's initiation. Symptoms include muscle stiffness, cogwheel rigidity, shuffling gait, stooped posture, and drooling. The pill-rolling tremor of idiopathic parkinsonism is rare, but a regular, coarse tremor similar to essential tremor may be present. *Rabbit syndrome* is a focal, perioral tremor that resembles the other parkinsonian effects of antipsychotics but can occur late in treatment. The masklike facies, bradykinesia, and akinesia of the parkinsonian syndrome are often misdiagnosed as being part of the negative symptom picture of schizophrenia and are, therefore, not treated.

Women are affected about twice as often as men, and the syndrome can occur at all ages, although most frequently after age 40. All antipsychotics can cause the symptoms, especially high-potency drugs with low anticholinergic activity. Chlorpromazine and thioridazine are less likely to be involved. The blockade of dopaminergic transmission in the nigrostriatal tract is the cause of drug-induced parkinsonism. Because not all patients have the syndrome, those who do seem not to be able to compensate for the presence of antipsychotic blockade in the nigrostriatal tract. The differential diagnosis should also include other causes of idiopathic parkinsonism, other organic causes of parkinsonism, and depression. The syndrome can be treated with anticholinergic agents, amantadine (Symadine, Symmetrel), or diphenhydramine. Although amantadine may have fewer side effects, it may be less effective at reducing muscular rigidity. Levodopa does not work in these cases, and it may exacerbate the psychosis. Anticholinergics should be withdrawn after four to six weeks to assess whether the patient has a tolerance to the parkinsonian efffects; approximately 50 percent of patients need continued treatment. Even after the antipsychotics are withdrawn, parkinsonian symptoms may last for up to two weeks and even up to three months in elderly patients. In such patients it is reasonable to continue the anticholinergic drug after stopping the antipsychotic.

Akathisia. Akathisia is a subjective feeling of muscular discomfort that can cause the patient to be agitated, pace relentlessly, stand and sit continually, and feel dysphoric. The symptoms are primarily motor and cannot be controlled by the patient's will. Akathisia can appear at any time during treatment. It is probably underdiagnosed, because the symptoms are mistakenly attributed to psychosis, agitation, or lack of cooperation. The mechanism underlying akathisia is poorly understood, although it presumably involves dopamine receptor blockade. The antipsychotic dosage should be reduced and treatment with anticholinergics or amantadine attempted, although that approach is often not effective. Propranolol (Inderal) (30 to 120 mg a day), benzodiazepines, and clonidine (Catapres) have been shown to be effective in several research studies (Table 19–5). In some cases of akathisia, no treatment seems to be effective.

Tardive dyskinesia. Tardive dyskinesia is a delayed effect of antipsychotics, rarely occurring until after six months of treatment. The syndrome consists of abnormal, involuntary, irregular, choreoathetoid movements of muscles of the head, limbs, and trunk. The severity of the movements ranges from minimal—often missed by patients and their families—to grossly incapacitating. Perioral movements are the most common and include darting, twisting, and protruding movements of the tongue; chewing and lateral jaw movements; lip puckering; and facial grimacing. Finger movements and hand clenching are also common. Torticollis, retrocollis, trunk twisting, and pelvic thrusting are seen in severe cases. Respiratory dyskinesias have also been reported. Dyskinesias are exacerbated by stress and disappear during sleep. Other tardive or late-occurring syndromes may include tardive dystonias, tardive parkinsonism, and tardive behavioral syndromes, although the last is quite controversial.

All the antipsychotics have been associated with causing tardive dyskinesia, although some evidence indicates that thioridazine is less likely to be involved. The longer patients are taking antipsychotics, the more likely they are to have tardive dyskinesia. Women are more affected than men, and patients over 50 years of age, patients with brain damage, and patients with mood disorders also seem to be at high risk. The incidence increases by approximately 3 to 4 percent a year after four to five years of treatment. Approximately 50 to 60 percent of chronically institutionalized patients have the syndrome. It is an interesting observation that 1 to 5 percent of schizophrenic patients had similar abnormal movements before the introduction of antipsychotics in the early 1950s. Tardive dyskinesia is hypothesized to be caused by dopaminergic receptor supersensitivity in the basal ganglia resulting from chronic blockade of dopamine receptors by antipsychotics. That hypothesis, however, has not been proved.

The three basic approaches to tardive dyskinesia are prevention, diagnosis, and management. Prevention is best achieved by using antipsychotic medications only when clearly indicated and in the lowest effective dosages. Patients receiving antipsychotics should be checked regularly for the appearance of abnormal movements, preferably by using a standardized rating scale (Table 19–6). When abnormal movements are detected, a differential diagnosis should be considered (Table 19–7).

Once a diagnosis of tardive dyskinesia is made, it becomes imperative to complete regular objective ratings of the movement disorder. Although tardive dyskinesia often emerges while the patient is taking a steady dosage of medication, it is even more likely to emerge when the dosage is reduced. Some investigators have called the latter dyskinesias ''withdrawal dyskinesias.'' Once tardive dyskinesia is recognized, consideration should be given to reducing or stopping the antipsychotic if at all possible. Consideration should also be given to treating the patient with clozapine (Chapter 15). Between 5 and 40 percent of all tardive dyskinesias eventually remit, and between 50 and 90 percent of mild cases remit. It is not thought at this time that tardive dyskinesia is a progressive condition.

There is no single effective treatment for tardive dyskinesia. If the movement disorder is severe, an attempt should be made to decrease or stop the antipsychotic. Lithium (Eskalith), carbamazepine (Tegretol), or benzodiazepines may be effective in reducing both the psychotic symptoms and the movement disorder. Various studies have reported that cholinergic agonists and antagonists, dopaminergic agonists, and γ-aminobutyric acid (GABA)-ergic drugs (for example, valproic acid [Depakene]) may be useful.

Neuroleptic malignant syndrome.   Neuroleptic malignant syndrome is a life-threatening complication of antipsychotic treatment, with a variable time of onset during treatment (Table 19–8). Symptoms include muscular rigidity and dystonia, akinesia, mutism, obtundation, and agitation. Autonomic symptoms include hyperpyrexia (up to 107°F), sweating, and increased pulse and blood pressure. Laboratory findings include increased white blood cell count (WBC), blood creatinine phosphokinase, liver enzymes, and myoglobin in plasma resulting in renal shutdown. The symptoms usually evolve over 24 to 72 hours, and the untreated syndrome lasts 10 to 14 days. The diagnosis is often missed in the early stages, and the withdrawal or agitation may be mistakenly considered increased psychosis. Men are affected more frequently than women, and the mortality rate is between 15 and 25 percent. The pathophysiology is unknown, although it may be related to hyperthermic crises that were seen in psychotic patients before the advent of antipsychotic drugs.

The treatment is the immediate discontinuation of antipsychotic drugs, medical support to cool the patient, and the monitoring of vital signs and renal output. Dantrolene (Dantrium), a skeletal muscle relaxant (1 mg per kg PO four times a

TABLE 19–6
Abnormal Involuntary Movement Scale (AIMS) Examination Procedure

Patient Identification		Date
Rated by		

Either before or after completing the examination procedure, observe the patient unobtrusively at rest (e.g., in waiting room).

The chair to be used in this examination should be a hard, firm one without arms.

After observing the patient, rate him or her on a scale of 0 (none), 1 (minimal), 2 (mild), 3 (moderate) and 4 (severe) according to the severity of symptoms.

Ask the patient whether there is anything in his or her mouth (i.e., gum, candy, etc.) and, if so, to remove it.

Ask the patient about the *current* condition of his or her teeth. Ask patient if he or she wears dentures. Do teeth or dentures bother patient *now*.

Ask patient whether he or she notices any movement in mouth, face, hands or feet. If yes, ask patient to describe and indicate to what extent they *currently* bother patient or interfere with his or her activities.

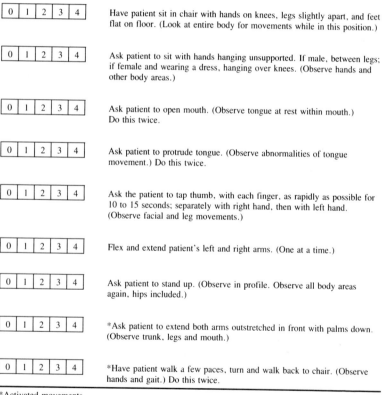

0	1	2	3	4	Have patient sit in chair with hands on knees, legs slightly apart, and feet flat on floor. (Look at entire body for movements while in this position.)
0	1	2	3	4	Ask patient to sit with hands hanging unsupported. If male, between legs; if female and wearing a dress, hanging over knees. (Observe hands and other body areas.)
0	1	2	3	4	Ask patient to open mouth. (Observe tongue at rest within mouth.) Do this twice.
0	1	2	3	4	Ask patient to protrude tongue. (Observe abnormalities of tongue movement.) Do this twice.
0	1	2	3	4	Ask the patient to tap thumb, with each finger, as rapidly as possible for 10 to 15 seconds; separately with right hand, then with left hand. (Observe facial and leg movements.)
0	1	2	3	4	Flex and extend patient's left and right arms. (One at a time.)
0	1	2	3	4	Ask patient to stand up. (Observe in profile. Observe all body areas again, hips included.)
0	1	2	3	4	*Ask patient to extend both arms outstretched in front with palms down. (Observe trunk, legs and mouth.)
0	1	2	3	4	*Have patient walk a few paces, turn and walk back to chair. (Observe hands and gait.) Do this twice.

*Activated movements.

TABLE 19–7
Differential Diagnosis for Tardive Dyskinesialike Movements

Common—Schizophrenic mannerisms and stereotypies
  Dental problems (e.g., ill-fitting dentures)
  Meige's syndrome and other senile dyskinesias

Drug-induced—Antidepressants
  Antihistamines
  Antimalarials
  Antipsychotics
  Diphenylhydantoin
  Heavy metals
  Levodopa
  Sympathomimetics

CNS—Anoxia-induced
  Hepatic failure
  Huntington's chorea
  Parathyroid hypoactivity
  Postencephalitic
  Pregnancy (chorea gravidarum)
  Renal failure
  Sydenham's chorea
  Systemic lupus erythematosus
  Thyroid hyperactivity
  Torsion dystonia
  Tumors
  Wilson's disease

TABLE 19–8
Operational Criteria for Diagnosis of Neuroleptic Malignant Syndrome

The following three items are all required for a definite diagnosis:

1. Hyperthermia: Oral temperature of at least 38.0°C in the absence of another known cause.
2. Severe extrapyramidal effects characterized by two or more of the following: lead-pipe muscle rigidity, pronounced cogwheeling, sialorrhea, oculogyric crisis, retrocollis, opisthotonos, trismus, dysphagia, choreiform movements, festinating gait, and flexor-extensor posturing
3. Autonomic dysfunction characterized by two or more of the following: hypertension (at least 20-mm rise in diastolic pressure above baseline), tachycardia (at least 30 beats/minute), prominent diaphoresis, and incontinence

In retrospective diagnosis, if one of those three items has not been specifically documented, a probable diagnosis is still permitted if the remaining two criteria are clearly met and the patient displays one of the following characteristic signs: clouded consciousness as evidenced by delirium, mutism, stupor, or coma; leukocytosis (more than 15,000 white blood cells/mm); and serum creatinine kinase level greater than 1,000 IU/mL.

Table from A F Schatzberg, J O Cole: *Manual of Clinical Psychopharmacology*, ed 2, p 126. American Psychiatric Press, Washington, 1991. Used with permission.

day, 1 to 5 mg per kg IV) may reduce the muscle spasms, and bromocriptine (Parlodel) (Chapter 8) has also been reported to be of some benefit in treating neuroleptic malignant syndrome.

Prevention and treatment of some neurological adverse effects. A variety of drugs (Table 19–5) may be used to prevent and treat extrapyramidal adverse effects caused by antipsychotics. The drugs include anticholinergics (Chapter 4), amantadine (Chapter 3), antihistamines (Chapter 5), benzodiazepines (Chapter 7), β-adrenergic receptor antagonists (Chapter 2), and clonidine (Chapter 14). Most acute dystonias and parkinsonlike symptoms are effectively treated by those drugs, and akathisia may also respond in some cases. It is not known whether prophylactic treatment with the drugs is warranted when starting to give a patient an antipsychotic. The proponents of prophylactic treatment argue that the increased likelihood of avoiding adverse neurological effects is more humane to the patient and increases the possibility of future compliance. The opponents of the practice argue that the increased likelihood of anticholinergic adverse effects from the drugs offsets any possible gain. A reasonable compromise is to give the drugs to patients under age 45 who are more at risk of neurological adverse effects and not to use the drugs prophylactically in patients over 45 who are at increased risk for anticholinergic toxicity. If a patient does have dystonias, parkinsonlike symptoms, or akathisia, a trial of the drugs is warranted.

Once a patient has started taking the drugs, he or she should be treated for four to six weeks. Then the clinician should attempt to taper and stop the medication over one month. Many patients become tolerant to the neurological adverse effects and no longer require the drug. Some patients experience the return of neurological symptoms and have to start taking the drugs again. Other patients state that they feel less anxious or depressed while taking the medications, so it may be reasonable to give the medications again, even in the absence of neurological symptoms.

Most clinicians use one of the anticholinergic drugs or diphenhydramine to provide prophylaxis or treatment for neurological adverse effects. Of those drugs, diphenhydramine is the most sedating; biperiden (Akineton) is neutral; and trihexyphenidyl (Artane, Pipanol) may be slightly stimulating. In fact, trihexyphenidyl, benztropine (Cogentin, Tremin), and diphenhydramine can be abused, as some patients report obtaining a euphoria from those drugs. Amantadine is most often used when one of the anticholinergic drugs does not work. Although amantadine does not typically exacerbate the psychosis of schizophrenia, some patients become tolerant of its antiparkinsonian effects. Amantadine is also a sedating drug in some patients.

DRUG-DRUG INTERACTIONS

Antacids

Antacids and cimetidine (Tagamet), administered in intervals of one to two hours of antipsychotic administration, reduce the absorption of antipsychotic drugs.

Anticholinergics

Anticholinergics may decrease the absorption of antipsychotics. The additive anticholinergic activity of antipsychotics, anticholinergics, and tricyclic antidepressants may result in anticholinergic toxicity.

Anticonvulsants

Phenothiazines, especially thioridazine, may decrease the metabolism of diphenylhydantoin, resulting in toxic levels of the latter. Barbiturates may increase the metabolism of antipsychotics, and antipsychotics may lower the seizure threshold.

Antidepressants

Tricyclic antidepressants and antipsychotics may decrease each other's metabolism, resulting in increased plasma concentrations of both. The anticholinergic, sedative, and hypotensive effects of the drugs may also be additive.

Antihypertensives

Antipsychotics may inhibit the uptake of guanethidine (Esimil, Ismelin) into the synapse and may also inhibit the hypotensive effects of clonidine and α-methyldopa (Aldomet). Conversely, antipsychotics may have an additive effect on some hypotensives. Antipsychotics have a variable effect on clonidine.

CNS Depressants

Antipsychotics potentiate the CNS depressant effects of sedatives, antihistamines, opiates, and alcohol, particularly in patients with an impaired respiratory status. When those agents are taken with alcohol, the risk of heat stroke may be increased.

Other Drugs

Cigarette smoking may decrease the plasma levels of antipsychotic drugs. Epinephrine has a paradoxical hypotensive effect in patients taking antipsychotics. The coadministration of lithium and antipsychotics may result in symptoms similar to those of lithium intoxication and neuroleptic malignant syndrome. There is no reason to believe that those two syndromes are more common with coadministration than when the agents are administered alone; the interaction is no more common with one antipsychotic than with another. Propranolol coadministration with antipsychotics increases the blood concentrations of both. Antipsychotics decrease the blood concentration of warfarin (Coumadin), resulting in decreased bleeding time. Phenothiazines and pimozide should not be coadministered with other agents that prolong the QT interval. Table 19–9 gives a summary of important drug-drug interactions.

RESERPINE

Although it is not a dopamine receptor antagonist, reserpine (Serpalan, Serpasil) does have antipsychotic effects. It is an indole alkaloid obtained from the root of *Rauwolfia serpentina*; it produces its antipsychotic effect by depleting the presynaptic stores of serotonin and catecholamines, rather than by the blockade of postsynaptic receptors. Reserpine is most commonly used as a hypotensive agent; it is rarely used as an antipsychotic. Its use is associated with the adverse side effect of depression, with significant suicide risk.

TABLE 19–9
Important Drug Interactions with Dopamine Receptor Antagonist Medications*

Agent	Possible Effect
Anesthetics	Potentiate hypotension
Antacid	Decrease absorption of antipsychotic
Anticholinergics	Decrease absorption
Anticoagulants	Increase bleeding time
Anticonvulsants	Increase anticonvulsant levels, effect on seizures variable; decrease antipsychotic levels
Antidepressants	Increase tricyclic and antipsychotic levels, additive hypotension effects
Antihypertensives	Generally potentiate hypotension
β-Blockers (propranolol)	Potentiate hypotension
Clonidine	Variable
Diuretics and smooth-muscle blockers	May potentiate hypotension
Guanethidine	Antagonizes antihypertensive effect
α-Methyldopa	May potentiate hypotension; ? organic brain syndrome with haloperidol
Barbiturates	
Long-term use	Decrease antipsychotic level
Short-term use	Increase CNS depressant effect
Carbamazepine	Decreases plasma levels of haloperidol and possibly all antipsychotics
Digitalis	Thioridazine may nullify inotropic effect
Estrogens	May increase antipsychotic blood level
Levodopa	Mutual antagonism
Lithium	Possible toxic synergism, ? decreased chlorpromazine levels
Narcotics	Potentiate analgesia, increased respiratory depression
Oral hypoglycemics	Variable
Pressor agents	
α-Agonists (norepinephrine)	Antagonize pressor effect
β-Agonists (isoproterenol)	Marked hypotension
Quinidine	May potentiate cardiac effect
Sedative-hypnotics	Additive CNS depressant effects

*Adapted from R B Lydiard, J S Carman, M S Gold: Antipsychotics: Predicting effect/maximizing efficacy. In *Advances in Psychopharmacology: Predicting and Improving Treatment Response*, M S Gold, R B Lydiard, J S Carman, editors. CRC Press, Boca Raton, Fla., 1964.
Table adapted from A Beebee, G Bartzokis: Neuroleptic antipsychotic medications. In *The Handbook of Psychiatry*, Residents of the UCLA Department of Psychiatry, p 366. Year Book Medical Publishers, Chicago, 1990. Used with permission.

References

Baldessarini R J, Cohen B M, Teicher M H: Significance of neuroleptic plasma level in the pharmacological treatment of psychoses. Arch Gen Psychiatry 45: 79, 1988.

Boyer P, Lecrubier Y, Puech A J: Treatment of positive and negative symptoms: Pharmacologic approaches. Mod Probl Pharmacopsychiatry 24: 152, 1990.

Chang W-H: Reduced haloperidol: A factor in determining the therapeutic benefit of haloperidol treatment? Psychopharmacology, 106: 289, 1992.

Davis J M, Barter J T, Kane J M: Antipsychotic drugs. In *Comprehensive Textbook of Psychiatry*, ed 5, H I Kaplan, B J Sadock, editors, p 1591. Williams & Wilkins, Baltimore, 1989.

Dixon L, Weiden P J, Frances A J, Rapkin B: Management of neuroleptic-induced movement disorders: Effects of physician training. Am J Psychiatry 146: 104, 1989.

Feinberg S S, Kay S R, Elijovich L R, Fiszbein A, Opler L A: Pimozide treatment of the negative schizophrenic syndrome: An open trial. J Clin Psychiatry 49: 235, 1988.

Jann M W, Lam Y W, Chang W H: Reversible metabolism of haloperidol and reduced haloperidol in Chinese schizophrenic patients. Psychopharmacology 101: 107, 1990.

Kane J M: The current status of neuroleptic therapy. J Clin Psychiatry 50: 322, 1989.

Keck P E, Cohen B M, Baldessarini R J, McElroy S L: Time course of antipsychotic effects of neuroleptic drugs. Am J Psychiatry 146: 1289, 1989.

Keck P E, Pope H G, Cohen B M, McElroy S L, Nierenberg A A: Risk factors for neuroleptic malignant syndrome: A case-control study. Arch Gen Psychiatry *46*: 914, 1989.

Kellam A M P: The neuroleptic malignant syndrome, so-called: A survey of world literature. Br J Psychiatry *150*: 752, 1987.

Miller L G, Jankovic J: Neurologic approach to drug-induced movement disorders: A study of 125 patients. South Med J *83*: 525, 1990.

Ochitill H, Dilley J, Kohlwes J: Psychotropic drug prescribing for hospitalized patients with acquired immunodeficiency syndrome. Am J Med *90*: 601, 1991.

Owen R R, Cole J O: Molindone hydrochloride: A review of laboratory and clinical findings. J Clin Psychopharmacol *9*: 268, 1989.

Rearson G T, Rifkin A, Schwartz A, Myerson A, Siris S G: Changing patterns of neuroleptic dosage over a decade. Am J Psychiatry *146*: 726, 1989.

Richelson E: Psychopharmacology of classical and atypical antipsychotics. Yakubutsu Seishin Koda *11*: 71, 1991.

Rosebush P, Steward T: A prospective analysis of 24 episodes of neuroleptic malignant syndrome. Am J Psychiatry *146*: 717, 1989.

Schneider I S, Pollock V E, Lyness S A: A metaanalysis of controlled trials of neuroleptic treatment in dementia. J Am Geriatr Soc *38*: 553, 1990.

Williams R, Dalby J T, Kennedy J: Long term use of neuroleptics by schizophrenic patients. Prog Neuropsychopharmacol Biol Psychiatry *15*: 221, 1991.

Yadalam K G, Simpson G M: Changing from oral to depot fluphenazine. J Clin Psychiatry *49*: 346, 1988.

20

Fenfluramine

In psychiatry fenfluramine (Pondimin), a sympathomimetic amine (an amphetamine cogener), has been studied and used as a treatment for autism. Because of its anorectic effect, it has also been used for obesity. The pharmacological activity of fenfluramine differs from that of the amphetamines in that fenfluramine produces more central nervous system (CNS) depression than stimulation. The molecular structure of fenfluramine is given in Figure 20–1.

PHARMACOLOGICAL ACTIONS

Fenfluramine may alter the brain levels or the turnover rates of serotonin. It is a serotonin releaser. Fenfluramine may stimulate the ventromedial nucleus of the hypothalamus, thus inhibiting appetite. Fenfluramine is well absorbed from the gastrointestinal (GI) tract. Maximal anorectic effect is seen after two to four hours. The half-life of fenfluramine is about 20 hours. Fenfluramine is lipid-soluble and crosses the placenta.

INDICATIONS

Fenfluramine has been well studied in autistic disorder. Overall, it has been ineffective, but some patients have shown improvement. It may be most useful in autistic children with significant agitation and an intelligence quotient (I.Q.) over 40.

CLINICAL GUIDELINES

In autism the dosage should be increased gradually to 1.0 to 1.5 mg per kg a day in divided doses. Fenfluramine's therapeutic effects include improved sleep pattern and relatedness, with decreased aggression, tantrums, irritability, self-mutilation, and hyperactivity. Fenfluramine is supplied as 20 mg tablets.

ADVERSE EFFECTS

Drowsiness, diarrhea, and dry mouth are the most common adverse effects of fenfluramine. Other adverse effects include dizziness, confusion, incoordination, headache, elevated mood, depressed mood, anxiety, nervousness or tension, insomnia, weakness or fatigue, agitation, dysarthria, and altered libido. Fenfluramine has not been studied in pregnant women. It is not known whether fenfluramine passes into breast milk.

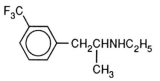

Figure 20–1. Molecular structure of fenfluramine.

DRUG-DRUG INTERACTIONS

Patients should be advised to avoid alcoholic beverages during fenfluramine therapy. There may be additive effects when fenfluramine is used with CNS depressants. Fenfluramine may increase the effect of some antihypertensives.

References

du Verglas G, Banks S R, Guyer K E: Clinical effects of fenfluramine on children with autism: A review of the research. Ann Prog Child Psychiatry Child Dev *22*: 471, 1989.

Ekman G, Miranda-Linne F, Gillberg C, Garle M: Fenfluramine treatment of twenty children with autism. J Autism Dev Disord *19*: 511, 1989.

Lichtenberg P, Shapira B, Blacker M, Gropp C, Calev A, Larer B: Effect of fenfluramine on mood: A double-blind placebo-controlled trial. Biol Psychiatry *31*: 351, 1992.

Sherman J, Factor D C, Swinson R, Darjes R W: The effects of fenfluramine (hydrochloride) on the behaviors of fifteen autistic children. J Autism Dev Disord *19*: 533, 1989.

Stern L M, Walker M K, Sawyer M G, Oades R D: A controlled crossover trial of fenfluramine in autism. J Child Psychol Psychiatry *31*: 569, 1990.

Varley C K, Holm V A: A two-year follow-up of autistic children treated with fenfluramine. J Am Acad Child Adolesc Psychiatry *29*: 137, 1990.

21

Flumazenil

Flumazenil (Mazicon) is a benzodiazepine receptor antagonist. It reverses the psychophysiological action of the benzodiazepine class of drugs. It is for emergency room use only.

PHARMACOLOGICAL ACTIONS

Flumazenil competitively inhibits the activity at the benzodiazepine recognition site (omega receptor) on the γ-aminobutyric acid (GABA)-benzodiazepine receptor complex. Its molecular structure is given in Figure 21–1.

Pharmacokinetics

After intravenous (IV) administration, plasma concentrations of flumazenil have a half-life of 7 to 15 minutes and a terminal half-life of 41 to 79 minutes. Peak concentration of flumazenil is proportional to dosage. Protein binding is approximately 50 percent, and the drug shows no preferential partitioning into red blood cells. Clearance of flumazenil occurs primarily by hepatic metabolism and depends on hepatic blood flow. The major metabolites of flumazenil identified in the urine are the de-ethylated free acid and its glucuronide conjugate. Elimination of the drug is essentially complete within 72 hours. The pharmacokinetics of flumazenil are not significantly affected by gender, age, renal failure, or hemodialysis but are affected by liver dysfunction, which prolongs the half-life.

Pharmacodynamics

Intravenous flumazenil antagonizes sedation, impairment of recall, and psychomotor impairment produced by benzodiazepines. Flumazenil does not antagonize the central nervous system (CNS) effects of drugs affecting GABA-ergic neurons by means other than the benzodiazepine (omega) receptor. The drugs include ethanol, barbiturates, and general anesthetics. Flumazenil does not reverse the effects of opioids.

INDICATIONS

Flumazenil is used to reverse the effects of benzodiazepines in conscious sedation, general anesthesia, and the management of benzodiazepine overdose. It has also been reported to be useful in the reduction of benzodiazepine withdrawal symptoms during benzodiazepine discontinuation.

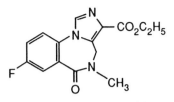

Figure 21–1. Molecular structure of flumazenil.

CLINICAL GUIDELINES

Benzodiazepine Overdose

For initial management of a known or suspected benzodiazepine overdose, the recommended initial dose of flumazenil is 0.2 mg (2 mL) administered intravenously over 30 seconds. If the desired level of consciousness is not obtained after waiting 30 seconds, a further dose of 0.3 mg (3 mL) can be administered over 30 seconds. Further doses of 0.5 (5 mL) can be administered over 30 seconds at one-minute intervals up to a cumulative dose of 3.0 mg. The clinician should not rush the administration of flumazenil. A secure airway and intravenous access should be established before administration of the drug. Patients should be awakened gradually.

Most patients with benzodiazepine overdose respond to a cumulative dose of 1 to 3 mg of flumazenil; doses beyond 3 mg do not reliably produce additional effects. If a patient has not responded five minutes after receiving a cumulative dose of 5 mg flumazenil, the major cause of sedation is probably not due to benzodiazepines, and additional flumazenil is likely to have no effect.

Return of Sedation

The clinician must be aware that resedation can occur in 1 to 3 percent of patients. Resedation can be treated by giving repeated doses at 20-minute intervals. For repeat treatment, no more than 1.0 mg (given as 0.5 mg per minute) should be given at any one time, and no more than 3.0 mg should be given in any one hour. Serious side effects may occur in the form of seizures in those patients who took overdoses of cyclic antidepressants. In those cases it is assumed that the benzodiazepines were protective against tricyclic-induced seizures and arrhthymias. Fatalities may occur in such situations.

ADVERSE EFFECTS

The most common effects of flumazenil are nausea, vomiting, dizziness, agitation, emotional lability, cutaneous vasodilation, injection-site pain, injection-site reaction, fatigue, abnormal vision, and headache.

DRUG-DRUG INTERACTIONS

No deleterious interactions have been noted when flumazenil is administered after narcotics, inhalation anesthetics, muscle relaxants, and muscle relaxant antagonists administered in conjunction with sedation or anesthesia. In cases of mixed-drug overdose, the toxic effects (such as convulsions and cardiac dysrhythmias) of other drugs taken in overdose (especially cyclic antidepressants) may emerge with flumazenil's reversal of the benzodiazepine effect.

References

Curran H V, Birch B: Differentiating the sedative, psychomotor and amnesic effects of benzodiazepines: A study with midazolam and the benzodiazepine antagonist flumazenil. Psychopharmacology *103*: 519, 1991.

Lader M, Morton S: Benzodiazepine withdrawal syndrome. Br J Psychiatry *158*: 435, 1991.

Nutt D J, Glue P, Lawson C, Wilson S: Flumazenil provocation of panic attacks: Evidence for altered benzodiazepine receptor sensitivity in panic disorder. Arch Gen Psychiatry *47*: 917, 1990.

Woods S W, Charney D S, Silver J M, Krystal J H: Behavioral, biochemical, and cardiovascular responses to the benzodiazepine receptor antagonist flumazenil in panic disorder. Psychiatry Res *36*: 115, 1991.

22

Lithium

Lithium (Eskalith, Lithobid) is an element and is the lightest of the alkali metals (group IA of the periodic table), similar to sodium, potassium, magnesium, and calcium. Lithium is a monovalent ion and is available as a carbonate (Lithane) (Li_2CO_3) for oral use in both rapidly acting and slow-release tablets and capsules. Lithium citrate (Cibalith) is available in a liquid form of oral administration.

PHARMACOLOGICAL ACTIONS

Pharmacokinetics

After ingestion, lithium is completely absorbed by the gastrointestinal tract. Serum levels peak in 0.5 to 2 hours for standard preparations and in 4 to 4.5 hours for the slow-release preparations. Lithium does not bind to plasma proteins and is distributed nonuniformly throughout body water. The half-life of lithium is about 20 hours, and equilibrium is reached after five to seven days of regular intake. Lithium is almost entirely eliminated by the kidneys. Renal clearance of lithium is decreased with renal insufficiency and in the puerperium and is increased during pregnancy. Lithium is excreted in breast milk and in insignificant amounts in feces and sweat.

Pharmacodynamics

The therapeutic mechanism of action for lithium remains uncertain. The most accepted current theory is that lithium works by blocking the enzyme inositol-1-phosphatase within neurons. That inhibition results in decreased cellular responses to neurotransmitters that are linked to the phosphatidylinositol second-messenger system.

INDICATIONS

Bipolar Disorder

Lithium has been proved effective in both the short-term treatment and the prophylaxis of bipolar disorder in approximately 70 to 80 percent of patients. Both manic and depressive episodes often respond to lithium treatment alone. However, because treatment with lithium alone can take a relatively long time, manic episodes are usually treated with both lithium and an antipsychotic, and depressive episodes are treated with a combination of lithium and an antidepressant. The clinician should be aware of the risk of inducing a manic episode or rapid cycling with antidepressant treatment. Most studies have reported that lithium maintenance halves the number of recurrences and that the recurrences that do occur are less severe. The prophylactic effect of lithium, however, does not develop for several months. Consequently, a recurrence of symptoms before that time should not be taken as an indication that the lithium is not effective. In severe cases of cyclothymia, treatment with lithium may be indicated.

Schizoaffective Disorder

The use of lithium for schizoaffective disorder (bipolar type) is certainly indicated. If a patient's schizoaffective disorder (depressive type) demonstrates a particularly cyclic nature, a lithium trial may also be warranted.

Major Depression

The chief indication for lithium in depression is as an adjuvant treatment to tricyclics, tetracyclics, or monoamine oxidase inhibitors (MAOIs) to convert an antidepressant nonresponder into a responder. Lithium alone may also be an effective treatment for depressed patients who are actually bipolar disorder patients who have not yet had their first manic episode. Moreover, lithium has been reported to be effective in major depression patients whose illness has a marked cyclicity.

Schizophrenia

The symptoms of approximately one fifth to one half of schizophrenic patients are further reduced when lithium is coadministered with their antipsychotic drug. Some schizophrenic patients who cannot take antipsychotics may benefit from lithium treatment. Intermittent angry outbursts in schizophrenic patients may also be reduced by lithium.

Impulse Control Disorders

The impulse control disorders include episodic violence and rage. Patients whose episodes are not premeditated and are seemingly untriggered may respond to lithium. Episodic angry outbursts in patients with mental retardation may also be reduced with lithium.

Other Disorders

A few studies have reported that the episodic disorder characterizing the premenstrual syndrome, the intermittent behaviors seen in borderline personality disorder, bulimia nervosa, and episodes of binge drinking respond to lithium treatment. Lithium may be useful in treating aggressive or self-injurious behavior in children with conduct disorder, pervasive developmental disorders, and mental retardation.

CLINICAL GUIDELINES

Lithium is the drug of first choice to treat bipolar disorder unless there is a specific reason not to use lithium or a specific reason to use another drug.

Initial Medical Workup

Before starting to administer lithium, the clinician should conduct a routine laboratory and physical examination. The laboratory examination should include a serum creatinine level (or a 24-hour urine creatinine if there is any reason to be concerned about renal function), an electrolyte screen, thyroid function tests (T_4, T_3RU, FT_4I, and thyroid-stimulating hormone [TSH]), complete blood count (CBC), electrocardiogram (ECG), and a pregnancy test if there is any risk of the patient's being pregnant.

Dosage

A variety of lithium preparations are available (Table 22–1). Regular-release capsules or tablets are usually used first, and the syrup or slow-release preparations are used if noncompliance or nausea occurs. If a patient has previously been treated with lithium and the former dosage is known, it is reasonable to use that dosage in the current episode unless there have been changes in the patient's pharmaco-kinetic parameters for lithium clearance. For most adult patients, it is reasonable to start lithium at 300 mg three times daily. The starting dosage in patients who are elderly or who have renal impairment should be 300 mg once or twice daily. The usual eventual dosage range is between 900 and 2,100 mg a day. Serum concentrations of lithium can be obtained after five days, and the dosage can be adjusted to obtain a serum level between 0.8 and 1.2 mEq per L during the acute episode. Lithium levels should be obtained 12 hours after the last dose. Lithium levels in patients treated with slow-release preparations are approximately 30 percent higher than the levels obtained with other preparations. The use of divided doses (three to four doses a day) reduces gastric upset and avoids a single large peak in lithium levels. There is currently a debate over whether multiple small daily peaks are less likely than a single large daily peak to cause adverse effects. Single daily dosing, however, is not considered standard practice at this time. Slow-release lithium preparations can be given two to three times daily and result in lower peak levels of lithium, but that procedure has not yet been demonstrated to be of special value. A therapeutic trial of lithium should last a minimum of four to six weeks. If there is some response within that time, improvement may continue for another five months. If the lithium treatment has been successful, it should be

TABLE 22–1
Lithium Carbonate Preparations

Regular-release capsules 150, 300, 600 mg (Eskalith, Lithonate, generic)
Regular-release tablets 300 mg (Eskalith, Lithane, Lithotabs)
Slow-release tablets 300, 450 mg (Eskalith, Lithobid)
Syrup 8 mEq per 5 mL (lithium citrate) (Cibalith-S, generic)

continued for a minimum of six to nine months, then tapered over a month unless the patient is to receive maintenance on lithium prophylaxis.

Lithium Levels

The patient's lithium level should be monitored weekly for the first month and then biweekly for another two months. After six months it may be appropriate to check the patient's lithium level every two months. If a patient has been stable for a year, checking lithium levels three or four times a year may be sufficient.

Patient Education

The patient should be advised that changes in the body's water and salt content can affect the amount of lithium excreted, resulting in either increases or decreases in lithium levels. Excessive intake of sodium (for example, a dramatic dietary change) lowers lithium levels. Conversely, too little sodium (for example, fad diets) can lead to potentially toxic levels of lithium. Decreases in body fluid (for example, excessive sweating) can lead to dehydration and lithium intoxication.

Failure of Drug Treatment

If the drug produces no clinical response after four weeks at therapeutic levels, slightly higher serum levels (up to 1.4 mEq per L) may be tried if there are no severe adverse effects. If after two weeks at a higher serum concentration the drug is still ineffective, the patient should be tapered off the drug over one to two weeks. Other drugs should be given therapeutic trials at that point. Rapid cycling not adequately controlled by lithium may respond to the addition of T_4, 25 to 50 μg a day. The substitution or the addition of carbamazepine or valproic acid may also be useful.

Maintenance

The decision to maintain a patient on lithium prophylaxis is based on the severity of the patient's illness, the risk of adverse effects from lithium, and the quality of the patient's support systems. Maintenance serum levels of lithium can be lower than those needed for short-term treatment. Such levels are usually kept between 0.6 and 0.8 mEq per L, although some researchers have reported successful prophylaxis with serum levels as low as 0.4 mEq per L. In addition to periodic measurements of lithium levels, serum creatinine and TSH levels should be monitored every three to six months.

ADVERSE EFFECTS

The most common adverse effects from lithium treatment are gastric distress, weight gain, tremor, fatigue, and mild cognitive impairment (Table 22–2). Gastric

TABLE 22-2
Side Effects of Lithium and Their Management*

Side Effect	Management
Gastrointestinal complaints	Give lithium after meals, give smaller doses more often, try slow-release preparation, lower the dosage
Tremor	Lower the dosage, give propranolol (40–100 mg/day), consider adding a benzodiazepine
Polyuria-diabetes insipidus	Try slow-release preparation, lower the dosage, add amiloride (5–10 mg/day), careful monitoring of lithium levels
Acne	Benzoyl peroxide (5–10%) topical solution, erythromycin (1.5–2%) topical solution
Muscular weakness, fasciculations, headaches	Usually resolve with first few weeks of treatment
Hypothyroidism	Levothyroxine (0.05 mg qd), follow TSH level and increase to 0.2 mg qd as needed
T wave inversion	Benign, no treatment needed
Cardiac dysrhythmias	Usually must discontinue lithium
Psoriasis, alopecia areata	Dermatology consult, reversible if lithium stopped
Weight gain	Difficult to treat, diet, may be partially reversible if lithium stopped
Edema	Consider spironolactone (50 mg PO qd); if severe, monitor lithium levels; resolves when lithium stopped
Leukocytosis	Benign, no treatment needed

*qd = every day.
Table from A Doupe, M Szuba: Lithium and other antimanic agents. In *The Handbook of Psychiatry*, Residents of the UCLA Department of Psychiatry, p 386. Year Book Medical Publishers, Chicago, 1990. Used with permission.

distress may include nausea, vomiting, and diarrhea and can often be reduced by further dividing up the dosage, administering the lithium with food, or switching among the various lithium preparations. Weight gain and edema can be impossible to treat other than by encouraging the patient to eat less and to exercise moderately. The tremor affects mostly the fingers and sometimes can be worse at peak levels of the drug. It can be reduced by further dividing the dosage. Propranolol (Inderal) (30 to 160 mg a day in divided doses) reduces the tremor significantly in most patients. The fatigue and mild cognitive impairment may decrease with time. Rare neurological adverse effects include symptoms of mild parkinsonism, ataxia, and dysarthria. Patients with organic brain impairment are at risk of neurotoxicity. Lithium may exacerbate Parkinson's disease. Lithium should be used with caution in diabetic patients, as it may induce seizures or exacerbate a seizure disorder. Dehydrated, debilitated, and medically ill patients are susceptible to side effects and toxicity. Leukocytosis is a common benign effect of lithium treatment.

Renal Effects

The most common adverse renal effect of lithium is polyuria with secondary polydipsia. The symptom is particularly a problem in 20 to 25 percent of treated patients. The polyuria is secondary to the decreased resorption of fluid from the distal tubules of the kidneys. When polyuria is a significant problem, the patient's renal function should be carefully evaluated and followed with 24-hour urine collections for creatinine clearance and with consultation with a nephrologist.

Lithium-induced nephrogenic diabetes insipidus is not responsive to vasopressin treatment and results in urine volumes up to 8 L a day and difficulty in maintaining adequate lithium levels. The syndrome can be treated with chlorothiazide 500 mg a day, hydrochlorothiazide (Aldoril) (50 mg a day), or amiloride (5 to 10 mg a day). The lithium dosage should be halved and the diuretic not started for five days, because the diuretic is likely to increase the retention of lithium.

The most serious renal adverse effects that were originally thought to be associated with lithium administration were minimal change glomerulopathy, interstitial nephritis, and renal failure. The original concern about those adverse effects was based on postmortem studies of kidneys from patients who had been treated with lithium. Although it is now generally thought that serious renal disorders are not associated with lithium administration, the clinician should vigorously explore any clinical changes in renal function.

Thyroid Effects

Lithium also affects thyroid function, causing a generally benign and often transient diminution in the concentrations of circulating thyroid hormones. Reports have also attributed goiter (5 percent), benign reversible exophthalmos, and hypothyroidism (3 to 4 percent) to lithium treatment. About 50 percent of patients receiving long-term lithium treatment have an abnormal thyrotropin-releasing hormone (TRH) response, and approximately 30 percent have elevated levels of TSH. If laboratory values of thyroid hormone indicate dysfunction, thyroid supplementation can be administered safely. TSH levels should be measured and checked periodically. Lithium-induced hypothyroidism should be considered when evaluating depressive episodes that emerge during lithium therapy. Hyperthyroidism has been reported rarely.

Cardiac Effects

The cardiac effects of lithium, which resemble those of hypokalemia on the ECG, are caused by displacement of intracellular potassium by the lithium ion. The most common changes on the ECG are T wave flattening or inversion. The changes are benign and disappear after the lithium is excreted from the body. Nevertheless, baseline ECGs are essential and should be repeated yearly.

Because lithium depresses the sinus node's pacemaking activity, lithium treatment is strongly contraindicated in patients with sick sinus syndrome. In rare cases, ventricular arrhythmias and congestive heart failure have been associated with lithium therapy.

Dermatological Effects

Several cutaneous adverse effects, which may be dose-dependent, have been associated with lithium treatment. The most prevalent effects include acneiform, follicular, and maculopapular eruptions; pretibial ulcerations; and worsening of psoriasis. Alopecia has also been reported. Many of those conditions respond to changing to another lithium preparation or the usual dermatological measures. Lithium levels should be monitored if tetracycline is used because of several reports of its increasing the retention of lithium. Occasionally, the aggravated psoriasis or acneiform eruptions may force the discontinuation of lithium treatment.

Use in Pregnancy

Lithium should not be administered to pregnant women in the first trimester because of the increased incidence of birth defects, specifically Ebstein's anomaly, which occurs in 3 percent of babies exposed to lithium in utero. Administration of lithium to the mother during the final months of pregnancy can result in babies who are lithium-toxic at birth. The syndrome consists of lethargy, cyanosis, ab-

TABLE 22–3
Signs and Symptoms of Lithium Toxicity

Mild to moderate intoxication
(lithium level, 1.5–2.0 mEq per L)

Gastrointestinal:
  Vomiting
  Abdominal pain
  Dryness of mouth
Neurological:
  Ataxia
  Dizziness
  Slurred speech
  Nystagmus
  Lethargy or excitement
  Muscle weakness

Moderate to severe intoxication
(lithium level, 2.0–2.5 mEq per L)

Gastrointestinal:
  Anorexia nervosa
  Persistent nausea and vomiting
Neurological:
  Blurred vision
  Muscle fasciculations
  Clonic limb movements
  Hyperactive deep tendon reflexes
  Choreoathetoid movements
  Convulsions
  Delirium
  Syncope
  Electroencephalographic changes
  Stupor
  Coma
Circulatory failure (lowered blood pressure, cardiac arrhythmias, and conduction abnormalities)

Severe intoxication
(lithium level, > 2.5 mEq per L)

Generalized convulsions
Oliguria and renal failure
Death

Table from Psychopharmacology and electroconvulsive therapy. In *The American Psychiatric Press Textbook of Psychiatry*, J A Talbott, R E Hales, S C Yudofsky, editors, p 826. American Psychiatric Association Press, Washington, 1988. Used with permission.

normal reflexes, and sometimes hepatomegaly. Lithium is excreted in breast milk and should not be used while a woman is breast-feeding.

Lithium Toxicity

The symptoms of lithium toxicity are severe manifestations of the aforementioned pharmacodynamic organ interactions (Table 22–3): vomiting, abdominal pain, profuse diarrhea, severe tremor, ataxia, coma, and seizures. Initial neurological signs of mental confusion, hyperreflexia, focal neurological signs, and dysarthria can proceed to coma and death. Cardiac arrhythmias may also occur. Lithium toxicity requires immediate medical attention (Table 22–4).

Overdoses

Overdoses of lithium result in symptoms of severe lithium toxicity. Treatment should include lavage with a wide-bore tube because of the drug's clumping in the stomach. Activated charcoal does not help in this condition. Osmotic diuresis, intravenous sodium bicarbonate, and peritoneal or hemodialysis can also be used.

DRUG-DRUG INTERACTIONS

Most diuretics (for example, thiazides, potassium-sparing, and loop) and prostaglandin synthetase inhibitors (for example, indomethacin [Indocin]) can increase lithium levels to toxic levels. Osmotic diuretics, carbonic anhydrase inhibitors, and xanthines (including caffeine) may reduce lithium levels to below therapeutic levels.

When coadministered, antipsychotics and lithium may result in a synergistic increase in the symptoms of lithium-induced neurological adverse effects. The interaction is not, as initially thought, specifically associated with the coadmin-

TABLE 22–4
Management of Lithium Toxicity

1. The patient should immediately contact his or her personal physician or go to a hospital emergency room.
2. Lithium should be discontinued, and the patient should be instructed to ingest fluids, if possible.
3. Physical examination, including vital signs, and a neurological examination with complete formal mental status examination should be completed.
4. Lithium level, serum electrolytes, renal function tests, and electrocardiogram should be obtained as soon as possible.
5. For significant acute ingestions, residual gastric contents should be removed by induction of emesis, gastric lavage, and absorption with activated charcoal.
6. Vigorous hydration and maintenance of electrolyte balance is essential.
7. For any patient with a serum lithium level greater than 4.0 mEq per L within six hours of ingestion or for any patient with serious manifestations of lithium toxicity, hemodialysis should be initiated.
8. Repeat dialysis may be required every 6 to 10 hours until the lithium level is within nontoxic range and the patient has no signs or symptoms of lithium toxicity.

Table from Psychopharmacology and electroconvulsive therapy. In *The American Psychiatric Press Textbook of Psychiatry*, J A Talbott, R E Hales, S C Yudofsky, editors, p 827. American Psychiatric Association Press, Washington, 1988. Used with permission.

istration of lithium and haloperidol (Haldol). The coadministration of lithium with anticonvulsants, including carbamazepine (Tegretol), may also aggravate neurological symptoms. Although it is reasonable to stop drug administration if serious symptoms of toxicity are noted, it is usually possible to restart both medications at lower dosages without the recurrence of the adverse effects. Delirium may occur if electroconvulsive therapy (ECT) and lithium are coadministered. Therefore, lithium should be discontinued two days before beginning ECT.

A summary of drug interactions with lithium is given in Table 22–5, and the effects of lithium on laboratory values is given in Table 22–6.

TABLE 22–5
Drug Interactions with Lithium

Class and Generic Name	Effect on Plasma Lithium Concentration	Significance
Antibiotics		
Tetracycline	Possible increase	Case reports: possibly from
Spectinomycin	Possible increase	nephrotoxic effect of antibiotics; tetracycline may be safe
Tricyclic antidepressants	Unknown	May cause switch to mania; increase in tremors
Anti-inflammatory agents		
Ibuprofen	Increase	Case reports of piroxicam and
Indomethacin	Increase	diclofenac sodium increasing
Naproxen	Increase	lithium concentrations;
Phenylbutazone	Increase	sulindac may have minimal effect
Antipsychotics		
Chlorpromazine	Possibly increase red blood cell (RBC) lithium	All antipsychotics may increase lithium's neurotoxicity
Fluphenazine	Possibly increase RBC lithium	
Haloperidol	Possibly increase plasma lithium	
Perphenazine	Possibly increase RBC lithium	
Thioridazine	Possibly increase RBC lithium	
Cardiovascular drugs		
Digoxin	Unknown	Case report of CNS confusion and bradycardia
ACE inhibitors	Increase	Case reports of toxicity, renal insufficiency
Methyldopa	Unknown	Case reports neurological toxicity
Diltiazem	Unknown	Case report of neurological toxicity
Verapamil	Unknown	Case report of neurological toxicity
Diuretics		
Carbonic anhydrase inhibitors	Decrease	Increase lithium excretion
Acetazolamide		
Loop diuretics		
Furosemide	Unclear	May increase lithium concentrations
Ethacrynic acid	Unclear	
Distal tubule diuretics		
Thiazides	Increase	Well-documented interaction
Metolazone	Increase	with increase in lithium
Chlorthalidone	Increase	concentrations

(Continued)

TABLE 22–5
Drug Interactions with Lithium (Continued)

Class and Generic Name	Effect on Plasma Lithium Concentration	Significance
Osmotic diuretics		
Mannitol	Decrease	Increase lithium excretion
Urea	Decrease	
Potassium-sparing diuretics		
Triamterene	Increase	May increase lithium concentrations
Spironolactone	Increase	
Amiloride	Unclear	May be used to treat lithium-induced polyuria
Xanthines		
Theophylline	Decrease	Increase lithium excretion
Caffeine	Decrease	
Neuromuscular blocking drugs		
Succinylcholine	Unknown	May prolong neuromuscular blockade
Pancuronium bromide	Unknown	
Miscellaneous		
Sodium chloride	Decrease	Increase lithium excretion
Sodium bicarbonate	Decrease	Alkalinization of urine increases lithium excretion
Metronidazole	Increase	Reports of toxicity, renal damage
Metoclopramide	Unknown	Case report of extrapyramidal symptoms
Carbamazepine	Unknown	May have synergistic effect in treating mania and depression; case reports of neurotoxicity
Iodides	Unknown	May have additive or synergistic hypothyroid effect
Alcohol	Unknown	Increased lithium toxicity in animals; acute alcohol ingestion may increase peak lithium concentration
Phenytoin	Possible increase	Case reports of lithium toxicity and changes in phenytoin concentrations

Table adapted from J L Kinney-Parker, M P Fankhauser: Bipolar disorder. In *Pharmacotherapy: A Pathophysiologic Approach*, J T DiPiro, R L Talbert, P E Hayes, G C Yee, L M Posey, editors, p 741. Elsevier, New York, 1989. Used with permission.

TABLE 22–6
Possible Effects of Lithium on Laboratory Values

Laboratory Value	Possible Effect of Lithium
White blood cells (WBCs)	Increased count
Serum glucose	Increased level
Serum magnesium	Increased level
Serum potassium	Decreased level
Serum uric acid	Decreased level
Serum thyroxine	Decreased
Serum cortisol	Decreased AM levels
Serum parathyroid hormone	Increased level due to adenoma
Serum calcium	Increased level due to increased parathyroid hormone level
Serum phosphorus	Decreased level due to increased parathyroid hormone level

Table from A Doupe, M Szuba: Lithium and other antimanic agents. In *The Handbook of Psychiatry*, Residents of the UCLA Department of Psychiatry, p 386. Year Book Medical Publishers, Chicago, 1990. Used with permission.

References

Aagaard J, Vestergaard P: Predictors of outcome in prophylactic lithium treatment: A 2-year prospective study. J Affective Disord *18*: 259, 1990.

Baraban J M, Worley P F, Snyder S H: Second messenger systems and psychoactive drug action: Focus on the phosphoinositide system and lithium. Am J Psychiatry *146*: 1251, 1989.

Di Costanzo E, Schifano F: Lithium alone or in combination with carbamazepine for the treatment of rapid-cycling bipolar affective disorder. Acta Psychiatr Scand *83*: 456, 1991.

Freeman T: A double-blind comparison of valproate and lithium in the treatment of acute mania. Am J Psychiatry *149*: 108, 1992.

Friedberg R C, Spyker D A, Herold D A: Massive overdoses with sustained-release lithium carbonate preparations: Pharmacokinetic model based on two case studies. Clin Chem *37*:1205, 1991.

Gitlin M J, Cochran S D, Jamison H R: Maintenance lithium treatment: Side effects and compliance. J Clin Psychiatry *50*: 127, 1989.

Hsu L K, Clement L, Santhouse R, Ju E S: Treatment of bulimia nervosa with lithium carbonate: A controlled study. J Nerv Ment Dis *179*: 351, 1991.

Jefferson J W: Lithium: A therapeutic magic wand. J Clin Psychiatry *50*: 81, 1989.

Jefferson J W, Greist J H: Lithium therapy. In *Comprehensive Textbook of Psychiatry*, ed 5, H I Kaplan, B J Sadock, editors, p 1655. Williams & Wilkins, Baltimore, 1989.

Maarbjerg K, Aagaard J, Vestergaard P: Adherence to lithium prophylaxis: I. Clinical predictors and patient's reasons for nonadherence. Pharmacopsychiatry *21*: 121, 1988.

McDougle C J, Price L H, Goodman W K, Charney D S, Heninger G R: A controlled trial of lithium augmentation in fluvoxamine-refractory obsessive-compulsive disorder: Lack of efficacy. J Clin Psychopharmacol *11*: 175, 1991.

Nierenberg A A, Price L H, Charney D S, Henlinger G R: After lithium augmentation: A retrospective follow-up of patients with antidepressant-refractory depression. J Affective Disord *18*: 167, 1990.

Schou M: Lithium prophylaxis: Myths and realities. Am J Psychiatry *146*: 573, 1989.

23

Methadone

Methadone hydrochloride (Dolophine, Methadose) is a synthetic diphenylheptane-derivative opiate agonist. The primary use of methadone in psychiatry is the detoxification and maintenance therapy of adolescents and adults addicted to opiates. The molecular structure of methadone is given in Figure 23–1.

PHARMACOLOGICAL ACTIONS

Methadone is well absorbed from the gastrointestinal (GI) tract and has an initial duration of action of four to six hours. The duration of action increases to 22 to 48 hours with repeated administration and is elevated in persons who have been abusing opiate agonists. Methadone is metabolized by the liver and is excreted by the kidneys. Methadone is an agonist at mu, kappa, and, probably, delta opiate receptors.

INDICATIONS AND CLINICAL GUIDELINES

Methadone is used for the short-term detoxification (30 days), long-term detoxification (180 days), and maintenance of opiate addicts. Methadone is a schedule II drug, the administration of which is governed by specific federal laws and regulations. Those regulations are currently in a state of flux because of the increase in efforts to place intravenous drug abusers in methadone programs. The aim of such efforts is to reduce the spread of acquired immune deficiency syndrome (AIDS), which can be contracted by the use of contaminated needles.

Methadone is supplied in tablets of 5, 10, and 40 mg; a solution of 5 mg per 5 mL, 10 mg per 5 mL, and 10 mg per mL; and a parenteral form of 10 mg per mL.

In maintenance programs, methadone is usually administered dissolved in water or fruit juices. For short-term detoxification, an initial dose of 15 to 20 mg usually

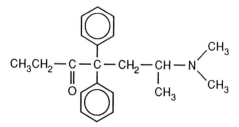

Figure 23–1. Molecular structure of methadone.

148

suppresses withdrawal symptoms, and additional doses can be given if the initial dose is insufficient. A dosage of 40 mg a day in single or divided doses is usually sufficient to control withdrawal symptoms in most patients. After stabilization, the methadone dosage is tapered at a rate that depends on the type of program, on whether the patient is an inpatient or an outpatient, and on the patient's level of tolerance for withdrawal symptoms. If withdrawal takes more than 180 days, the treatment program is officially described as methadone maintenance. Maintenance should be at the lowest possible dosage of methadone, and, generally, the patient should eventually be withdrawn completely from methadone. The administration of methadone for both withdrawal and maintenance must follow the strict federal guidelines, generally requiring patients to receive the methadone in person to avoid its abuse by persons other than the patient.

Pregnancy

Methadone should be administered to pregnant women only if the potential benefits outweigh the possible risks. Detoxification is not recommended for pregnant women; maintenance methadone may be appropriate in some circumstances. Whether methadone treatment is harmful to the fetus is not known. A significant number of infants born to mothers receiving methadone show withdrawal symptoms. Women should not breast-feed their babies if they are taking methadone.

ADVERSE EFFECTS

An overdose of methadone can cause respiratory and circulatory depression, leading to respiratory arrest, cardiac arrest, and death. Methadone is also capable of inducing tolerance, psychological dependence, and physical dependence. Other adverse effects on the central nervous system (CNS) include dizziness, depression, sedation, euphoria, dysphoria, agitation, and seizures. Delirium and insomnia have also been reported in rare cases. Methadone has significant effects on the GI system, where it can cause biliary spasm or colic, nausea, vomiting, and constipation. It can also cause urinary retention and oliguria. Systemically, methadone is associated with sweating, flushing, pruritis, and urticaria. It should be used with caution in patients with respiratory disease, hepatic or renal dysfunction, and seizure disorders.

Methadone Withdrawal

Abrupt cessation of methadone results in withdrawal symptoms in three to four days, with peak symptoms appearing at the sixth day. Withdrawal symptoms include weakness, anxiety, anorexia, insomnia, gastric distress, headache, sweating, and hot and cold flashes. The withdrawal symptoms usually resolve after two weeks; however, a protracted abstinence syndrome is possible.

DRUG-DRUG INTERACTIONS

Methadone can potentiate the CNS depressant effects of other opiate agonists, barbiturates, benzodiazepines, and alcohol. Antipsychotics, especially low-potency agents; tricyclic and tetracyclic antidepressants; and monoamine oxidase inhibitors (MAOIs) should be used very cautiously with methadone. Two other opiate agonists, meperidine (Demerol) and fentanyl, have been associated with fatal drug-drug interactions with the MAOIs.

References

Ball J C, Corty E: Basic issues pertaining to the effectiveness of methadone maintenance treatment. NIDA Res Monogr 86: 178, 1988.

Cooper J R: Methadone treatment and acquired immunodeficiency syndrome. JAMA 262: 1664, 1989.

Gossop M, Strang J: A comparison of the withdrawal responses of heroin and methadone addicts during detoxification. Br J Psychiatry 158: 697, 1991.

Jaffe J H: Drug dependence: Opiods, nonnarcotics, nicotine (tobacco), and caffeine. In *Comprehensive Textbook of Psychiatry*, ed 5, H I Kaplan, B J Sadock, editors, p 642. Williams & Wilkins, Baltimore, 1989.

Ladewig D: Opiate maintenance and abstinence: Attitudes, treatment modalities and outcome. Drug Alcohol Depend 25: 245, 1990.

Liappas J A, Jenner F A, Vicente B: Literature on methadone maintenance clinics. Int J Addict 23: 927, 1988.

Loimer N, Lenz K, Schmid R, Presslich O: Technique for greatly shortening the transition from methadone to haltrexone maintenance of patients addicted to opiates. Am J Psychiatry 148: 933, 1991.

Maddux J F, Desmond D P: Methadone maintenance and recovery from opioid dependence. Am Drug Alcohol Abuse 18: 63, 1992.

Nunes E V, Quitkin F M, Brady R, Stewart J W: Imipramine treatment of methadone maintenance patients with affective disorder and illicit drug use. Am J Psychiatry 148: 667, 1991.

Segest E, Mygind O, Bay H: The influence of prolonged stable methadone maintenance treatment on mortality and employment: An 8-year follow-up. Int J Addict 25: 53, 1990.

Wolff K, Hay A, Raistrick D, Calvert R, Feely M: Measuring compliance in methadone maintenance patients: Use of a pharmacologic indicator to estimate methadone plasma levels. Clin Pharmacol Ther 50: 199, 1991.

24

Monoamine Oxidase Inhibitors

The monoamine oxidase inhibitors (MAOIs) are probably as effective as the tricyclic antidepressants in treating depression. When MAOIs were first introduced into clinical practice, there was a lack of awareness of the risk of tyramine-induced hypertensive crises, leading to fatalities and the temporary withdrawal of the drugs from the market. It is now appreciated that the drugs are as safe as tricyclic antidepressants, provided reasonable dietary precautions are followed. Some clinicians believe that MAOIs are underused as effective antidepressant treatment.

CLASSIFICATION

There are four commonly used MAOIs in the United States (Figure 24–1). Phenelzine (Nardil) and isocarboxazid (Marplan) are derivatives of hydrazine (-CNN is the hydrazine moiety), and tranylcypromine (Parnate) is a derivative of amphetamine. Selegiline (Eldepryl, Deprenyl) is a specific inhibitor of MAO_B (enzyme subtype more specific for dopamine [Table 24–1]) and is approved for use in the treatment of parkinsonism. It has not been established whether it is an effective antidepressant.

Clorgyline is a specific inhibitor of MAO_A (enzyme subtype more specific for norepinephrine and serotonin). Clorgyline may be particularly effective in treating depression in rapid-cycling bipolar disorder patients, but it is not available for clinical use in the United States.

PHARMACOLOGICAL ACTIONS

Pharmacokinetics

MAOIs are readily absorbed when administered orally. The hydrazine MAOIs are metabolized by acetylation. About one half of North American and European persons and an even higher proportion of Asians are slow acetylators, which may explain why, when given the drugs, some patients have more adverse effects than do others.

Pharmacodynamics

MAOIs irreversibly inhibit monoamine oxidase (MAO), reaching maximum inhibition after 5 to 10 days. Antidepressant effects, however, take three to six weeks to develop. The measurement of MAO activity in platelets can be used as an indicator of MAO inhibition. Platelet MAO activity needs to be reduced 80 percent to achieve a therapeutic response. Because platelet MAO is of the B type,

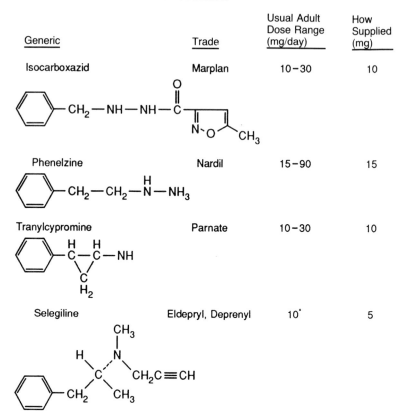

Generic	Trade	Usual Adult Dose Range (mg/day)	How Supplied (mg)
Isocarboxazid	Marplan	10–30	10
Phenelzine	Nardil	15–90	15
Tranylcypromine	Parnate	10–30	10
Selegiline	Eldepryl, Deprenyl	10*	5

Figure 24–1. Molecular structures of the monoamine oxidase inhibitors.
*Therapeutic dosage for the treatment of parkinsonism. See text regarding use and dosage for depression.

TABLE 24–1
Comparison of Monoamine Oxidase A and B

Type	Location	Preferred Substrates	Selective Inhibitors
A	Central nervous system, sympathetic terminals, liver, gut, skin	Norepinephrine, serotonin, dopamine, tyramine, octopamine, tryptamine	Clorgyline
B	Central nervous system, liver, platelets	Dopamine, tyramine, tryptamine, phenylethylamine, benzylamine, N-methylhistamine	*Selegiline (Deprenyl)

*Selectivity lost at higher doses (≥ 10 mg/day)
Table from G W Arana, S E Hyman: *Handbook of Psychiatric Drug Therapy*, ed 2, p 68. Little, Brown, Boston, 1991. Used with permission.

that measurement cannot be used if the effects of clorgyline are being studied. Because the MAO inhibition by MAOIs is irreversible, the body takes approximately two weeks after their discontinuation to synthesize enough new MAO to restore its baseline concentrations.

INDICATIONS

The indications for MAOIs are similar to those for tricyclic and tetracyclic antidepressants (Chapter 29). MAOIs may be particularly effective in agoraphobia with panic attacks, posttraumatic stress disorder, eating disorders, social phobia, and pain syndromes. Some investigators have reported that MAOIs may be preferable to tricyclic antidepressants in the treatment of atypical depression, characterized by hypersomnia, hyperphagia, anxiety, and the absence of vegetative symptoms. Those depressions are often less severe than major depression, and the patients present with less functional impairment. A trial of MAOIs may be indicated for any depressed patient if a trial of a tricyclic antidepressant has been unsuccessful.

Although depression is not an approved indication for selegiline, some positive results have been reported. Several studies have found statistically significant improvement, as compared with a placebo. An advantage of selegiline is that it functions to conserve dopamine through selective inhibition of MAO_B and thus is not as likely to cause hypertensive reactions. However, the antidepressant effects of selegiline have been noted at higher dosages than those recommended for use in Parkinson's disease, and at those higher dosages (20 to 60 mg a day) hypertensive episodes have been noted. Because dosages above 10 to 20 mg a day for selegeline diminish its selectivity for MAO_B, there is the potential for inhibition of MAO_A. Patients on those higher dosages must follow tyramine-restricted diets and avoid sympathomimetic agents.

CLINICAL GUIDELINES

There is no definitive rationale for choosing one MAOI over another, except that tranylcypromine may be the most activating of the drugs. Phenelzine should be started with a test dose of 15 mg on the first day. On an outpatient basis, the dosage can be increased to 45 mg a day during the first week and increased by 15 mg a day each week thereafter until 90 mg a day is reached by the end of the fourth week. Tranylcypromine and isocarboxazid should begin with a test dose of 10 mg and may be increased to 30 mg a day by the end of the first week. Upper limits of 50 mg for isocarboxazid and 40 mg for tranylcypromine have been suggested by some researchers. If an MAOI trial is not successful after six weeks, lithium or L-triiodothyronine (T_3 or liothyronine) (Cytomel) augmentation is warranted. The combined treatment of MAOIs and tricyclic antidepressants is described in Chapter 29.

Liver function tests should be monitored periodically because of possible hepatotoxicity. The elderly may be more sensitive to MAOI side effects than are younger adults. MAOI use in children has not been studied.

ADVERSE EFFECTS

The most frequent adverse effects of MAOIs are orthostatic hypotension, weight gain, edema, sexual dysfunction, and insomnia. The orthostatic hypotension, if severe, may respond to treatment with fludrocortisone (Florinef), a mineralocorticoid, 0.1 to 0.2 mg a day; support stockings; corsets; hydration; and increased salt intake. Weight gain, edema, and sexual dysfunction are often not responsive to any treatment and may warrant switching from a hydrazine to a nonhydrazine MAOI or vice versa. When switching from one MAOI to another, the clinician should taper and stop the first one for 10 to 14 days before beginning the second one. Insomnia and behavioral activation can be treated by dividing the dose, not giving medication after dinner, and using a benzodiazepine hypnotic if necessary. Insomnia may paradoxically be accompanied by sedation during the day. Myoclonus, muscle pains, and parathesias are also occasionally seen in patients treated with MAOIs. Parasthesias may be secondary to MAOI-induced pyridoxine deficiency, which may respond to supplementation with pyridoxine, 50 to 150 mg orally each day. Occasionally, patients complain of feeling drunk or confused, perhaps indicating that the dosage should be reduced and then increased more gradually. There are uncommon reports that the hydrazine MAOIs are associated with hepatoxic effects. MAOIs are less cardiotoxic and less epileptogenic than tricyclic and tetracyclic antidepressants.

MAOIs should be used with caution in patients with renal disease, seizure disorders, cardiovascular disease, or hyperthyroidism. MAOIs may exacerbate symptoms of Parkinson's disease or alter the hypoglycemic agent requirements in diabetic patients. MAOIs may provoke a manic switch in bipolar disorder patients or exacerbate psychotic symptoms in patients with schizophrenia. MAOIs are contraindicated during pregnancy. MAOIs pass into the breast milk.

Tyramine-Induced Hypertensive Crisis

When patients taking MAOIs ingest foodstuffs rich in tyramine (Table 24–2), they may have a hypertensive reaction that can be life-threatening (for example, cerebrovascular disorder). Patients should also be warned that bee stings may cause a hypertensive crisis. The mechanism is MAO inhibition in the gastrointestinal (GI) tract, resulting in the increased absorption of tyramine, which then acts as a false neurotransmitter. Increased concentrations of norepinephrine in presynaptic endings is a result of MAO_A inhibition and may be an even more significant mechanism in producing the hypertensive effect.

Patients should be warned about the dangers of ingesting tyramine-rich foods while taking MAOIs, and they should be advised to continue the dietary restrictions for two weeks after they stop MAOI treatment in order to allow the body to resynthesize the enzyme. The prodromal symptoms of a hypertensive crisis may include headache, stiff neck, sweating, nausea, and vomiting. If those symptoms occur, a patient should seek immediate medical treatment. An MAOI-induced hypertensive crisis can be treated with nifedipine (Procardia); however, some controversy exists regarding that practice because it produces a rapid drop in arterial pressure. The standard dose is 10 mg. To enhance therapeutic response, the clinician

TABLE 24–2
Tyramine-Rich Foods to Be Avoided while Taking MAOIs

Very high tyramine content:
Alcohol (particularly beer and wines, especially Chianti; a small amount of scotch, gin, vodka, or
sherry is permissible)
Fava or broad beans
Aged cheese (e.g., Camembert, Liederkranz, Edam, and cheddar; cream cheese and cottage cheeses
are permitted)
Beef or chicken liver
Orange pulp
Pickled or smoked fish, poultry, or meats
Soups (packaged)
Yeast vitamin supplements
Meat extracts (e.g., Marmite, Bovril)
Summer (dry) sausage

Moderately high tyramine content (no more than one or two servings a day):
Soy sauce
Sour cream
Bananas (green bananas can be included only if cooked in their skins; ordinary peeled bananas are fine)
Avocados
Eggplant
Plums
Raisins
Spinach
Tomatoes
Yogurt

should tell the patient to bite the capsule and swallow its contents with water.
Treatment should include the administration of α-adrenergic blockers, such as
phentolamine (Regitine). Chlorpromazine (Thorazine) may also be used, and some
clinicians give their patients several 50 mg tablets of chlorpromazine to use in an
emergency. A headache from the hypotensive effects of MAOIs may confuse the
patient, however, and taking the chlorpromazine could result in more severe hypotension, fainting, and possibly injury.

Overdose Attempts

In general, intoxication caused by MAOIs is characterized by agitation that
progresses to coma with hyperthermia, hypertension, tachypnea, tachycardia, dilated pupils, and hyperactive deep tendon reflexes. Involuntary movements may
be present, particularly in the face and the jaw.

There is often an asymptomatic period of one to six hours after the ingestion
of the drugs before the occurrence of toxicity. Acidification of the urine markedly
hastens the excretion of MAOIs, and dialysis may be of some use. Phentolamine
and chlorpromazine may be useful if hypertension is a problem.

DRUG-DRUG INTERACTIONS

The inhibition of MAO can cause severe and even fatal interactions with various
other drugs (Table 24–3). Patients should be instructed to tell any other physicians
who are treating them that they are taking an MAOI. MAOIs may potentiate the
action of or be additive with central nervous system (CNS) depressants, including

TABLE 24-3
Drugs to Be Avoided during MAOI Treatment

Never use:
Anesthetic—never spinal anesthetic or local anesthetic containing epinephrine (lidocaine and procaine are safe)
Antiasthmatic medications
Antihypertensives (α-methyldopa, guanethidine, reserpine, pargyline)
Diuretics
L-Dopa, L-tryptophan
Fluoxetine
Paroxetine
Narcotics (especially meperidine [Demerol]; morphine or codeine may be less dangerous)
Over-the-counter cold, hay fever, and sinus medications, especially those containing dextromethorphan (aspirin, acetaminophen, and menthol lozenges are safe)
Sympathomimetics (amphetamine, cocaine, methylphenidate, dopamine, metaraminol, epinephrine, norepinephrine, isoproterenol)

Use carefully:
Antihistamines
Disulfiram
Hydralazine (Apresoline)
Propranolol (Inderal)
Terpin hydrate with codeine

alcohol. A serotonin syndrome—including autonomic instability, hyperthermia, rigidity, myoclonus, confusion, delirium, and coma—may occur when serotonergic drugs are given concurrently with MAOIs.

References

Birkmayer W: Deprenyl (selegiline) in the treatment of Parkinson's disease. Acta Neurol Scand Suppl 95: 103, 1983.
Davis J M, Glassman A H: Antidepressant drugs. In *Comprehensive Textbook of Psychiatry*, ed 5, H I Kaplan, B J Sadock, editors, p 1627. Williams & Wilkins, Baltimore, 1989.
Georgotas A, McCue R E, Cooper T B: A placebo-controlled comparison of nortriptyline and phenelzine in maintenance therapy of elderly depressed patients. Arch Gen Psychiatry 46: 783, 1989.
Kahn D, Silver J M, Opler L A: The safety of switching rapidly from tricyclic antidepressants to monoamine oxidase inhibitors. J Clin Psychopharmacol 9: 198, 1989.
Kennedy S H, Piran N, Warsh J J, Prendergast P, Mainprize E, Whynot C, Garfinkel P E: A trial of isocarboxazid in the treatment of bulima nervosa. J Clin Psychopharmacol 8: 391, 1989.
Liebowitz M: Phenelzine vs atenolol in social phobia: A placebo-controlled comparison. Arch Gen Psychiatry 49: 290, 1992.
Mann J J, Aarons S F, Wilner P J, Keilp J G, Sweeney J A, Pearlstein T, Frances A J, Kocsis J H, Brown R P: A controlled study of the antidepressant efficacy and side effects of (−)-deprenyl: A selective monoamine oxidase inhibitor. Arch Gen Psychiatry 46: 45, 1989.
Mann J J, Frances A, Kaplan R D, Kocsis J, Peselow E D, Gershon S: The relative efficacy of l-deprenyl, a selective monoamine oxidase type B inhibitor, in endogenous and nonendogenous depression. J Clin Psychopharmacol 2: 54, 1982.
Quitkin F M, McGrath P J, Stewart J W, Harrison W, Wager S G, Nunes E, Rabikin J G, Tricamo E, Markowitz J, Klein D F: Phenelzine and imipamine in mood reactive depressives. Arch Gen Psychiatry 46: 787, 1989.
Shulman K I, Walker S E, MacKenzie S, Knowles S: Dietary restriction, tyramine, and the use of monoamine oxidase inhibitors. J Clin Psychopharmacol 9: 397, 1989.
Thase M E, Mallinger A G, McKnight D, Himmelhoch J M: Treatment of imipramine-resistant recurrent depression: IV. A double-blind crossover study of tranylcypromine for anergic bipolar depression. Am J Psychiatry 149: 195, 1992.

25

Serotonin-Specific Reuptake Inhibitors

Since 1989 three serotonin-specific reuptake inhibitors (fluoxetine [Prozac], paroxetine [Paxil], and sertraline [Zoloft]) have been introduced for the treatment of depression in the United States. An additional drug in this category, fluvoxamine, is likely to be approved by the U.S. Food and Drug Administration (FDA) soon. Although this chapter unites the drugs under the heading of their primary mechanism of action, the four drugs are discussed separately within the chapter because knowledge of the drugs is still too limited to discuss them together, as is now possible with dopaminergic antagonists and tricyclic drugs. Despite their widespread clinical use, these are new drugs, and information about their clinical use, adverse effects, and drug-drug interactions is incomplete.

FLUOXETINE

Fluoxetine (Prozac) is a phenylpropylamine-derivative drug with antidepressant activity (Figure 25–1). It has the fewest adverse effects of any antidepressant drug currently available and is generally given at the same dosage (20 mg a day) during the entire course of treatment. There is usually no need for dose titration. Those features have made fluoxetine the largest-selling antidepressant in the United States.

Pharmacological Actions

Fluoxetine is well absorbed from the gastrointestinal (GI) tract and reaches peak plasma levels in approximately four to eight hours. Fluoxetine is metabolized in the liver to norfluoxetine, an active metabolite, which is eventually excreted by the kidneys. The half-life of fluoxetine is two to three days; the half-life of norfluoxetine is seven to nine days. Because of the very long half-life, steady-state plasma levels are not attained until after two to three weeks at a steady dosage.

The therapeutic effects of fluoxetine result from a highly selective blockade of the reuptake of serotonin into the presynaptic neurons. Fluoxetine has almost no effects on norepinephrine or dopamine neurotransmission. It also lacks anticholinergic, antihistaminergic, and anti-α_1-adrenergic activities; thus, it is associated with almost none of the adverse effects that are associated with the standard antidepressants—tricyclic and tetracyclic antidepressants and monoamine oxidase inhibitors (MAOIs).

Indications

Depression. Fluoxetine is as effective as the standard antidepressant drugs in the short-term treatment of major depression. Whether it can be used for the

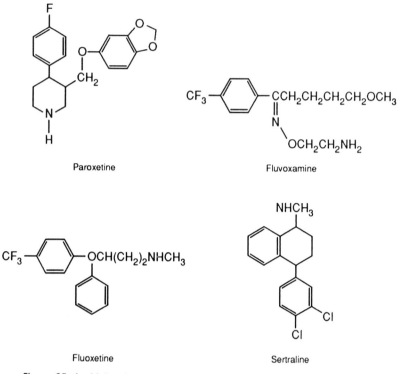

Paroxetine

Fluvoxamine

Fluoxetine

Sertraline

Figure 25–1. Molecular structures of serotonin-specific reuptake inhibitors

prevention of depressive episodes is being examined in long-term, controlled studies. Fluoxetine is regularly used as a major drug for the treatment of depression; however, many clinicians still prefer tricyclic or tetracyclic antidepressants for the treatment of depression. Fluoxetine is also effective for the treatment of depression associated with bipolar disorder. Fluoxetine may provoke a switch into mania in some patients, but it is less likely to do so than are the tricyclics. It may be of particular use in treatment-refractory bipolar II disorder patients.

Dysthymia. Several reports indicate that fluoxetine is useful in the treatment of mild depressive episodes and possibly of dysthymia. No data, however, concern the long-term outcome of such treatments.

Other disorders. As with most new drugs, there are many reports of its successful application in a wide range of disorders. It is known that serotonin is involved in the regulation of eating, and, in fact, fluoxetine very often has the effect of reducing appetite and weight. Fluoxetine has been reported to be useful in the treatment of obesity, anorexia nervosa, and bulimia nervosa. Serotonin is also implicated in the pathophysiology of anxiety and impulse control disorders, and fluoxetine has been reported to be useful in the treatment of obsessive-compulsive disorder and panic disorder. Several recent studies have suggested that fluoxetine may be useful as an adjunct to antipsychotics for the treatment of depression in schizophrenia.

Clinical Guidelines

Fluoxetine is available in 20 mg capsules and 20 mg per 5 mL liquid. The initial dosage is 20 mg orally (PO) a day, usually given in the morning, because insomnia is a potential adverse effect of the drug. Fluoxetine should be taken with food to minimize possible nausea. The long half-life of the drug causes the drug to accumulate in the body over a period of two to three weeks. As with all available antidepressants, the antidepressant effects may be seen in the first one to three weeks, but it is much more reasonable to wait to evaluate the antidepressant activity until the patient has been taking the drug for four to six weeks. Several studies have suggested that 20 mg a day is as effective as higher dosages. There may be a therapeutic window for the drug. The maximum daily dosage recommended by the manufacturer is 80 mg a day. A reasonable strategy is to maintain a patient with 20 mg a day for three weeks; if the patient shows no signs of clinical improvement, an increase to 20 mg PO two times a day may be warranted. The second dose is usually given at noon to avoid problems with insomnia. Occasionally, fluoxetine is associated with sedation, in which case the drug can be given in the evening.

To minimize early side effects of anxiety and restlessness, some clinicians initiate fluoxetine at doses of 5 to 10 mg a day by instructing patients to dissolve the contents of a capsule in water or juice. The mixture should be refrigerated. The newly available liquid preparation can also be used for lower dosage titration. Alternatively, fluoxetine can be initiated in an every-other-day regimen. Panic disorder patients may be particularly sensitive to the side effects and may benefit from low-dosage strategies. They may have a therapeutic response at dosages of 10 mg a day or less.

In obsessive-compulsive disorder, dosages of 80 mg a day are generally used. Eight to twelve weeks at that dosage constitutes an adequate trial. In partial responders or nonresponders, augmentation with buspirone (BuSpar) or combination therapy with clomipramine (Anafranil) can be considered. In treating patients with clomipramine and fluoxetine, the clinician should use lower dosages and careful titration, as fluoxetine raises the tricyclic levels and toxicity can result.

In treatment-resistant depressions, combinations of fluoxetine with a tricyclic (for example, desipramine [Norpramin]) may be useful. Again, caution should be applied. Fluoxetine augmented with stimulants (for example, pemoline [Cylert] or dextroamphetamine [Dexedrine]), buspirone, or lithium carbonate (Eskalith) may be another useful regimen in the treatment of refractory depression. Two weeks should elapse between the discontinuation of MAOIs and the initiation of fluoxetine. Fluoxetine must be discontinued for five weeks before initiating MAOI therapy.

Fluoxetine has not been studied in elderly adults or children.

Adverse Effects

The most common adverse effects of fluoxetine involve the central nervous system (CNS) and the GI system (Tables 25–1 and 25–2). Anorgasmia and delayed orgasm may affect approximately 5 percent of patients. That side effect may respond to cyproheptadine (Periactin), 4 to 8 mg PO taken one to two hours before sexual

TABLE 25–1
Common Adverse Effects of Fluoxetine

	Patients (%)
Central nervous system	
Headache	20
Nervousness	15
Insomnia	14
Drowsiness	12
Anxiety	9
Tremor	8
Dizziness	6
Gastrointestinal system	
Nausea	21
Diarrhea	12
Dry mouth	10
Anorexia	9
Stomach upset	6
Other	
Excessive sweating	8
Weight loss > 5% body weight	13
Increase in suicidal ideation or violent behavior (six cases reported)	

activity is planned. Various types of rashes may appear in 4 percent of patients. There have been rare reports of extrapyramidal side effects. Akathisia may be responsive to the usual pharmacological interventions (for example, dosage reduction, β-blockers, and benzodiazepines). Seizures have been reported in 0.2 percent of patients, approximately the incidence with standard antidepressants. Fluoxetine, like almost all antidepressants, suppresses rapid eye movement (REM) sleep, although it is arguable whether that is an adverse therapeutic effect of the drug. Most notable about fluoxetine is the absence of the anticholinergic adverse effects associated with standard antidepressants. Fluoxetine has no recognized adverse effects on the cardiovascular system, although it is associated with a decrease in heart rate of approximately three beats a minute. Because experience with fluoxetine is still limited, fluoxetine should be used with caution in patients with preexisting cardiac disorders, as there have been reports of arrhythmias, palpitations, syncopy, and hypotension.

There has been only one report of a lethal overdose of fluoxetine taken by itself. That makes the drug very safe to give to suicidal patients compared with tricyclic and tetracyclic antidepressants, which are highly lethal in overdose and have a high suicide potential. There have been a number of reports of fatal overdoses of fluoxetine when taken with other psychotropic drugs. The symptoms of overdose include agitation, restlessness, insomnia, tremor, nausea, vomiting, tachycardia, and seizures. The clinician should try to ascertain whether other drugs were taken with the fluoxetine. The first steps in the treatment of overdose are gastric lavage and emesis.

In a few cases, patients who were taking fluoxetine experienced suicidal ideation, self-mutilation, and violent behavior, but the significance of those findings for fluoxetine use is questionable and unclear. The FDA does not attribute those adverse effects to fluoxetine.

Fluoxetine has not been studied in pregnant women. It may pass into the breast

TABLE 25–2
Side Effects with an Incidence of ≥ 19 Percent Reported for Selected Serotonin Reuptake Inhibitors, Imipramine, and Placebo

Side Effect	Sertraline N=1,568	Placebo N=851	Fluoxetine N=1,378	Fluvoxamine N=222	Paroxetine N=1,387	Imipramine N=599
Nausea and vomiting	21%	—	25%	37%	29%	—
Headache	—	20%	—	22%	20%	19%
Dry mouth	—	—	—	26%	20%	76%
Sedation	—	—	—	26%	24%	30%
Nervousness, restlessness, and anxiety	—	—	21%	—	—	—
Dizziness	—	—	—	—	—	27%
Insomnia	—	—	19%	—	—	—
Sweating	—	—	—	—	—	21%

Table adapted from K Rickels, E Schweizer: Clinical overview of serotonin reuptake inhibitors. J Clin Psychiatry *51*: 10, 1990. Used with permission.

milk. Fluoxetine should be used with caution in patients with hepatic or renal disease, diabetes, or seizure disorders.

Drug-Drug Interactions

Experience with fluoxetine is still limited. The coadministration of fluoxetine with tricyclic antidepressants, trazodone (Desyrel), or benzodiazepines increases the plasma levels of the antidepressants or the benzodiazepines. Fluoxetine cannot be used with MAOIs because of the risk of a serotonin syndrome. Toxic reactions may occur if fluoxetine is combined with selegiline (Eldepryl) or L-tryptophan. Fluoxetine may change levels of carbamazepine (Tegretol), lithium, or digitalis. The coadministration of fluoxetine with buspirone has been reported to decrease the therapeutic efficacy of buspirone and may precipitate extrapyramidal symptoms; however, in some cases a positive synergistic effect occurred.

FLUVOXAMINE

Fluvoxamine is currently available in Canada and Europe as an antidepressant drug and is being investigated in the United States as a potential treatment for depression and obsessive-compulsive disorder. Fluvoxamine is a potent specific inhibitor of neuronal serotonin reuptake with few adverse effects, as compared with tricyclic antidepressants. The molecular structure of fluvoxamine is given in Figure 25–1.

Pharmacological Actions

The antidepressant and antiobsessive actions of fluvoxamine are believed to be related to its selective inhibition of presynaptic serotonin reuptake in brain neurons. There is minimum interference with noradrenergic activity and very little affinity for adrenergic, dopaminergic, histaminergic, and muscarinic receptors.

Fluvoxamine is well absorbed after oral administration. After a single dose, peak plasma levels are attained in 1.5 to 8 hours. The mean plasma half-life is 15 hours after a single dose and 17 to 22 hours during repeated dosing. Steady-state plasma levels are usually achieved within 10 to 14 days.

Fluvoxamine undergoes extensive hepatic transformation, mainly through oxidative demethylation to at least nine metabolites that are excreted by the kidneys. The two major metabolites show negligible pharmacological activity.

Indications

Fluvoxamine appears to be effective in the treatment of depression and obsessive-compulsive disorder.

Clinical Guidelines

Fluvoxamine should be administered within a range of 50 to 300 mg a day. A starting dosage of 100 mg daily is recommended for the first week, after which the dosage can be adjusted as dictated by adverse effects and patient response. A tapered reduction of the dosage may be necessary if nausea develops over the first two weeks of therapy. Fluvoxamine can be administered as a single evening dose to minimize its adverse effects. Tablets should be swallowed with water and, preferably, food without chewing the tablet. Fluvoxamine is available in 50 and 100 mg tablets in Europe. It is in phase III clinical trials in the United States.

The safety of fluvoxamine during pregnancy and lactation has not been established.

Adverse Effects

The most commonly observed adverse events associated with fluvoxamine administration are nausea (sometimes accompanied by vomiting), drowsiness, constipation, nervousness, anorexia, insomnia, and tremor.

Drug-Drug Interactions

The use of fluvoxamine together with monoamine oxidase inhibitors (MAOIs) should be avoided. At least two weeks should elapse after the discontinuation of MAOI therapy before fluvoxamine treatment is initiated. Potentiation of the effects of alcohol, including increased psychomotor impairment, have been noted. Prolongation of the elimination of drugs (such as warfarin [Coumadin], phenytoin [Dilantin], and theophylline) that are metabolized by oxidation in the liver has been noted, and a clinically significant interaction is likely when the second agent has a narrow therapeutic index. Increases in plasma levels of propranolol (Inderal) may occur during concurrent administration of fluvoxamine.

PAROXETINE

Paroxetine (Paxil) is a phenylpiperidine derivative that acts as a potent and selective-serotonin reuptake inhibitor. It is structurally unrelated to the other selective-serotonin reuptake inhibitors, with the most in vitro inhibition of serotonin reuptake in that class of drugs. Paroxetine has been shown to be effective in the treatment of depression and the treatment of anxiety and agitation associated with depression. Paroxetine has been shown to be as effective as tricyclic and other standard antidepressants in severely depressed outpatients. The molecular structure of paroxetine is given in Figure 25–1.

Pharmacological Actions

Paroxetine is well absorbed from the gastrointestinal tract. Absorption is unaffected by the presence or the absence of food or by the concurrent use of antacids.

After a single dose, maximum plasma concentrations are reached in approximately five hours. Steady-state concentrations are reached in 4 to 14 days after starting therapy or changing the dosage. Concentrations are elevated in patients with severe hepatic or renal disease. Paroxetine has lipophilic properties and has wide tissue distribution. It is estimated to be 95 percent protein-bound. The half-life is variable, with a mean of 24 hours; it is prolonged in the elderly. Paroxetine is almost completely metabolized in the liver to sulfate and glucuronide metabolites that are inactive. Those metabolites are excreted in both the urine and the feces; only 1 to 2 percent of a dose is excreted unchanged in the urine.

In vitro studies have shown paroxetine to be a more potent inhibitor than fluoxetine, fluvoxamine, or sertraline. It has a low affinity for α-adrenoreceptors, histamine type 1 (H_1), 5-hydroxytryptamine (5-HT_2), and dopamine type 2 (D_2) receptors, which results in a reduced tendency to cause autonomic and central nervous system side effects.

Indications

Paroxetine is as effective as the standard antidepressants in treating major depressive illness. Data indicate that paroxetine is effective in the long-term treatment of depressed patients and that it reduces the possibility of relapse in patients with a history of recurrent depression. Based on experiences with other antidepressants and the favorable side effect profile of paroxetine, the drug should be useful in the treatment of mild depressive episodes and dysthymia.

Paroxetine is also being studied in obsessive-compulsive disorder, other compulsive behaviors and panic.

Clinical Guidelines

The optimal dosage for most patients is 20 mg a day. Some patients may require higher dosages. Therapy should be initiated at 20 mg a day. An increase in the dosage should be considered for patients who do not show an adequate response in one to three weeks. At that point, upward dose titration in 10 mg increments at weekly intervals to a maximum of 50 mg a day can be initiated. Patients who experience gastrointestinal upset may benefit by taking the drug with food. Paroxetine should be taken as a single daily dose in the morning. Patients with melancholia may be likely to require doses greater than 20 mg a day. No differences in safety or efficacy have been shown in elderly and young patients. The suggested therapeutic dosage range for elderly patients is 20 to 40 mg a day, as they have been found to have higher mean plasma concentrations than do young adults. A lower starting dosage should be considered for debilitated patients. Paroxetine is available in 20 and 30 mg tablets. Compliance appears to be facilitated by the ability to give paroxetine in a single daily dose and by the fact that 20 mg is both the starting dose and the optimal dose for most patients.

Adverse Effects

The most commonly reported adverse effects of paroxetine are nausea, dry mouth, headache, somnolence, asthenia, insomnia, diarrhea, constipation, and tremor. Paroxetine has no effect on psychomotor skills and does not induce new anxiety symptoms. Side effects are usually mild and well tolerated. The drug does not lower the seizure threshold. It does not have the typical anticholinergic side effects that are associated with tricyclic antidepressants.

Paroxetine has no clinically significant cardiovascular effects, and it is relatively safe in overdose. It should be used with caution in patients with hepatic or renal disease. Its safe use in pregnancy has not been established. The drug has a similar adverse effect profile in both elderly and young patients. No clinically significant effects on cardiovascular variables, laboratory safety data, and vital signs have been reported when paroxetine is used by elderly patients.

Drug-Drug Interactions

At least two weeks should elapse between the use of paroxetine and MAOIs. The coadministration of paroxetine and phenytoin (Dilantin) may result in decreased plasma concentrations of paroxetine. Paroxetine appears to have no adverse psychomotor effects when used in combination with other CNS depressants, such as alcohol. Paroxetine has no significant interaction with digoxin and propranolol.

SERTRALINE

Sertraline (Zoloft) is a naphthylamino compound that is structurally unrelated to other available drugs with antidepressant activity. It has as few adverse effects as any other antidepressant drug in clinical use. However, because it is a new drug, information about its clinical use, adverse effects, and drug-drug interactions is incomplete. The molecular structure of sertraline is given in Figure 25–1.

Pharmacological Actions

Maximum plasma concentrations of sertraline occur about five to eight hours after an initial dose. Sertraline has an average plasma elimination half-life of 26 hours, which allows for once-daily dosing. Sertraline undergoes extensive first-pass metabolism. Less than 0.2 percent of unchanged sertraline is detected in the urine. The drug undergoes biotransformation through N-demethylation to form a primary amine. That desmethyl metabolite is substantially less active than sertraline. The pharmacokinetics of sertraline in patients with significant hepatic or renal dysfunction have not been determined. Sertraline clearance is approximately 40 percent less in the elderly than in younger patients. Steady-state plasma levels of sertraline should be achieved within seven days in young adults and after two to three weeks in elderly patients.

Sertraline is a potent inhibitor of serotonin reuptake, has only weak effects on norepinephrine and dopamine uptake, and has a negligible affinity for muscarinic, cholinergic, histaminergic, and α-adrenergic receptors. Because of the selective effect on central neurotransmission, sertraline has almost none of the adverse effects that are associated with tricyclic and tetracyclic antidepressants and monoamine oxidase inhibitors (MAOIs). In animal models, sertraline is about 14 times more potent than fluoxetine in enhancing serotonergic neurotransmission.

Indications

Depression. Sertraline is comparable to standard tricyclic agents in antidepressant efficacy. It is effective in patients with moderate or severe depression, those with or without melancholia, those with low or high anxiety, those with psychomotor agitation and psychomotor retardation, and those with or without insomnia. After an initial response, sertraline is effective when used as continuation therapy. Sertraline is also an effective antidepressant in elderly patients.

Other disorders. As a new drug, sertraline has been thoroughly studied only as an antidepressant. However, it may be useful in treating obsessive-compulsive disorder and panic disorder, in view of another serotonin-specific reuptake inhibitor's (fluoxetine's) use in those illnesses.

Clinical Guidelines

For the initial treatment of depression, sertraline should be initiated with a dosage of 50 mg once daily. Patients not responding to a 50 mg dose may benefit from dosage increases up to a maximum of 200 mg once daily. Given the elimination half-life of sertraline (about one day), dosage changes can be made, if necessary, at intervals of one week or more.

Sertraline can be administered once daily either in the morning or in the evening, without regard to meals. The therapeutic effect usually occurs two to four weeks after treatment is started. Care should be used in patients with renal or hepatic impairment. Sertraline is available in 50 and 100 mg tablets.

Adverse Effects

Compared with therapy with tricyclics, sertraline is associated with a significantly lower incidence of a number of anticholinergic, antihistaminergic, and antiadrenergic side effects. Side effects that occur with a significantly greater incidence with sertraline compared with tricyclics are insomnia, diarrhea, and nausea.

In therapeutic doses, sertraline has no clinically significant effect on the electrocardiogram (ECG) findings in patients with depressive illness. Although sertraline is not associated with cardiovascular side effects, it has not yet been used to any appreciable extent in patients with heart disease. Although sertraline has rarely been discontinued because of weight loss, significant weight loss may be an undesirable result of treatment for some patients.

It is recommended that sertraline not be used in combination with an MAOI. At least 14 days should elapse between the discontinuation of an MAOI and the initiation of treatment with sertraline. In addition, at least 14 days should elapse between the discontinuation of sertraline and the administration of an MAOI.

Sertraline has not been evaluated in patients with seizure disorders. As with other antidepressants, sertraline therapy should be initiated with care in epileptic patients. During clinical trials, three patients took overdoses of sertraline; all recovered completely.

Drug-Drug Interactions

Sertraline is tightly bound to plasma protein. The use with other drugs tightly bound to protein (for example, warfarin, digitoxin [Crystodigin]) may cause a shift in plasma concentrations, potentially resulting in an adverse effect. Adverse effects may also result from the displacement of protein-bound sertraline by other tightly bound drugs. Sertraline may increase prothombin time after dosing with warfarin. Accordingly, prothrombin time should be carefully monitored when sertraline therapy is initiated or stopped during warfarin therapy.

Sertraline does not significantly alter steady-state lithium levels or the renal clearance of lithium, but plasma lithium levels should be monitored after the initiation of sertraline therapy. Sertraline may decrease the clearance of tolbutamide. No clinical studies have established the risks or the benefits of the combined use of electroconvulsive therapy (ECT) and sertraline.

References

Boyer W F, Feighner J P: An overview of paroxetine. J Clin Psychiatry *53*: 3, 1992.

Ciraulo D A, Shader R I: Fluoxetine drug-drug interactions: I. Antidepressants and antipsychotics. J Clin Psychopharmacol *10*: 48, 1990.

Davis J M, Glassman A H: Antidepressant drugs. In *Comprehensive Textbook of Psychiatry*, ed 5, H I Kaplan, B J Sadock, editors, p 1627. Williams & Wilkins, Baltimore, 1989.

de Jonghe F, Swinkels J, Tuynman Qua H: Randomized double-blind study of fluvoxamine and maprotiline in treatment of depression. Pharmacopsychiatry *24*: 21, 1991.

Doogan D P, Caillard V: Sertraline: A new antidepressant. J Clin Psychiatry *49* (8, Suppl): 46, 1988.

Dunbar G C, Stoker M J: Paroxetine in the treatment of severe (melancholic) depression. Biol Psychiatry *25*: 55, 1991.

Fabre L F, Scharf M B, Itil T M: Comparative efficacy and safety of nortriptyline and fluoxetine in the treatment of major depression: A clinical study. J Clin Psychiatry *52* (6, Suppl): 62, 1991.

Feighner J P, Boyer W F: Paroxetine in the treatment of depression: A comparison with imipramine and placebo. J Clin Psychiatry *53*: 22, 1992.

Goff D C, Midha K K, Brotman A W, Waites M, Baldessarini R J: Elevation of plasma concentrations of haloperidol after the addition of fluoxetine. Am J Psychiatry *148*: 790, 1991.

Goodman W K, Price L H, Rasmussen S A, Heninger G R, Charney D S: Fluvoxamine as an antiobsessional agent. Psychopharmacol Bull *25*: 31, 1989.

Guthrie S K: Sertraline: A new specific serotonin reuptake blocker. DICP Ann Pharmacother *25*: 952, 1991.

Herman J B, Brotman A W, Pollack M H, Falk W E, Biederman J, Rosenbaum J F: Fluoxetine-induced sexual dysfunction. J Clin Psychiatry *51*: 25, 1990.

Heym J, Koe B K: Pharmacology of sertraline: A review. J Clin Psychiatry *49* (8, Suppl): 40, 1988.

Liebowitz M R, Hollander E, Schneier F, Campeas R, Hatterer J, Papp L, Fairbanks J, Sandberg D, Davies S, Stein M: Fluoxetine treatment of obsessive-compulsive disorder: An open clinical trial. J Clin Psychopharmacol *9*: 423, 1989.

Rickels K, Amsterdam J, Clary C: A placebo-controlled, double-blind, clinical trial of paroxetine in depressed outpatients. Acta Psychiatr *80*: 117, 1989.

Roth D, Mattes J, Sheehan K H, Sheehan D V: A double-blind comparison of fluvoxamine, desipramine and placebo in outpatients with depression. Prog Neuropsychopharmacol Biol Psychiatry *14*: 929, 1990.

Simpson S G, DePaulo J R: Fluoxetine treatment of bipolar II depression. J Clin Psychopharmacol *11*: 52, 1991.

Teicher M H, Glod C, Cole J O: Emergence of intense suicidal preoccupation during fluoxetine treatment. Am J Psychiatry *147*: 207, 1990.

26

Sympathomimetics

The sympathomimetic drugs used in psychiatry are dextroamphetamine (Dexedrine), methylphenidate (Ritalin), and pemoline (Cylert). Those drugs are also known as psychostimulants and analeptics. The sympathomimetics are approved for use in narcolepsy and attention-deficit hyperactivity disorder; the drugs are also sometimes used to treat depression. The molecular structure of methylphenidate is similar to that of amphetamine, whereas pemoline is unrelated to amphetamine (Figure 26–1).

PHARMACOLOGICAL ACTIONS

Dextroamphetamine is well absorbed from the gastrointestinal (GI) tract. Because it has a half-life of 8 to 12 hours, dextroamphetamine must be given two or three times a day. Dextroamphetamine is partially metabolized in the liver and partially excreted unchanged by the kidneys. Methylphenidate is well absorbed from the GI tract and reaches peak plasma levels in one to two hours. Because it has a short half-life of three to four hours, methylphenidate must be given three or four times a day. Methylphenidate is metabolized in the liver. Pemoline has the advantage of a long half-life and, therefore, can be given once daily.

The sympathomimetics are indirectly acting catecholamine stimulants. Amphetamine causes catecholamines, particularly dopamine, to be released from presynaptic neurons and also inhibits the reuptake of released catecholamines back into the presynaptic neurons. The net result is stimulation of several brain regions, particularly the ascending reticular activating system. Short-term use of the sympathomimetics induces a euphoric feeling; however, tolerance develops to both the euphoric feeling and the sympathomimetic activity. Tolerance does not develop to the therapeutic effects in attention-deficit hyperactivity disorder.

INDICATIONS

The major indications for sympathomimetics are attention-deficit hyperactivity disorder and narcolepsy. Sympathomimetics are an effective treatment in 70 to 80 percent of patients with attention-deficit hyperactivity disorder. Although methylphenidate is the most commonly used drug for that indication, dextroamphetamine is equally effective. The data on the efficacy of pemoline are somewhat less robust; however, some clinicians prefer to use pemoline because of its lower abuse potential. The symptoms of narcolepsy include excessive daytime sleepiness and transient, irresistible attacks of daytime sleep. Unfortunately, patients with narcolepsy, unlike patients with attention-deficit hyperactivity disorder, experience tolerance to the therapeutic effects of sympathomimetics.

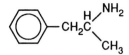

Dextroamphetamine

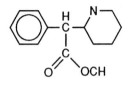

Methylphenidate

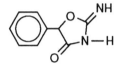

Pemoline

Figure 26–1. Molecular structures of sympathomimetics.

Sympathomimetics may be used to treat depression. Possible indications for their use include treatment-resistant depressions; depression in the elderly, who are at increased risk for adverse effects from tricyclic and tetracyclic antidepressants and monoamine oxidase inhibitors (MAOIs); depression in medically ill patients (especially acquired immune deficiency syndrome [AIDS] patients); and clinical situations in which a rapid response is important but for which electroconvulsive therapy (ECT) is contraindicated. Dextroamphetamine may be useful in differentiating pseudodementia of depression from dementia. A depressed patient generally responds to a 5 mg dose with increased alertness and improved cognition; a primarily demented patient responds with increased alertness and worsened cognition. Sympathomimetics usually provide only short-term benefit (two to four weeks) for depression, because tolerance to the antidepressant effects of the drugs develops rapidly in most patients. Long-term treatment of chronic depression with sympathomimetics has been useful in carefully monitored situations, although that use is controversial because of the abuse potential of the drugs.

Sympathomimetics were previously used in the treatment of obesity because of their anorexia-inducing effects. Because tolerance develops to the anorectic effects and because the drugs are associated with abuse, that treatment is no longer indicated.

CLINICAL GUIDELINES

Sympathomimetics are schedule II drugs and in some states require triplicate prescriptions. Many clinicians initiate treatment with pemoline, because it is associated with somewhat less abuse potential than either amphetamine or methylphenidate. Pretreatment evaluation should include an evaluation of cardiac function, with particular attention to the presence of hypertension or tachyarrhythmias. Patients should also be examined for the presence of movement disorders, such as tics and dyskinesias, because those conditions can be exacerbated by the administration of sympathomimetics. Liver function and renal function should be assessed, and dosages of sympathomimetics should be reduced if their metabolism is impaired. There is virtually no justifiable indication for the use of sympathomimetics during pregnancy. Dextroamphetamine and methylphenidate pass into the breast milk. It is not known whether pemoline passes into the breast milk. The dose ranges for sympathomimetics are given in Table 26–1.

When treating children for attention-deficit hyperactivity disorder, the clinician gives dextroamphetamine and methylphenidate at 8 AM and 12 noon. Pemoline is given at 8 AM. The dosage of dextroamphetamine is 2.5 to 40 mg a day up to 0.5 mg per kg a day. Methylphenidate is given in dosages of 10 to 60 mg a day up to 0.5 mg per kg a day. Pemoline is given in dosages of 37.5 to 112.5 mg daily. Liver function tests should be monitored when using pemoline. Children are more sensitive to side effects than are adults. The medications have not been studied specifically in elderly adults.

Many psychiatrists believe that amphetamine use has been overly regulated by governmental authorities. Amphetamines and narcotics are listed as schedule II drugs by the U.S. Drug Enforcement Agency. In addition, in New York State, for example, physicians must use triplicate prescriptions for such drugs, one copy of which is filed with a state government agency. Such mandates worry both patients and physicians about breaches in confidentiality; and physicians are concerned that their prescribing practices may be misinterpreted by official agencies. Consequently, some physicians may withhold amphetamines, even from a patient who may benefit from the medication.

The outstanding psychopharmacologist Donald Klein and associates in their 1980 book *Diagnosis and Drug Treatment of Psychiatric Disorders* (and reaffirmed in a personal communication [1990]) summarized the use of stimulant medication in the practice of psychiatry as follows:

> The use of stimulant medication, e.g., dextroamphetamine, methylphenidate, and magnesium pemoline, has been energetically discouraged in our present social climate, the reason being that such drugs may be abused, in common with cocaine, their illegal relative. In addition, there is the frightening possibility that prolonged use of stimulants in high doses may result in a paranoid psychosis or the exacerbation of a schizophrenic disorder. In view of these two considerations, it is not surprising that the prescription of these agents is attended by considerable anxiety and that many doctors simply refuse to use them. In certain jurisdictions, e.g., Sweden, they are outlawed.
>
> . . . Short-term use of stimulant medication is often of marked value in helping demoralized people to get going by overcoming their hampering appetitive inhibition. A daily dose of dextroamphetamine (5 to 15 mg) may

TABLE 26–1
Sympathomimetics

Generic Name	Trade Name	Preparations	Adult Starting Dose (mg a day)	Adult Average Daily Dose (mg)	Adult Maximum Daily Dose (mg)
Dextroamphetamine	Dexedrine	5, 10 mg tablets 5 mg per 5 mL elixer 5, 10, 15 mg sustained-release tablets	2.5–10	10–20	40
Methylphenidate	Ritalin	5, 10, 20 mg tablets 20 mg sustained-release tablets	5–10	20–30	60–80
Pemoline	Cylert	18.75, 37.5, 75 mg tablets 37.5 mg chewable tablet	18.75–37.5	56.25–75	112.5

enable a patient to start constructive activity, such as searching for a job or becoming socially active. . . .

A much more difficult question is whether chronic administration of stimulant medication is ever justified, in view of the risks of addiction and psychosis.

We have treated a number of patients who seem in chronically "low gear," have difficulty mustering energy and initiative, have a variety of neurasthenic complaints and, despite high intelligence, are underachievers, with chronic small doses of dextroamphetamine (5 to 15 mg) daily. The potential development of tolerance and dependence and the conceivable psychotogenic effects are thoroughly discussed with these patients, and the utilization of the medication is closely monitored. Strikingly, some have been able to maintain the use of amphetamines, at a level that has never exceeded 15 mg daily, for years. During this period their mood has remained consistently improved and their ability to muster energy and function effectively has been clearly benefited. They have been able to cease taking the medication on numerous occasions, such as during vacations, when a high level of focused attention was not necessary and the circumstances were rewarding, so that the mood-elevating effects were superfluous. Several of these patients have been switched from dextroamphetamine to a MAOI with good results.

ADVERSE EFFECTS

The most common adverse effects associated with sympathomimetics are anxiety, irritability, insomnia, and dysphoria. Sympathomimetics cause a decreased appetite, although tolerance develops to that effect. They can also cause an increase in heart rate and blood pressure and may cause palpitations. Less common adverse effects include the induction of movement disorders, such as tics, Tourette's disorderlike symptoms, and dyskinesias. In children, sympathomimetics may cause a transient suppression of growth. The most limiting adverse effect of sympathomimetics is their association with psychological and physical dependence. Sympathomimetics may exacerbate glaucoma, hypertension, cardiovascular disorders, hyperthyroidism, anxiety disorders, psychotic illnesses, and seizure disorders.

High doses of sympathomimetics can cause dry mouth, pupillary dilation, bruxism, formication, and emotional lability. Long-term use of high dosages can cause a delusional disorder that can be indistinguishable from paranoid schizophrenia. Overdoses of sympathomimetics present with hypertension, tachycardia, hyperthermia, toxic psychosis, delirium, and occasionally seizures. Overdoses of sympathomimetics can also result in death. Seizures can be treated with benzodiazepines, cardiac effects with propranolol (Inderal), fever with cooling blankets, and delirium with dopamine receptor antagonists. The treatment of common adverse effects in attention-deficit hyperactivity disorder are given in Table 26–2.

DRUG-DRUG INTERACTIONS

The coadministration of sympathomimetics with tricyclic or tetracyclic antidepressants, warfarin (Coumadin), primidone (Mysoline), phenobarbital, phenytoin (Dilantin), or phenylbutazone (Butazolidin) decreases the metabolism of those

TABLE 26–2
Management of Common Stimulant-Induced Adverse Effects in Attention-Deficit Hyperactivity Disorder

Adverse Effect	Management
Anorexia, nausea, weight loss	• Administer stimulant with meals. • Use caloric-enhanced supplements. Discourage forcing meals. • If using pemoline, check liver function tests.
Insomnia, nightmares	• Administer stimulants earlier in day. • Change to short-acting preparations. • Discontinue afternoon or evening dosing. • Consider adjunctive treatment (e.g., antihistamines, clonidine, antidepressants).
Dizziness	• Monitor blood pressure. • Encourage fluid intake. • Change to long-acting form.
Rebound phenomena	• Overlap stimulant dosing. • Change to long-acting preparation or combine long- and short-acting preparations. • Consider adjunctive or alternative treatment (e.g., clonidine, antidepressants).
Irritability	• Assess timing of phenomena (during peak or withdrawal phase). • Evaluate comorbid symptoms. • Reduce dose. • Consider adjunctive or alternative treatment (e.g., lithium, antidepressants, anticonvulsants).
Growth impairment	• Attempt weekend and vacation holidays. • If severe, consider nonstimulant treatment.
Dysphoria, moodiness, agitation	• Consider comorbid diagnosis (e.g., mood disorder). • Reduce dose or change to long-acting preparation. • Consider adjunctive or alternative treatment (e.g., lithium, anticonvulsants, antidepressants).

Table from T E Wilens, J Biederman: The stimulants. In *The Psychiatric Clinics of North America: Pediatric Psychopharmacology*, D Shaffer, editor. Saunders, Philadelphia, 1992. Used with permission.

compounds, resulting in increased plasma levels. Sympathomimetics decrease the therapeutic efficacy of many hypertensives, especially guanethidine (Esimil, Ismelin). Methylphenidate should be used with caution in patients treated with MAOIs. Amphetamines should not be used during treatment with MAOIs or within two weeks of taking MAOIs.

References

Aaron C K: Sympathomimetics. Emerg Med Clin North Am *8*: 513, 1990.
Campbell M: Pharmacotherapy. In *Comprehensive Textbook of Psychiatry*, ed 5, H I Kaplan, B J Sadock, editors, p 1933. Williams & Wilkins, Baltimore, 1989.
Chirarello R J, Cole J O: The use of psychostimulants in general psychiatry: A reconsideration. Arch Gen Psychiatry *44*: 286, 1987.
Fawcett J, Kravitz H M, Zajecka J M, Schaff M R: CNS stimulant potentiation of monoamine oxidase inhibitors in treatment-refractory depression. J Clin Psychopharmacol *11*: 127, 1991.
Harvey J A: Behavioral pharmacology of central nervous system stimulants. Neuropharmacology *26*: 887, 1987.
Lingam V R, Lazarus L W, Groves L, Oh S H: Methylphenidate in treating poststroke depression. J Clin Psychiatry *49*: 151, 1988.

Rosenberg P B, Ahmed I, Hurwitz S: Methylphenidate in depressed medically ill patients. J Clin Psychiatry *52*: 263, 1991.

Sallee F R, Stiller R L, Perel J M: Pharmacodynamics of pemoline in attention deficit disorder with hyperactivity. J Am Acad Child Adolesc Psychiatry *31*: 244, 1992.

Satel S L, Nelson J C: Stimulants in the treatment of depression: A critical overview. J Clin Psychiatry *50*: 241, 1989.

27

Thyroid Hormones

Thyroid hormones (Figure 27–1) are used in psychiatry as adjuvants to antidepressants, often in an attempt to convert an antidepressant-nonresponsive patient into an antidepressant-responsive patient. The most commonly used thyroid hormone is L-triiodothyronine (T_3 or liothyronine) (Cytomel); thyroxine (T_4 or levothyroxine) (Levoxine, Levothroid, Synthroid) is also sometimes used for the same purpose. Endogenous thyroxine and exogenous thyroxine are converted into triiodothyronine in the body.

PHARMACOLOGICAL ACTIONS

Thyroid hormones are administered orally, and their absorption from the gastrointestinal (GI) tract is variable. Absorption is increased if the drug is administered while the patient's stomach is empty. The half-life of thyroxine is six to seven days, and the half-life of triiodothyronine is one to two days. The mechanism of action for thyroid hormone effects on antidepressant efficacy is unknown, although interactions with the β-adrenergic receptors have been hypothesized.

INDICATIONS AND CLINICAL GUIDELINES

The major indication for thyroid hormones in psychiatry is as an adjuvant to antidepressants. There is no correlation between the laboratory measures of thyroid function and the response to thyroid hormone supplementation of antidepressants. If a patient has been nonresponsive to a six-week course of antidepressants at appropriate dosages, adjuvant therapy with either lithium (Eskalith) or a thyroid hormone is an alternative. Most clinicians use adjuvant lithium before trying a thyroid hormone. The available clinical data suggest that triiodothyronine is more effective than thyroxine. Although several controlled trials have indicated that the use of triiodothyronine converts 33 to 75 percent of antidepressant nonresponders to responders, several other studies have failed to support that finding.

The dosage of triiodothyronine is 25 or 50 μg a day added to the patient's antidepressant regimen. Triiodothyronine has been used as an adjuvant for all the tricyclic and tetracyclic antidepressants, the monoamine oxidase inhibitors (MAOIs), and trazodone (Desyrel). Clinical data regarding its use with either bupropion (Wellbutrin) or fluoxetine (Prozac) are very limited. An adequate trial of triiodothyronine supplementation should last 7 to 14 days. If triiodothyronine supplementation is successful, it should be continued for two months, then tapered at the rate of 12.5 μg a day every three to seven days.

Thyroid hormones have not been shown to cause particular problems in pediatric

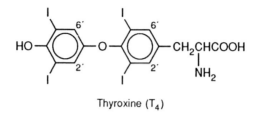

Thyroxine (T$_4$)

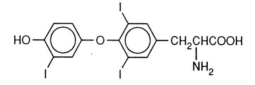

L-Triiodothyronine (T$_3$)

Figure 27–1. Molecular structures of the thyroid hormones.

or geriatric patients; however, the hormones should be used with caution in the elderly, who may have occult heart disease.

Triiodothyronine is available in 5, 25, and 50 μg tablets. Thyroxine is available in 12.5, 25, 50, 75, 88, 100, 112, 125, 150, 175, 200, and 300 μg tablets; it is also available in a 200 and 500 μg parenteral form.

ADVERSE EFFECTS

Thyroid hormones should not be administered to patients with cardiac disease, angina, or hypertension. The hormones are contraindicated in thyrotoxicosis and uncorrected adrenal insufficiency and in patients with acute myocardial infarctions. Thyroid hormones can be administered safely to pregnant women, because the thyroid hormones do not cross the placenta. Thyroid hormones are minimally excreted in the breast milk and have not been shown to cause problems in nursing babies. The most common adverse effects associated with thyroid hormones are weight loss, palpitations, nervousness, diarrhea, abdominal cramps, sweating, tachycardia, increased pulse and blood pressure, tremors, headache, and insomnia. Osteoporosis may also occur. Overdoses can lead to cardiac failure and death.

DRUG-DRUG INTERACTIONS

Thyroid hormones can potentiate the effects of warfarin (Coumadin) and other anticoagulants by increasing the catabolism of clotting factors. Thyroid hormones may increase the insulin requirement for diabetic patients. Sympathomimetics and thyroid hormones should not be coadministered because of the risk of cardiac decompensation.

References

Bauer M S, Whybrow P C: Rapid cycling bipolar affective disorder: II. Treatment of refractory rapid cycling with high-dose levothyroxine: A preliminary study. Arch Gen Psychiatry *47*: 435, 1990.

Joffe R T: Triiodothyronine potentiation of fluoxetine in depressed patients. Can J Psychiatry *37*: 48, 1992.

Joffe R T: Triiodothyronine potentiation of the antidepressant effect of phenelzine. J Clin Psychiatry *49*: 409, 1988.

Kaplan P M, Boggiano W E: Anticonvulsants, noradrenergic drugs, and other organic therapies. In *Comprehensive Textbook of Psychiatry*, ed 5, H I Kaplan, B J Sadock, editors, p 1681. Williams & Wilkins, Baltimore, 1989.

Stein D, Anvi A: Thyroid hormones in the treatment of affective disorders. Acta Psychiatr Scand *77*: 623, 1988.

Thase M E, Kupfer D K, Jarrett D B: Treatment of imipramine-resistant recurrent depression: I. An open clinical trial of adjunctive L-triiodothyronine. J Clin Psychiatry *50*: 385, 1989.

28

Trazodone

Trazodone (Desyrel) is a triazolopyridine derivative that is used primarily for the treatment of depression (Figure 28–1). Trazodone shares the triazolo ring structure with alprazolam (Xanax), a benzodiazepine with possible antidepressant effects. Trazodone is structurally unrelated to the tricyclic antidepressants, tetracyclic antidepressants, and monoamine oxidase inhibitors (MAOIs). It differs from those other antidepressants in having almost no anticholinergic adverse effects.

PHARMACOLOGICAL ACTIONS

Trazodone is readily absorbed from the gastrointestinal (GI) tract, reaches peak plasma levels in one to two hours, and has a half-life of 6 to 11 hours. Trazodone is metabolized in the liver, and 75 percent of its metabolites are excreted in the urine.

Trazodone has its therapeutic effects as a specific inhibitor of serotonin reuptake. One active metabolite of trazodone, m-chlorophenyl-piperazine, also possesses some postsynaptic serotonin agonist activity. The adverse effects of trazodone are partially mediated by α_1-adrenergic antagonism and antihistaminergic activity.

INDICATIONS

The primary indication for the use of trazodone is major depression. Trazodone is as effective as standard antidepressants in the short-term and long-term treatment of major depression. Trazodone is particularly effective at improving sleep quality. Trazodone increases total sleep time, decreases the number and the duration of nighttime awakenings, and decreases rapid eye movement (REM) sleep amount. Unlike tricyclic antidepressants, trazodone does not decrease stage 4 sleep.

There are a few case reports and uncontrolled trials of trazodone for the treatment of depression with marked anxiety symptoms and for panic disorder and agoraphobia. Final evaluation of the use of trazodone for those disorders requires further clinical research.

Trazodone may be useful in low dosages for controlling severe agitation in elderly patients. Preliminary reports have evaluated the use of low doses, 25 to 75 mg, of trazodone as a hypnotic. Those reports have found that the drug is effective for that indication and can be of use for patients taking nonsedating psychotropic drugs.

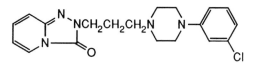

Figure 28–1. Molecular structure of trazodone.

CLINICAL GUIDELINES

Trazodone is available in tablets that can be divided into 50, 100, 150, and 300 mg amounts. The usual starting dose is 50 mg orally (PO) the first day. That dose can be increased to 50 mg PO twice daily on the second day and possibly 50 mg PO three times daily on the third or fourth day if there are no problems with sedation or orthostatic hypotension. The therapeutic range for trazodone is 200 to 600 mg a day in divided doses. Some reports indicate that dosages of 400 to 600 mg a day are required for maximal therapeutic effects; other reports suggest that 300 to 400 mg a day is sufficient. The dosage may be titrated up to 300 mg a day and then evaluated for the need for further dosage increases on the basis of the presence or the absence of signs of clinical improvement. Elderly adults are more sensitive to side effects than are younger adults. Trazodone has not been studied in children.

ADVERSE EFFECTS

The most common adverse effects associated with trazodone are sedation, orthostatic hypotension, dizziness, headache, and nausea. As a result of α-adrenergic blockade, dry mouth is present in some patients. Trazodone may cause gastric irritation. Trazodone is not associated with the usual anticholinergic adverse effects, such as urinary retention and constipation. There have been no reported fatalities from trazodone overdoses when the drug was taken alone; however, there have been fatalities when trazodone was taken with other drugs. Symptoms of an overdose include loss of muscle coordination, nausea and vomiting, and drowsiness. Trazodone does not have the quinidinelike antiarrhythmic effects of imipramine (Tofranil). There have been a few case reports of an association between trazodone and arrhythmias in patients with preexisting premature ventricular contractions or mitral valve prolapse. The use of trazodone is contraindicated in pregnant and nursing women. Trazodone should be used with caution in patients with hepatic and renal diseases.

Trazodone is associated with the rare occurrence of priapism, the symptom of prolonged erection in the absence of sexual stimuli. Patients should be advised to report if erections are gradually becoming more frequent or prolonged; in such cases physicians should consider another antidepressant medication. Untreated priapism can lead to impotence. A patient who has priapism while taking trazodone should stop taking the drug and consult a physician immediately. One effective treatment for priapism involves the intracavernosal injection of a 1 μg per mL solution of epinephrine (an α-adrenergic agonist). Other forms of sexual dysfunction may occur with trazodone.

DRUG-DRUG INTERACTIONS

Trazodone has been reported to be useful in treating fluoxetine (Prozac)-induced insomnia. The usual dose range is 50 to 100 mg at bedtime. Fluoxetine raises trazodone levels. Trazodone potentiates the central nervous system depressant effects of other centrally acting drugs and alcohol. The combination of monoamine oxidase inhibitors and trazodone should be avoided. Concurrent use of trazodone and antihypertensives may cause hypotension. Electroconvulsive therapy (ECT) concurrent with trazodone administration should be avoided.

References

Beasley C M Jr, Dornseif B E, Pultz J A, Bosomworth J C, Sayler M E: Fluoxetine versus trazodone: Efficacy and activating-sedating effects. J Clin Psychiatry 52: 294, 1991.

Bryant S G, Hokanson J A, Brown C S: A drug utilization review of prescribing patterns for trazodone versus amitriptyline. J Clin Psychiatry 51:(9, Suppl): 27, 1990.

Davis J M, Glassman A H: Antidepressant drugs. In Comprehensive Textbook of Psychiatry, ed 5, H I Kaplan, B J Sadock, editors, p 1627. Williams & Wilkins, Baltimore, 1989.

Fabre L F, Feighner J P: Long-term therapy for depression with trazodone. J Clin Psychiatry 44: 17, 1983.

Greenblatt D J, Friedman H, Burstein E S, Scavone J M, Blyden G T, Ochs H R, Miller L G, Harmatz J S, Shader R I: Trazodone kinetics: Effects of age, gender, and obesity. Clin Pharmacol Ther 42: 193, 1987.

Himmelhoch J M: Cardiovascular effects of trazodone in humans. J Clin Psychopharmacol 1(6, Suppl): 76S, 1981.

Mouret J, Lemoine P, Minuit M P, Benkelfat C, Renardet M: Effects of trazodone on the sleep of depressed subjects: A polygraphic study. Psychopharmacology 95: S37, 1988.

Nierenberg A: Possible trazodone potentiation of fluoxetine: A case series. J Clin Psychiatry 53: 83, 1992.

Sakulscripong M, Curran H V, Lader M: Does tolerance develop to the sedative and amnesic effects of antidepressants? A comparison of amitryptiline, trazodone and placebo. Eur J Clin Pharmacol 40: 43, 1991.

Scharf M B, editor: Insights in the use of trazodone in depressed patients. J Clin Psychiatry 51(9, Suppl): 2, 1990.

Thompson J W Jr, Ware M R, Blashfield R K: Psychotropic medication and priapism: A comprehensive review. J Clin Psychiatry 51: 430, 1990.

29

Tricyclics and Tetracyclics

The tricyclic antidepressants (also known as the tricyclics) and the monoamine oxidase inhibitors (MAOIs) are often considered the classic antidepressant drugs. The indications for the drugs, however, have expanded beyond depression to include anxiety disorders, eating disorders, and chronic pain syndromes. The tricyclic antidepressants share many pharmacokinetic and pharmacodynamic properties and similar adverse effect profiles. Three tetracyclic drugs were initially introduced as being significantly different from the tricyclics. Further study and clinical use have demonstrated that the tetracyclic and tricyclic drugs can best be conceptualized as one family of drugs. The heterocyclic antidepressants generally include the monocyclic, dicyclic, tricyclic, and tetracyclic antidepressants. The term "heterocyclic antidepressant" is not used in this textbook because it is an overinclusive classification for a diverse group of drugs with no single side effect profile or therapeutic profile.

For the treatment of depression, the drugs available as alternatives to the tricyclics and tetracyclics include the MAOIs (Chapter 24), serotonin-specific reuptake inhibitors (Chapter 25), trazodone (Desyrel) (Chapter 28), bupropion (Wellbutrin) (Chapter 9), and the sympathomimetics (Chapter 26).

CLASSIFICATION

All tricyclics have a three-ring nucleus in their molecular structures (Figure 29–1). Imipramine (Tofranil), amitriptyline (Elavil), clomipramine (Anafranil), trimipramine (Surmontil), and doxepin (Adapin, Sinequan) are called *tertiary amines*, because there are two methyl groups on the nitrogen atom of the side chain. Desipramine (Norpramin, Pertofrane), nortriptyline (Pamelor, Aventyl), and protriptyline (Vivactil) are called *secondary amines*, because there is only one methyl group in that position. The tertiary amines are metabolized into their corresponding secondary amines in the body.

The classification of tetracyclic is somewhat arbitrarily based on a gross count of the number of rings in the molecular structure. Amoxapine (Asendin), actually a dibenzoxazepine, is a derivative of the antipsychotic drug loxapine (Loxitane) and has a cyclic side chain off the three-ring nucleus, for a total of four rings. Maprotiline (Ludiomil) is a tetracyclic with the same side chain as desipramine; its fourth ring actually bridges the center of the standard tricyclic nucleus. Mianserin is a tetracyclic drug whose side chain has been cyclicized to form a fourth ring; mianserin is not currently available for clinical use in the United States.

PHARMACOLOGICAL ACTIONS

Pharmacokinetics

Absorption from oral administration of most tricyclics and tetracyclics is incomplete, and there is a significant metabolism from the first-pass effect. Imipramine pamoate is a depot form of the drug for intramuscular (IM) administration; indications for the use of the preparation are limited. Protein binding is usually over 75 percent; the lipid solubility is quite high; and the volume of distribution ranges from 10 to 30 L per kg for tertiary amines to 20 to 60 L per kg for secondary amines. The tertiary amines are demethylated to form the related secondary amines. The ratio of methylated to demethylated forms varies widely from person to person. The tricyclic nucleus is oxidized in the liver, conjugated with glucuronic acid, and excreted. The 7-hydroxymetabolite of amoxapine has potent dopamine-blocking activity, thus causing the antipsychoticlike neurological and endocrinological adverse effects that are seen with the drug. The half-lives vary from 10 to 70 hours, although nortriptyline, maprotiline, and particularly protriptyline can have longer half-lives. The long half-lives allow for all the compounds to be given once daily and means that five to seven days are needed to reach steady-state plasma levels.

Pharmacodynamics

The short-term effects of tricyclics and tetracyclics are to reduce the reuptake of norepinephrine and serotonin and to block muscarinic acetylcholine and histamine receptors. The different tricyclics and tetracyclics vary in their pharmacodynamic effects (Table 29–1). Amoxapine, nortriptyline, desipramine, and maprotiline have the least anticholinergic activity, and doxepin has the most antihistaminergic activity. Clomipramine is the most serotonin-selective of the tricyclics and tetracyclics. The reuptake blockade of norepinephrine and serotonin by the drugs and the monoamine oxidase inhibition by the MAOIs led to the development of the monoamine hypothesis of mood disorders. Long-term administration of tricyclics and tetracyclics results in a decrease in the number of β-adrenergic receptors and, perhaps, a similar decrease in the number of serotonin type 2 receptors. That down-regulation of receptors after repeated administration most closely correlates with the time that clinical effects appear in patients. The down-regulation of β-adrenergic receptors occurs whether the initial effect is blocking noradrenergic or serotonin receptors. Research with animals has demonstrated, however, that intact noradrenergic and serotonergic systems are required for the down-regulation to occur.

INDICATIONS

Major Depressive Episode

A major depressive episode in both major depression patients and bipolar disorder patients is the principal indication for using tricyclic and tetracyclic drugs.

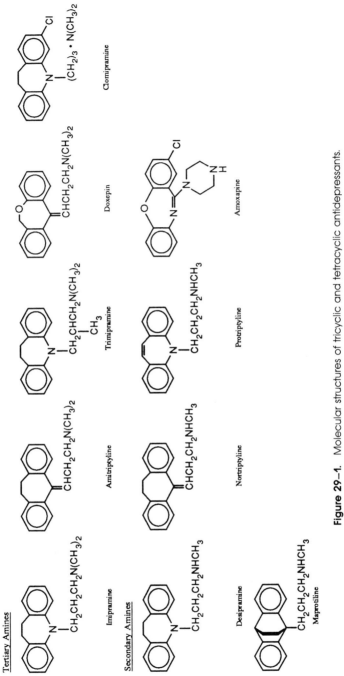

Figure 29–4. Molecular structures of tricyclic and tetracyclic antidepressants.

TABLE 29–1
Neurotransmitter Effects of Tricyclic and Tetracyclic Antidepressants

	Reuptake Blockade		Receptor Blockade		
	NE	5-HT	Muscarinic ACh	H_1	H_2
Imipramine	+	+	+ +	±	±
Desipramine	+ + +	±	±	−	−
Trimipramine	±	±	+ +	+ +	?
Amitriptyline	±	+ +	+ + +	+ +	+ +
Nortriptyline	+ +	±	+	±	±
Protriptyline	+ + +	±	+	+ + +	−
Amoxapine	+ +	±	+	±	?
Doxepin	+	±	+ +	+ + +	+
Maprotiline	+ + +	−	+	±	?
Clomipramine	±	+ +	+	?	?

Symptoms of melancholia and prior episodes of depression increase the likelihood of a therapeutic response.

Secondary Depression

Depressions associated with organic syndromes may respond to tricyclic and tetracyclic drugs. They include depressions after cerebrovascular disorders and central nervous system (CNS) trauma and the depressive symptoms seen in some dementias and movement disorders, such as Parkinson's disease. Depression associated with acquired immune deficiency syndrome (AIDS) may also respond to the drugs.

Panic Disorder with Agoraphobia

Imipramine has been the tricyclic most studied for panic disorder with agoraphobia, although other tricyclics are also effective. Early reports suggested that small dosages of imipramine (50 mg a day) were often effective; however, recent studies indicate that the usual antidepressant dosages are usually required.

Generalized Anxiety Disorder

The use of doxepin for the treatment of anxiety is approved by the Food and Drug Administration (FDA). Some research data show that imipramine may also be useful, and some clinicians use a drug containing a combination of chlordiazepoxide and amitriptyline (marketed as Limbitrol) for mixed anxiety and depressive disorders.

Obsessive-Compulsive Disorder

Obsessive-compulsive disorder is classified under the anxiety disorders in the revised third edition of *Diagnostic and Statistical Manual of Mental Disorders* (DSM-III-R) and appears to respond somewhat specifically to clomipramine. It does not appear that any of the other tricyclics and tetracyclics are nearly as effective as clomipramine.

Eating Disorders

Both anorexia nervosa and bulimia nervosa have been successfully treated with imipramine and desipramine, although other tricyclics and tetracyclics may also be effective.

Pain

Chronic pain syndromes, including headaches (such as migraines), are often treated with tricyclics and tetracyclics.

Other Syndromes

Childhood enuresis is often treated with imipramine. Peptic ulcer disease, a psychosomatic condition, can be treated with doxepin, which has marked anti-histaminergic effects. Other indications for tricyclics and tetracyclics are narcolepsy, nightmares, and posttraumatic stress disorder. The drugs are sometimes used in children or adolescents with attention-deficit hyperactivity disorder, somnambulism, separation anxiety disorder, sleep terror disorder, eating disorders, and major depression.

CLINICAL GUIDELINES

Choice of Drug

The specific choice of which tricyclic or tetracyclic to use should be based on the general guidelines outlined in Chapter 1. All available tricyclic and tetracyclic drugs have been demonstrated to be equally effective in the treatment of depression. In the case of an individual patient, however, one tricyclic or tetracyclic may be effective, whereas another one may be ineffective. The adverse effects of the tricyclic and tetracyclic drugs differ (Table 29–2). The tertiary amine tricyclics tend to produce more adverse effects—including sedation, orthostatic hypotension, and anticholinergic effects (such as dry mouth)—whereas the secondary amines tend to produce fewer of those adverse effects. Among the secondary amine tricyclics, nortriptyline is associated with the least orthostatic hypotension, and desipramine is associated with the least anticholinergic activity. Among the tetracyclic drugs, amoxapine is sometimes recommended for the treatment of major depression with psychotic features because of its antidopaminergic activity.

Researchers have demonstrated differences among the tricyclics and tetracyclics in their relative ability to block either serotonin reuptake or norepinephrine reuptake. No study has demonstrated that the serotonin-to-norepinephrine ratio for each of the drugs can be used to help choose a specific drug to treat a particular patient. It is perhaps reasonable to switch from a strongly serotonergic drug to a strongly

TABLE 29–2
Side Effect Profile of Tricyclic and Tetracyclic Antidepressants

	Anticholinergic Effects	Sedation	Orthostatic Hypotension	Seizures	Conduction Abnormalities
Tertiary amines					
Amitriptyline	+ + + +	+ + + +	+ + +	+ + +	+ + + +
Clomipramine	+ + + +	+ + + +	+ + +	+ + +	+ + + +
Doxepin	+ + +	+ + + +	+ +	+ + +	+ +
Imipramine	+ + +	+ + +	+ + + +	+ + +	+ + + +
Trimipramine	+ + + +	+ + + +	+ + +	+ + +	+ + + +
Secondary amines					
Desipramine	+ +	+ +	+ + +	+ +	+ + +
Nortriptyline	+ + +	+ + +	+	+ +	+ + +
Protriptyline	+ + +	+	+ +	+ +	+ + + +
Tetracyclic					
Amoxapine	+ + +	+ +	+	+ + +	+ +
Maprotiline	+ + +	+ + +	+ +	+ + + +	+ + +

+ + + +, high; + + +, moderate; + +, low; +, very low.

noradrenergic drug or vice versa if the first drug is ineffective in relieving the patient's symptoms.

Clomipramine. Clomipramine is an effective antidepressant that is also the first-line drug in the treatment of obsessive-compulsive disorder and, therefore, may be the drug of choice for depressed patients with marked obsessive features. Clomipramine has its major effect as an inhibitor of serotonin reuptake but may also affect dopaminergic neurotransmission. Clomipramine has been shown to be more effective than a placebo, amitriptyline, imipramine, and doxepin in the treatment of obsessive-compulsive disorder. Several initial studies have shown that fluoxetine (Prozac) and possibly other serotonin-specific reuptake blockers may have as much efficacy as clomipramine in the treatment of obsessive-compulsive disorder. Improvement is usually seen in two to four weeks, but improvement may continue for the first four to five months of treatment. Similar to the standard tricyclic and tetracyclic drugs, clomipramine may also be effective in the treatment of panic attacks, phobias, and chronic pain.

Initiation of Treatment

A routine physical and laboratory examination of a patient to be administered tricyclics or tetracyclics should be conducted. The routine laboratory tests include a complete blood count (CBC) with differential, a white blood cell count (WBC), and serum electrolytes (SMA-6) with liver function tests (SMA-12). An electrocardiogram (ECG) should probably be obtained for all patients, especially women over 40 and men over 30. The initial dose should be small and should be raised gradually. The clinician can raise the dosage for inpatients more quickly than for outpatients because of the inpatients' closer clinical supervision.

It should be explained to patients that, although sleep and appetite may improve in one to two weeks, tricyclics and tetracyclics usually take three to four weeks to have antidepressant effects, and a complete trial should last six weeks. It may be important to explain to some patients what the drug treatment plan will entail if there is no clinical response at that time.

TABLE 29–3
Clinical Information for the Tricyclic and Tetracyclic Antidepressants

Generic Name	Trade Name	Usual Adult Dose Range (mg a day)	Therapeutic Plasma Levels* (μg per mL)
Imipramine	Tofranil	150–300†	150–300
Desipramine	Norpramin, Pertofrane	150–300†	150–300
Trimipramine	Surmontil	150–300†	?
Amitriptyline	Elavil, Endep	150–300†	100–250†
Nortriptyline	Pamelor, Aventyl	50–150	50–150 (maximum)
Protriptyline	Vivactil	15–60	75–250
Amoxapine	Asendin	150–400	?
Doxepin	Adapin, Sinequan	150–300†	100–250
Maprotiline	Ludiomil	150–225	150–300
Clomipramine	Anafranil	150–250	?

*Exact range may vary among laboratories.
†Includes parent compound and desmethyl metabolite.

The elderly and children are more sensitive to antidepressant side effects than are young adults. In children, ECG monitoring is needed. A baseline electroencephalogram (EEG) is recommended, as children are sensitive to the epileptogenic effects of antidepressants and are prone to medication-induced constipation.

Dosage

Imipramine, amitriptyline, doxepin, desipramine, clomipramine, and trimipramine can be started at 75 mg a day. Divided doses at first reduce the severity of the side effects, although most of the dosage should be given at night to help induce sleep if a sedating drug, such as amitriptyline, is used. Eventually, the entire dosage can be given at bedtime. Protriptyline and less-sedating drugs should be given not less than two to three hours before a patient goes to sleep. For outpatients the dosage can be raised to 150 mg a day the second week, 225 mg a day the third week, and 300 mg a day the fourth week. A common clinical mistake is to stop increasing the dosage when the patient is taking less than 250 mg a day and does not show clinical improvement. Doing so can result in a further delay in obtaining a therapeutic response, disenchantment with the treatment, and even premature discontinuation of the drug. The clinician should routinely assess the patient's baseline pulse and postural hypotension while the dosage is being raised.

Other tricyclics and tetracyclics have different guidelines for dosage. Nortriptyline should be started at 50 mg a day and raised to 150 mg a day over three or four weeks unless a response occurs at a lower dosage, such as 100 mg. Amoxapine should be started at 150 mg a day and raised to 400 mg a day. Protriptyline should be started at 15 mg a day and raised to 60 mg a day. Maprotiline has been associated with an increased incidence of seizures if the dosage is raised too quickly or is maintained at too high a level. Maprotiline should be started at 75 mg a day and maintained at that level for two weeks. The dosage can be increased over four weeks to 225 mg a day but should be kept at that level for only six weeks and then reduced to 175 to 200 mg a day (Table 29–3).

Panic disorder patients may be particularly sensitive to side effects when tricyclics are started. Therefore, it may be prudent to begin with low dosages that

TABLE 29–4
Tricyclic and Tetracyclic Antidepressant Preparations

	Tablets	Capsules	Parenteral	Solution
Imipramine	10, 25, 50 mg	75, 100, 125, 150 mg	12.5 mg/mL	—
Desipramine	10, 25, 50, 75, 100, 150 mg	25, 50 mg	—	—
Trimipramine	—	25, 50, 100 mg	—	—
Amitriptyline	10, 25, 50, 75, 100, 150 mg	—	10 mg/mL	—
Nortriptyline	—	10, 25, 50, 75 mg	—	10 mg/5 mL
Protriptyline	5, 10 mg	—	—	—
Amoxapine	25, 50, 100, 150 mg	—	—	—
Doxepin	—	10, 25, 50, 75, 100, 150 mg	—	10 mg/mL
Maprotiline	25, 50, 75 mg	—	—	—
Clomipramine	—	25, 50, 75 mg	—	—

are raised in small increments. Some clinicians coadminister benzodiazepines until the patients are stabilized on an antidepressant.

In children, imipramine can be initiated at 1.5 mg per kg a day. The dosage can be titrated to not more than 5 mg per kg a day. In functional enuresis the dosage is usually 50 to 100 mg taken at bedtime. Clomipramine can be initiated at 50 mg a day and increased to not more than 3 mg per kg a day or 200 mg a day.

The available preparations of tricyclic and tetracyclic antidepressants are given in Table 29–4.

Failure of Drug Trial and Treatment-Resistant Depression

If a tricyclic or tetracyclic has been used for four weeks at maximal dosages without a therapeutic effect, the clinician should obtain a plasma level and adjust the dosage accordingly. If plasma levels are adequate, supplementation with lithium or L-triiodothyronine (T_3) (Cytomel) should be considered.

Lithium. Lithium (Eskalith) (900 to 1,200 mg a day, serum level between 0.6 and 0.8 mEq per L) can be added to the tricyclic or tetracyclic dosage for 7 to 14 days. That approach converts a significant number of nonresponders into responders. The mechanism of action is not known, although it has been hypothesized that the lithium potentiates the serotonergic neuronal system.

L-Triiodothyronine. The addition of 25 to 50 μg a day of T_3 to the regimen for 7 to 14 days may convert tricyclic and tetracyclic nonresponders into responders. The adverse effects of T_3 are minor but may include a headache and feeling warm. The mechanism of action for T_3 augmentation is not known. Empirical data suggest that T_3 is more effective than thyroxine (T_4) as an adjunct to tricyclic and tetracyclic antidepressants. If T_3 augmentation is successful, the T_3 should be continued for two months and then tapered at the rate of 12.5 μg a day every three to seven days.

Buspirone. Augmentation of tricyclics with 30 mg a day of buspirone (BuSpar) has also been reported to convert nonresponders into responders.

MAOIs. MAOIs should be discontinued for two weeks before initiating treatment with a tricyclic. A minimum of a one-week washout is needed when switching from a tricyclic to an MAOI. Both classes of drugs are sometimes used in combination for resistant depressions. Certain precautions must be taken to avoid hypermetabolic crisis. Desipramine, imipramine, clomipramine, and tranylcypromine (Parnate) are to be avoided. A low dose of a tricyclic should be initiated after at least a one-week washout. The MAOI is then added. Every few days each medication is alternately increased while the patient is carefully monitored.

Maintenance

Tricyclics and tetracyclics effectively resolve the acute symptoms of depression. If treatment is stopped prematurely, symptom reemergence is likely to occur. To minimize the risk of recurrence or relapse, the clinician should continue tricyclics and tetracyclics at the acute-treatment dosage throughout the course of treatment. When treatment is discontinued, the clinician may reasonably reduce the dosage to three fourths the maximal dosage for another month. At that time, if no symptoms are present, the drug can be tapered by 25 mg (5 mg for protriptyline) every two to three days. The slow tapering process is indicated for most psychotherapeutic drugs, and, in the case of most tricyclics and tetracyclics, it avoids a cholinergic-rebound syndrome consisting of nausea, upset stomach, sweating, headache, neck pain, and vomiting. The appearance of that syndrome can be treated by reinstituting a small dosage of the drug and tapering more slowly. There are also several case reports of rebound mania or hypomania after the abrupt discontinuation of tricyclic and tetracyclic antidepressants. If a patient has been treated with lithium augmentation, it seems reasonable to taper and stop the lithium first and then the tricyclic or tetracyclic antidepressant. Clinical studies supporting that approach are lacking, however, and the guidelines may change as more physicians report their experience with that drug combination.

Tricyclics, tetracyclics, and lithium are useful in preventing the recurrence of depressive episodes. The decision to use a prophylactic treatment is based on the severity and the nature of the disorder in a particular patient. Some data suggest that the long-term use of antidepressants may induce a rapid-cycling bipolar disorder. Lithium prophylaxis, therefore, may be an alternative treatment in a patient who has frequent, episodic, and serious depressive episodes.

Several investigators have suggested that neuroendocrine tests may be a guide for deciding when to maintain the use of tricyclics, tetracyclics, and other antidepressants. Specifically, the normalization of previously abnormal results in a dexamethasone-suppression test or a thyrotropin-releasing hormone-stimulation test may indicate that a patient can safely discontinue drug treatment. That use of neuroendocrine monitoring is still being investigated.

Plasma Levels

Research has defined the dose-response curves for tricyclic and tetracyclic antidepressants. Clinical determinations of plasma levels should be conducted 8 to 12 hours after the last dose after five to seven days on the same dosage of medication. Because of variations in absorption and metabolism, there is a 30- to 50-fold difference in the plasma levels of humans given the same dose of a tricyclic or tetracyclic. The therapeutic ranges for plasma levels have been determined (Table 29–3). Nortriptyline is unique in its association with a therapeutic window; that is, plasma levels over 150 μg per mL may reduce its efficacy. Clinicians must follow the directions for collection from the testing laboratory and have confidence in the assay procedures used.

The use of plasma levels in clinical practice is still an evolving skill. Plasma levels may be useful in confirming compliance, assessing reasons for drug failures, and documenting effective plasma levels for future treatment. Clinicians should always treat the patient and never the plasma level. Some patients have adequate clinical responses with seemingly subtherapeutic plasma levels, and other patients have responses only at supratherapeutic plasma levels without experiencing adverse effects. The latter situation, however, should alert clinicians to carefully monitor the patient's condition with, for example, an ECG.

ADVERSE EFFECTS

Psychiatric Effects

A major adverse effect of all tricyclic and tetracyclic antidepressants is the possibility of inducing a manic episode in both bipolar disorder patients and patients without a previous history of bipolar disorder. The clinician should watch carefully for that effect in bipolar disorder patients, especially if drug-induced mania has been a problem in the past. It is prudent to use very low doses of tricyclic and tetracyclic antidepressants in such patients or to use an agent such as fluoxetine or bupropion, which may be less likely to have that effect. Tricyclics and tetracyclics can exacerbate psychotic disorders.

Anticholinergic Effects

Patients should be warned that anticholinergic effects are common but that they may have a tolerance to them with continued treatment. Amitriptyline, imipramine, trimipramine, and doxepin are the most anticholinergic; amoxapine, nortriptyline, and maprotiline are less anticholinergic; and desipramine may be the least anticholinergic. Anticholinergic effects include dry mouth, constipation, blurred vision, and urinary retention. Sugarless gum or candy or fluoride lozenges can alleviate the dry mouth. Bethanechol (Urecholine), 25 to 50 mg three or four times a day, may reduce urinary hesitancy and may be helpful for impotence when taken 30 minutes before sexual intercourse. Narrow-angle glaucoma can also be aggravated by anticholinergic drugs, and the precipitation of glaucoma requires emergency treatment with a miotic agent. Tricyclic and tetracyclic antidepressants can be used in patients with glaucoma, provided that pilocarpine eye drops are administered concurrently. More severe anticholinergic effects can lead to a CNS anticholinergic syndrome with confusion and delirium, especially if tricyclic and tetracyclic antidepressants are administered with antipsychotics and anticholinergics. Some clinicians have used IM or intravenous (IV) physostigmine (Antilirium, Eserine) as a diagnostic tool to confirm the presence of anticholinergic delirium.

Sedation

Sedation is a common effect of antidepressants and may be welcomed if sleeplessness has been a problem. The sedative effect of tricyclic and tetracyclic antidepressants is a result of serotonergic, cholinergic, and histaminergic (H_1) activity. Amitriptyline, trimipramine, doxepin, and trazodone are the most sedating agents; imipramine, amoxapine, nortriptyline, and maprotiline have some sedating effects; and desipramine and protriptyline are the least sedating agents.

Autonomic Effects

The most common autonomic effect, partly because of α_1-adrenergic blockade, is orthostatic hypotension, which can result in falls and injuries in affected patients. Nortriptyline may be the drug least likely to cause the problem, and some patients respond to fludrocortisone (Florinef), 0.025 to 0.05 mg twice a day. Other possible autonomic effects are profuse sweating, palpitations, and increased blood pressure.

Cardiac Effects

When administered in their usual therapeutic doses, the tricyclic and tetracyclic antidepressants may cause tachycardia, flattened T waves, prolonged QT intervals, and depressed ST segments in the ECG. Imipramine has been shown to have a quinidinelike effect at therapeutic plasma levels and, indeed, may reduce the number of premature ventricular contractions. Because the drugs prolong conduction time, their use in patients with preexisting conduction defects is contraindicated. In patients with a cardiac history, tricyclic and tetracyclic antidepressants should be initiated at low doses, with gradual increases in dosage and careful monitoring of cardiac functions. At high plasma levels, as seen in overdoses, the drugs become arrhythmogenic. The agents should be discontinued several days before elective surgery because of the occurrence of hypertensive episodes during surgery in patients receiving tricyclics.

Neurological Effects

In addition to the sedation induced by tricyclics and tetracyclics and the possibility of anticholinergic-induced delirium, two tricyclics—desipramine and protriptyline—are associated with psychomotor stimulation. Myoclonic twitches and tremors of the tongue and upper extremities are fairly common. Rarer effects include speech blockage, paresthesias, peroneal palsies, and ataxia.

Amoxapine is unique in causing parkinsonianlike symptoms, akathisia, and even dyskinesias because of the dopaminergic blocking activity of one of its metabolites. It may cause neuroleptic malignant syndrome. Maprotiline may cause seizures when the dosage is increased too quickly or is kept at high levels for too long. Clomipramine may lower the seizure threshold. Amoxapine may also be a bit more epileptogenic than the other tricyclics and tetracyclics. All tricyclics and tetracyclics, however, may induce seizures in patients who have epilepsy or organic brain lesions. Although tricyclics and tetracyclics can still be used in such patients, the initial doses should be lower and then raised more slowly than in other patients.

Allergic Effects

Exanthematous skin rashes are seen in 4 to 5 percent of all patients treated with maprotiline. Jaundice is rare. Agranulocytosis, leukocytosis, leukopenia, and eosinophilia are rare complications of tricyclic and tetracyclic treatment. However, a patient who has a sore throat or fever during the first few months of tricyclic or tetracyclic treatment should have a CBC done immediately.

Other Adverse Effects

Weight gain, primarily an effect of the blockade of histamine type 2 receptors, is common. If it is a major problem, changing to fluoxetine or trazodone may help. Impotence, an occasional problem, is perhaps most often associated with amoxapine because of its blockade of dopamine receptors in the tuberoinfundibular tract. Amoxapine can also cause hyperprolactinemia, galactorrhea, anorgasmia, and ejaculatory disturbances. Other tricyclic and tetracyclic antidepressants have also been associated with gynecomastia and amenorrhea. Inappropriate secretion of antidiuretic hormone has also been reported with tricyclic and tetracyclic antidepressants. Other effects include nausea, vomiting, and hepatitis. The agents should be avoided during pregnancy. They pass into the breast milk and have the potential to cause serious adverse reactions in nursing infants. They should be used with caution in patients with hepatic or renal disease.

Overdose Attempts

Overdose attempts with tricyclic and tetracyclic antidepressants are serious and can often be fatal. Prescriptions for tricyclic and tetracyclic antidepressants should be nonrefillable and for no longer than a week at a time. Amoxapine may be more likely than the other tricyclic and tetracyclic antidepressants to result in death when taken in an overdose attempt.

Symptoms of overdose include agitation, delirium, convulsions, hyperactive deep tendon reflexes, bowel and bladder paralysis, dysregulations of blood pressure and temperature, and mydriasis. The patient then progresses to coma and perhaps respiratory depression. Cardiac arrhythmias may not respond to treatment. Because of the long half-lives of tricyclic and tetracyclic antidepressants, the patients are at risk of cardiac arrhythmias for three to four days after the overdose attempt, and so they should be monitored carefully in an intensive care medical setting.

DRUG-DRUG INTERACTIONS

Antihypertensives

Tricyclic and tetracyclic antidepressants block the neuronal reuptake of guanethidine (Esimil, Ismelin), which is required for antihypertensive activity. The antihypertensive effects of propranolol (Inderal) and clonidine (Catapres) may also be blocked by tricyclic and tetracyclic antidepressants. Coadministration of tricyclic and tetracyclic antidepressants with α-methyldopa may cause behavioral agitation.

Antipsychotics

The plasma levels of tricyclic and tetracyclic antidepressants and antipsychotics are increased by their coadministration. Antipsychotics also add to the anticholinergic and sedative effects of the tricyclic and tetracyclic antidepressants.

CNS Depressants

Opioids, alcohol, anxiolytics, hypnotics, and over-the-counter cold medications have additive effects by causing CNS depression when coadministered with antidepressants.

Sympathomimetics

Tricyclic use with sympathomimetic drugs may cause serious cardiovascular effects.

Oral Contraceptives

Birth control pills may decrease tricyclic and tetracyclic plasma levels through the induction of hepatic enzymes.

Other Pharmacokinetic Interactions

Tricyclic and tetracyclic plasma levels may also be increased by acetazolamide, acetylsalicylic acid, cimetidine (Tagamet), thiazide diuretics, and sodium bicarbonate. Decreased plasma levels may be caused by ascorbic acid, ammonium chloride, barbiturates, cigarette smoking, chloral hydrate, lithium, and primidone (Mysoline). Fluoxetine increases tricyclic plasma levels.

Electroconvulsive therapy.   Tricyclics and tetracyclics should not be coadministered with electroconvulsive therapy (ECT).

References

Ancill R J, Holliday S G: Treatment of depression in the elderly: A Canadian view. Prog Neuropsycho-pharmacol Biol Psychiatry *14*: 655, 1990.

Aronson T A, Shukla S: Long-term continuation antidepressant treatment: A comparison study. J Clin Psychiatry *50*: 285, 1989.

Balsessarini R J: Current status of antidepressants: Clinical pharmacology and therapy. J Clin Psychiatry *50*: 117, 1989.

Cole J O: The drug treatment of anxiety and depression. Med Clin North Am *72*: 815, 1988.

Davis J M, Glassman A H: Antidepressant drugs. In *Comprehensive Textbook of Psychiatry*, ed 5, H I Kaplan, B J Sadock, editors, p 1627. Williams & Wilkins, Baltimore, 1989.

Dietch J T, Fine M: The effect of nortriptyline in elderly patients with cardiac conduction disease. J Clin Psychiatry *51*: 65, 1990.

Mavissakalian M, Perel j M: Clinical experiments in maintenance and discontinuation of imipramine therapy in panic disorder with agoraphobia. Arch Gen Psychiatry *49*: 318, 1992.

Peselow E D, Dunner D L, Fieve R R, DiFiglia C: The prophylactic efficacy of tricyclic antidepressants: A five-year followup. Prog Neuropsychopharmacol Biol Psychiatry *15*: 71, 1991.

Roose S P, Glassman A H, Dalack G W: Depression, heart disease, and tricyclic antidepressants. J Clin Psychiatry *50* (7, Suppl): 12, 1989.

Wehr T A, Goodwin F K: Can antidepressant cause mania and worsen the course of affective illness? Am J Psychiatry *144*: 1403, 1987.

30

L-Tryptophan

L-Tryptophan, the amino acid precursor to serotonin, has been used as an adjuvant to antidepressant drugs and has also been used as a hypnotic. In 1989 L-tryptophan and L-tryptophan-containing products were recalled in the United States because of an outbreak of eosinophilia-myalgia syndrome associated with those products. The symptoms of eosinophilia-myalgia syndrome include fatigue, myalgia, shortness of breath, rashes, and swelling of the extremities. Congestive heart failure and death can also occur. It has been determined that the syndrome was related to a contaminant in a single manufacturing plant. L-Tryptophan is described here because the drug is likely to be available again in the United States once the current problem is resolved. The molecular structure of L-tryptophan is given in Figure 30–1.

PHARMACOLOGICAL ACTIONS

L-Tryptophan is somewhat erratically absorbed from the gastrointestinal (GI) tract. A significant portion of the drug is metabolized by the liver in a first-pass effect. Absorption of L-tryptophan can be enhanced by taking the drug with a low-protein, high-carbohydrate meal. The half-life of L-tryptophan may be as little as one to two hours; therefore, unless the drug is used as a hypnotic, four times daily dosing is necessary to maintain plasma levels. L-Tryptophan has its effects because a portion of the ingested dose crosses the blood-brain barrier, is taken up by serotonergic neurons, and is converted into serotonin, thus raising serotonin concentrations in the central nervous system (CNS).

INDICATIONS AND CLINICAL GUIDELINES

The most common indication for L-tryptophan is insomnia, although that indication does not have Food and Drug Administration (FDA) approval. Doses of 1 to 15 g taken at bedtime have a hypnotic effect in a significant number of persons. Whether the hypnotic effects of L-tryptophan persist with long-term treatment is not certain. L-Tryptophan is not associated with visuospatial, cognitive, or memory deficits the day after drug ingestion. Low doses of L-tryptophan are not associated with any change in the sleep electroencephalogram (EEG) other than earlier sleep onset; high doses of L-tryptophan are associated with increases in slow-wave sleep.

L-Tryptophan has been used as an adjuvant to tricyclic and tetracyclic antidepressants for depressed persons who did not respond to the tricyclic or tetracyclic antidepressant alone. The use of either lithium (Eskalith) or L-triiodothyronine (T_3) (Cytomel) adjuvant therapy with antidepressant nonresponders is more often used than L-tryptophan supplementation. L-Tryptophan has also been used as an adjuvant

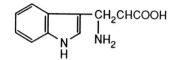

Figure 30–1. Molecular structure of L-tryptophan.

to lithium treatment for bipolar disorder patients who had incomplete symptom remission with lithium alone.

ADVERSE EFFECTS

Other than eosinophilia-myalgia syndrome, mentioned above, moderate doses of L-tryptophan are well tolerated by most patients. The only significantly reported adverse effect is nausea, which is sometimes compared to the nausea of pregnancy. L-Tryptophan may cause hepatotoxicity.

DRUG-DRUG INTERACTIONS

Much more significant are drug interactions when L-tryptophan is taken with either fluoxetine (Prozac) or monoamine oxidase inhibitors (MAOIs). Those combinations can cause diarrhea, insomnia, nausea, headaches, chills, agitation, and poor concentration. The symptoms are probably due to an excess serotonin concentration because of the additive effects of those compounds.

References

Flannery M T, Wallach P M, Espinoza L R, Dohrenwend M P, Moscisnski L C: A case of eosinophilia-myalgia syndrome associated with use of an L-tryptophan product. Ann Intern Med *112*: 300, 1990.

Gorman J M, Davis J M: Antianxiety drugs. In *Comprehensive Textbook of Psychiatry*, ed 5, H I Kaplan, B J Sadock, editors, p 1579. Williams & Wilkins, Baltimore, 1989.

Hajak G, Huether G, Blanke J, Blomer M, Freyer C, Poeggeler B, Reimer A, Rodenbeck A, Schulz-Varszegi M, Ruther E: The influence of intravenous L-tryptophan on plasma melatonin and sleep in men. Pharmapsychiatry *24*: 17, 1991.

Hedaya R J: Pharmacokinetic factors in the clinical use of tryptophan. J Clin Psychopharmacol *4*: 347, 1984.

Kamb M L, Murphy J J, Jones J L, Caston J L: Eosinophilia-myalgia syndrome in L-tryptophan-exposed patients. JAMA *267*: 77, 1992.

Maes M, Vandewoude M, Schotte C, Martin M, D'Hondt P, Scharpe S, Blockx P: The decreased availability of L-tryptophan in depressed females: Clinical and biological correlates. Prog Neuropsychopharmacol Biol Psychiatry *14*: 903, 1990.

Schneider-Helmert D, Spinweber C L: Evaluation of L-tryptophan for treatment of insomnia: A review. Psychopharmacology *89*: 1, 1986.

Steiner W, Fontaine R: Toxic reaction following the combined administration of fluoxetine and L-tryptophan: Five case reports. Biol Psychiatry *21*: 1067, 1986.

Zajecka J M, Fawcett J: Antidepressant combination and potentiation. Psychiatr Med *9*: 55, 1991.

31

Valproic Acid

Valproic acid and sodium valproate (both Depakene) and sodium divalproex (Depakote) are carboxylic acid-derivative anticonvulsants. Valproic acid is an anticonvulsant that joins the ranks of two other anticonvulsants—carbamazepine (Tegretol) (Chapter 12) and clonazepam (Klonopin) (Chapter 7)—as a potentially effective drug for the treatment of bipolar disorder (Figure 31–1). Lithium (Eskalith) and carbamazepine remain the first-line drugs for bipolar disorder, but valproic acid joins clonazepam and verapamil (Calan, Isoptin) (Chapter 11) as alternatives if lithium or carbamazepine is ineffective or cannot be tolerated by a particular patient.

PHARMACOLOGICAL ACTIONS

Sodium valproate is converted into valproic acid in the stomach and is then almost completely absorbed by the gastrointestinal (GI) tract. Peak plasma levels are reached in one to two hours if the drug is taken when the stomach is empty and in four to five hours if the drug is taken when the stomach is full. The presence of food, however, does not affect the amount of drug absorbed. The half-life of valproic acid is about eight hours, thus making three-times-daily dosing necessary to maintain stable plasma concentrations. The therapeutic effects of valproic acid for seizure control are probably mediated by a decrease in the catabolism of γ-aminobutyric acid (GABA), resulting in increased central nervous system (CNS) GABA concentrations. Whether that is the mechanism involved in the therapeutic effects for bipolar disorder is unknown.

INDICATIONS

Bipolar Disorder

Valproic acid has been shown to be effective in the treatment of both manic and depressive episodes in bipolar disorder patients. Valproic acid is also an effective prophylactic treatment in the control of manic and depressive episodes; however, it should be reserved for the treatment of patients who either do not respond to or cannot tolerate lithium or carbamazepine. Additional alternative drugs for the treatment of bipolar disorder include clonazepam and verapamil. Some studies have reported that the addition of valproic acid to lithium can convert a lithium-nonresponsive patient into a drug-responsive patient. Other reports have suggested that valproic acid may be especially effective in the treatment of rapid-cycling bipolar disorder and in mania or depression resulting from organic brain disease.

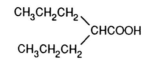

Figure 31–1. Molecular structure of valproic acid.

Other Disorders

A few reports have indicated that valproic acid may be effective in controlling psychotic symptoms of schizophrenic patients and organic mental disorder patients. The coadministration of valproic acid and antipsychotics may increase the plasma concentrations of both drugs. The effectiveness of valproic acid in drug-induced akathisia and atypical depression with marked hypersomnia has also been noted in some case reports.

CLINICAL GUIDELINES

Valproic acid is available in 250 mg capsules. It is best to initiate drug treatment gradually, so as to minimize the common adverse effects of nausea, vomiting, and sedation. The dose on the first day should be 250 mg administered with a meal. The dosage can be raised up to 250 mg orally (PO) three times daily over the course of three to six days. Plasma levels can be taken in the morning before the first daily dose of the drug is administered. Therapeutic plasma levels for the control of seizures are between 50 and 100 μg per mL, although some physicians use up to 125 μg per mL. It is reasonable to use the same range for the treatment of psychiatric disorders, although the data to support that practice are not yet available. Most patients attain those plasma levels on a dosage of valproic acid between 1,200 and 1,500 mg a day in divided doses. The drug should not be administered to patients with hepatic disease or to pregnant or nursing women. It is excreted in the breast milk. Children and the elderly are more sensitive to valproic acid's side effects than are younger adults. It should be used with caution in patients with renal disease.

ADVERSE EFFECTS

The most common adverse effects are nausea, vomiting, and sedation, although tolerance to those effects often develops. The adverse effects can be minimized by increasing the dosage slowly and by taking the drug with meals. Other uncommon neurological adverse effects include hand tremor, asterixis, and, more rarely, ataxia, headache, anxiety, and depression. Also uncommon are thrombocytopenia and platelet dysfunction, occurring most commonly at high dosages and resulting in the prolongation of bleeding times. Alopecia and generalized pruritus have been reported as rare adverse dermatological effects.

Serious adverse effects involve the pancreas and the liver. Rare cases of pancreatitis have been reported, occurring most often in the first six months of treatment and occasionally resulting in death. Transient increases in transaminases and lactate dehydrogenase occur in approximately 25 percent of patients. Liver chemistry levels should be monitored on a regular basis. The laboratory abnormalities usually do not evidence themselves clinically and usually resolve in the first six months of treatment. Rare cases of hepatitis have been reported, occurring in approximately 1 in 20,000 patients. Hepatitis occurs most often in the first three to six months of treatment in children with severe seizure disorders who are treated with multiple drugs. A modest increase seen in liver function tests does not correlate with the development of hepatitis; however, the emergence of malaise, anorexia, jaundice, lethargy, or weakness should prompt the clinician to evaluate the patient's hepatic status immediately.

DRUG-DRUG INTERACTIONS

There are complex drug-drug interactions between valproic acid and other anticonvulsants. The clinician should consult the treating neurologist before adding valproic acid to an existent antiepileptic drug regimen. Valproic acid has additive depressant effects with CNS depressants, including alcohol. The hematological effects of valproic acid may potentiate the anticoagulant effects of aspirin and warfarin (Coumadin). Valproic acid also interferes with at least two laboratory tests, resulting in falsely elevated urine ketones and abnormal thyroid test results. Valproic acid may potentiate the effects of monoamine oxidase inhibitors (MAOIs) and other antidepressants, possibly necessitating an antidepressant dosage reduction.

References

Calabrese J R, Delucchi G A: Spectrum of efficacy of valproate in 55 patients with rapid-cyclic bipolar disorder. Am J Psychiatry *147*: 431, 1990.

Fesler F A: Valproate in combat-related posttraumatic stress disorder. J Clin Psychiatry 52: 361, 1991.

Journal of Clinical Psychopharmacology: Valproate and mood disorders: Perspectives. J Clin Psychopharmacol *12*(1, Suppl): 2, 1992.

Kaplan P M, Boggiano W E: Anticonvulsants, noradrenergic drugs, and other organic therapies. In *Comprehensive Textbook of Psychiatry*, ed 5, H I Kaplan, B J Sadock, editors, p 1681. Williams & Wilkins, Baltimore, 1989.

McElroy S L, Keck P E, Pope H G: Sodium valproate: Its use in primary psychiatric disorders. J Clin Psychopharmacol 7: 16, 1987.

McElroy S L, Keck P E, Pope H G, Hudson J I: Valproate in the treatment of bipolar disorder: Literature review and clinical guidelines. J Clin Psychopharmacol *12*: 42S, 1992.

McElroy S L, Keck P E, Pope H G, Hudson J I: Valproate in the treatment of rapid-cycling bipolar disorder. J Clin Psychopharmacol 8: 275, 1988.

McFarland B H, Miller M R, Straumfjord A A: Valproate use in the older manic patient. J Clin Psychiatry *51*: 479, 1990.

Mitchell P, Cullen M J: Valproate for rapid-cycling unipolar affective disorder. J Nerv Ment Dis *179*: 503, 1991.

Pies R, Adler D A, Ehrenberg B L: Sleep disorders and depression with atypical features: Response to valproate. J Clin Psychopharmacol 9: 352, 1989.

Pope H G, McElroy S L, Keck P E, Hudson J I: Valproate in the treatment of acute mania. A placebo-controlled study. Arch Gen Psychiatry 48: 62, 1991.

Pope H G, McElroy S L, Satlin A, Hudson J, Keck P E, Kalish R: Head injury, bipolar disorder, and response to valproate. Compr Psychiatry 29: 34, 1988.

Post R M, editor: Emerging perspectives on valproate in affective disorders. J Clin Psychiatry *50*(3, Suppl): 2, 1989.

32

Yohimbine

Yohimbine (Yocon) is an α_2-adrenergic antagonist that has been used as a treatment for male sexual dysfunction. The use of the drug in psychiatry is controversial and highly questionable. Its molecular structure is shown in Figure 32–1.

PHARMACOLOGICAL ACTIONS

Yohimbine hydrochloride is derived from an alkaloid found in *Rubaceae* and related trees and in the *Rauwolfia serpentina* plant. Yohimbine produces effects on the peripheral blood vessels similar to the effects produced by reserpine. Yohimbine blocks presynaptic α_2-adrenergic receptors. Clinically, yohimbine produces increased parasympathetic (cholinergic) tone.

INDICATIONS

In psychiatry yohimbine has been used experimentally as a possible aphrodisiac and as a treatment of organic, psychogenic, and drug-induced erectile impotence. Its effect on male sexual performance is possibly related to its peripheral autonomic nervous system effect, which decreases sympathetic (adrenergic) activity, thereby increasing parasympathetic (cholinergic) tone. Penile erection has been linked to cholinergic activity and to α_2-adrenergic blockade, which theoretically results in increased penile inflow of blood or decreased penile outflow of blood or both. Urologists have also used yohimbine for the diagnostic classification of certain types of male impotence.

CLINICAL GUIDELINES

The dosage of yohimbine in the treatment of impotence is approximately 18 mg a day. The dosage range is 4 mg to 7.5 mg three times a day. In the event of significant adverse effects, dosage should first be reduced, then gradually increased again. Yohimbine should be used judiciously in psychiatric patients because it may have an adverse effect on their mental status. Yohimbine should not be used in female patients or in patients with renal disease, cardiac disease, glaucoma, and a history of gastric or duodenal ulcer. It has no consistent effects on erectile dysfunction, and its use for the disorder remains highly speculative. Yohimbine is available in 5.4 mg tablets.

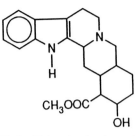

Figure 32–1. Molecular structure of yohimbine.

ADVERSE EFFECTS AND DRUG-DRUG INTERACTIONS

The side effects of yohimbine include elevated blood pressure and heart rate, increased psychomotor activity, irritability, tremor, headache, skin flushing, dizziness, urinary frequency, nausea, vomiting, and sweating. Patients with panic disorder show heightened sensitivity to yohimbine, experiencing increased anxiety, a rise in blood pressure, and increased plasma 3-methoxy-4-hydroxyphenylglycol (MHPG). Yohimbine also blocks the effect of clonidine (Catapres).

References

Gurguis G N, Uhde T W: Plasma 3-methoxy-4-hydroxyphenylethylene glycol (MHPG) and growth hormone responses to yohimbine in panic disorder patients and normal controls. Psychoneuroendocrinology *15*: 217, 1990.

Jacobsen F: Fluoxetine-induced sexual dysfunction and an open trial of yohimbine. J Clin Psychiatry *53*: 119, 1992.

Jenike M A: The pharmacological treatment of obsessive-compulsive disorders. Int Rev Psychiatry *2*: 411, 1990.

Morley M J, Bradshaw C M, Szabadi E: Effects of clonidine and yohimbine on the pupillary light reflex and carbachol-evoked sweating in healthy volunteers. Br J Clin Pharmacol *31*: 99, 1991.

Price J, Grunhaus L J: Treatment of clomipramine-induced anorgasmia with yohimbine: A case report. J Clin Psychiatry *51*: 32, 1990.

Sonda L P, Mazo R, Chancellor M B: The role of yohimbine for the treatment of erectile impotence. J Sex Marital Ther *16*: 15, 1990.

33

Combined Psychotherapy and Pharmacotherapy

Using drugs that affect the central nervous system in combination with psychotherapy is one of the fastest growing practices in American psychiatry. In this therapeutic approach, individual or group therapy is augmented by the use of pharmacological agents. It should not be a system in which the therapist meets with the patient on an occasional or irregular basis to monitor the effects of medication or to make notations on a rating scale to assess progress or side effects; rather, it should be a system in which both therapies are integrated and synergistic. In many cases it has been demonstrated that the results of combined therapy are superior to either type of therapy used alone. The term "pharmacotherapy-oriented psychotherapy" is used by some practitioners to refer to the combined approach. The methods of psychotherapy used can vary immensely, and all can be combined with pharmacotherapy.

HISTORY

With the introduction of antipsychotic medication in the 1950s, the value of using combined therapy became immediately apparent. For example, before that time the psychotherapy for schizophrenia was limited by two factors: (1) schizophrenic patients were unpredictable and sometimes had aggressive outbursts, often directed at the therapist, and (2) schizophrenic patients were often withdrawn, uncommunicative, and unable to talk about their thoughts and feelings. Consequently, many psychiatrists were fearful of starting psychotherapy because of the risk of physical assault. Moreover, the patient's inability to communicate interfered with the conduct of psychotherapy.

To some extent those two factors remain among the most significant reasons to use medication in combination with psychotherapy. Medication helps reduce aggression and enhances communication, regardless of the diagnosis.

QUALIFICATIONS OF THERAPISTS

In addition to having extensive training in one or more psychoanalytic or psychotherapeutic techniques, the psychiatrist who practices pharmacotherapy-oriented psychotherapy must have a comprehensive knowledge of psychopharmacology. That knowledge must include a thorough understanding of the indications for the use of each drug, the contraindications, the pharmacokinetics, the pharmacodynamics, the drug-drug interactions (with all pharmacological agents, not only the psychoactive agents), and the adverse effects. The psychiatrist must also be able to diagnose and treat the adverse effects. Nonpsychiatric physicians often use

Table 33–1
Countertransference Issues in Compliance

1. Overprescribing related to anger and helplessness
2. Inducing guilt in the patient
3. Colluding with noncompliance to demonstrate how ill the patient will get
4. Bullying the patient
5. Failures of empathy
6. Dread of the patient's anger

Table from G O Gabbard: Dynamic pharmacotherapy of depression. In *Psychiatric Times: Medicine and Behavior*, p 52. 1991. Used with permission.

psychoactive agents inaccurately (too small or too large a dose for too short or too long a course) because they lack the requisite psychopharmacological knowledge, training, and experience. Psychiatrists must have a high level of confidence and assurance in the combined-therapy approach. They must view emotional disorders as biopsychosocial events and must not separate mind from body. A unitary model in which illness is conceptualized as an interaction between biological and psychological processes allows the therapist to use combined therapy most effectively.

COUNTERTRANSFERENCE

As in all types of psychotherapy, psychiatrists must be aware of their conscious and unconscious feelings toward their patients, known as countertransference. When faced with a noncompliant patient, some psychiatrists may become angry. If unaware of that anger, the therapist may act in a way that is detrimental to the therapy by becoming punitive, authoritarian, or even rejecting. It is unwise, for example, to threaten a patient with termination because the patient will not take a prescribed drug. In those instances the resistance of the patient should be examined.

Psychiatrists must also be aware of their own psychological attitudes toward drugs (Table 33–1). Medications cannot replace the therapeutic alliance. They are not a shortcut to cure and are no substitute for the intense concentration and involvement on the part of the psychiatrist who is conducting psychotherapy. Therapists who are pessimistic about the value of psychotherapy or who misjudge the patient's motivation may prescribe medications out of their own nihilistic belief. Others may withhold medication if they overvalue psychotherapy or devalue pharmacological agents. Withholding medication is most likely to occur with borderline personality disorder patients, suicidal patients, and patients with a history of substance abuse. Each case must be evaluated individually, and the risk-benefit ratio must be carefully assessed so that the patient is not undeservedly punished, deprived, or mistreated.

INDICATIONS FOR COMBINED THERAPY

The primary indication for combined therapy is as a treatment for the specific disorder. As mentioned above, psychotropics reduce the hostility and the aggression that may be directed toward the therapist and, thus, improve the patient's capacity to communicate and to participate in the psychotherapeutic process. Another indication for combined therapy is to relieve distress when the signs and the symptoms of the patient's disorder are so prominent that they require more rapid amelioration than psychotherapy alone may be able to offer. In addition, each technique may facilitate the other; psychotherapy may enable the patient to accept a much-needed pharmacological agent, and the psychoactive drug may enable the patient to overcome resistance to entering or continuing psychotherapy.

TYPES OF PSYCHOTHERAPY

Psychoanalysis

The ability to tolerate frustration and to delay gratification is a part of all psychotherapies, but the ability must exist most especially in psychoanalysis, which requires that regressive patterns emerge in the form of a transference neurosis. This is the phenomenon in which the patient has a strong emotional attachment to the therapist because of the patient's feelings toward persons in his or her past. Many psychoanalysts are reluctant to use medication for fear that it will interfere with the development of the transference neurosis. However, if the analyst examines the meaning of the medication for the patient, it can provide material for further analysis. For example, in the technique of free association, one patient may view the analyst's prescribing medication as equivalent to receiving nurturance from an all-giving mother. Conversely, another patient may view the giving of medication as an act of control by an authoritarian father.

Analysts opposed to using medication believe that it violates, in theory, the rule of abstinence, in which patients are able to recognize their infantile needs only when they are not gratified. However, in actual practice, if interpretations of the patient's unconscious drives are timely and relevant and if the mental representation of the prescribed medication is explored, insights can be gained, often expeditiously. For example, transference may be expressed through the patient's attitude to the drug. In such cases, feelings are usually displaced from the therapist onto the medication and are subject to examination and interpretation. In some surveys 60 percent of psychoanalysts reported prescribing medication for some of their patients. Transference issues affecting compliance are listed in Table 33–2.

Psychoanalytic Psychotherapy

Psychoanalytic psychotherapy relies on psychoanalytic principles but focuses on current conflicts in the patient's life to a greater degree than does classic psychoanalysis. It is commonly divided into insight-oriented or expressive psychotherapy and supportive or relationship-oriented psychotherapy. Pharmacotherapy is used more often within this therapeutic framework than in psychoanalysis. Because this type of therapy is usually associated with guidance, advice giving, therapeutic leadership, and other relationship factors, both patients and therapists are generally less conflicted about using medication than they are in classic psychoanalysis. When the psychiatrist deals with issues related to the use of medications, many patients gain new insights into their behavior. For example, some patients are so frightened of becoming dependent on the therapist that they categorically refuse all medications.

Table 33–2
Transference Issues in Compliance

1. The doctor is experienced as authoritarian or controlling.
2. The doctor threatens the patient's counterdependent stance.
3. The patient experiences the doctor as a mothering figure who will take care of all needs, inducing passivity in the patient.
4. The patient rejects help as a way of defeating the doctor.
5. The doctor is experienced as giving up on psychotherapeutic approaches.
6. The patient develops transference to the medication itself.

Table from G O Gabbard: Dynamic pharmacotherapy of depression. In *Psychiatric Times: Medicine and Behavior*, p 51. 1991. Used with permission.

Behavior Therapy

The variety of behavior therapies include systematic desensitization, relaxation training, and social skills training. Various drugs have been used successfully to hasten the process in which the patient learns to decrease anxiety and to develop new patterns of behavior. With drugs such as methohexital (Brevital) and diazepam (Valium), almost all patients can become relaxed and in that state be exposed to the stimulus that elicits the anxiety response. As a result, they are desensitized to anxiety. Medications can also be used to increase assertiveness and overcome shyness, especially if such avoidant behavior is associated with depression or anxiety.

Cognitive Therapy

This short-term structured therapy has been used most often to treat patients with depression, including patients with suicidal ideation. Such patients can have their therapy augmented with antidepressants and psychostimulants to overcome apathy, anhedonia, abulia, and feelings of helplessness.

Interpersonal Therapy

This type of psychotherapy is used primarily to treat depression. The therapy consists of once-a-week meetings held over a three-to-four-month period. The therapist attempts to clarify feeling states and to improve interpersonal relations. Medication is often used to deal with the sense of hopelessness and the feelings of anxiety that frequently accompany the depression that the patients experience.

Group Therapy

The concomitant use of medication can reduce withdrawal, isolation, avoidance, shyness, hostility, and other signs and symptoms of psychiatric disorders that interfere with social interactions. These interactions are crucial if cohesiveness, interpersonal learning, instillation of hope, identification, and other therapeutic factors in group psychotherapy are to be effective.

Table 33–3
Resistance Issues in Compliance

1. Illness may be preferable to health.
2. Punishment is felt to be deserved.
3. Illness is denied because of stigmatization.
4. Unconscious identification with a depressed relative is being warded off.
5. Psychological factors override pharmacological effects.

Table from G O Gabbard: Dynamic pharmacotherapy of depression. In *Psychiatric Times: Medicine and Behavior*, p 52. 1991. Used with permission.

Triangular Therapy

Triangular therapy, also known as cotherapy, is a form of treatment in which one therapist (who may be a psychologist or a social worker) conducts psychotherapy while the other therapist (always a psychiatrist) prescribes medications. The method requires that the two therapists have regular exchanges of information. Some patients split the transference between the two; one therapist may be seen as giving and nurturing and the other as withholding and aloof. Similarly, countertransference issues, such as one therapist's identifying with the patient's idealized or devalued image of the other therapist, can interfere with therapy. Those issues must be worked out, and the cotherapists must be compatible and respectful of each other's orientation, so that the triangular therapy program can succeed.

THERAPEUTIC CONSIDERATIONS

Motivation for Psychotherapy

The reduction of symptoms, especially anxiety, does not decrease the patient's motivation for psychoanalysis or other insight-oriented psychotherapy. In practice, drug-induced symptom reduction improves communication and motivation. All therapies have a cognitive base, and anxiety generally interferes with the patient's ability to gain cognitive understanding of the illness. Drugs that decrease anxiety facilitate cognitive understanding. They also increase other functions of the ego, such as attention, concentration, memory, and learning. If resistance to combined therapy is persistent, the therapist should consider the factors listed in Table 33–3.

Self-Esteem

It may be a blow to the patient's self-esteem when the therapist introduces the need for a drug. Some patients may see themselves as sicker than they thought, and others may feel themselves to be failures who are not suitable for psychotherapy. If those reactions are explored, they usually lead to previously unexpressed fears and feelings of inadequacy and self-deprecation. In most instances drugs help raise the self-esteem of patients. As a result of improved functioning, patients are better able to cope with the stresses of life, and their self-esteem improves.

Symptom Substitution

According to Sigmund Freud, symptom formation is the result of a conflict between the id, the superego, and the ego that produces anxiety, which is then channeled into a symptom. Even though medication reduces the symptom, the conflict remains and can be analyzed; the drug does not cause symptom substitution. Thus, in a phobic patient whose phobia is diminished by medication, another symptom does not develop in its place; the insight-oriented therapy continues to make the unconscious conflict accessible to conscious reality.

Defense Mechanisms

Some processes relieve conflict and anxiety arising from one's impulses and drives. The ego uses defense mechanisms to guard against or to reduce the strength of an impulse, which is usually sexual or aggressive in nature. Mentally ill patients tend to use immature defense mechanisms to deal with those impulses. If a drug can lower instinctual anxiety, the patient may have more ability to use a mature defense mechanism in place of a primitive or immature defense. For example, a delusional patient using the immature defense of projection—that is, attributing to another person unacceptable thoughts or feelings—may be able to use the mature defense of suppression—that is, conscious controlling and inhibiting of unacceptable impulses or ideas—and thus eliminate those unwanted ideas from consciousness and function more normally as a result.

Linkage Phenomenon

At some point patients may view the improvement being made in therapy as the result of a conscious or unconscious linkage between the psychopharmacological agent and the therapist. In fact, after being weaned from medication, patients often carry a pill with them for reassurance. In that sense the pill acts as a transitional object between the patient and the therapist.

Some patients with anxiety disorders, for example, may carry a single benzodiazepine tablet, which they take when they think they are about to have an anxiety attack. Then the patient may report that the attack was aborted immediately—before the medication could even have been absorbed into the bloodstream. In other cases the pill is never taken because the patient knows that the pill is available and gains reassurance from that fact. The linkage phenomenon is usually not seen unless the patient is in a positive transference to the therapist. The therapist may use the phenomenon to his or her advantage by suggesting that the patient carry medication to use as needed. Eventually, the behavior has to be analyzed, and one often finds that the patient has attributed magical properties to the therapist that are then transferred to the medication. Some clinicians believe the effect to be the result of conditioning. After repeated trials the sight of the medicine can decrease anxiety.

CHOICE OF DRUG

The psychiatrist identifies and elicits from patients signs and symptoms of psychiatric disorders. *Signs* are objective findings observed by the clinician—for example, tachycardia and flat affect. *Symptoms* are subjective complaints listed by the patient—for example, palpitations and depressed mood. In many conditions, such as anxiety disorder, signs and symptoms overlap. The sign or the symptom can be targeted and used as a specific criterion that both the psychiatrist and the patient can use to determine whether the psychotropic agent is having the desired effect.

Placebo Effect

In pharmacology the *placebo effect* is that phenomenon in which a person exhibits a clinically significant response to a pill containing a physiologically inert substance. The response is not due to any psychopharmacological property of the drug but results from purely psychological effects. In some cases the placebo effect can be measured objectively. For example, not only does the patient state that he or she feels less anxious, but there is less autonomic nervous system arousal, such as lower blood pressure, and a decrease in heart rate. Placebo effects are common in patients with dissociative disorders, hypochondriasis, somatoform disorders, anxiety disorders, and sexual disorders.

COMPLIANCE AND PATIENT EDUCATION

Compliance is the degree to which a patient carries out the recommendations of the treating physician. Compliance is fostered when the doctor-patient relationship is a positive one, and the patient's refusal to take medication may provide insight into a negative transferential situation. In some cases the patient acts out hostilities by noncompliance, rather than becoming aware of and ventilating such negative feelings toward the doctor. Medication noncompliance may provide the psychiatrist with the first clue that a negative transference is present in an otherwise compliant patient who had appeared to be nothing but agreeable and cooperative.

Patients should know the target signs and symptoms that the drug is supposed to reduce, the length of time that they will be taking the drug, both the expected and the unexpected adverse effects, and the treatment plan to be followed if the current drug is unsuccessful. Although some psychiatric disorders interfere with patients' ability to comprehend that information, the psychiatrist should relay as much of the information as possible. The clear presentation of the material is often less frightening than are patients' fantasies about drug treatment. The psychiatrist should tell patients when they will begin to receive benefits from the drug. That information is perhaps most critical when the patient has a mood disorder and may not observe any therapeutic effects for three to four weeks (Table 33–4).

Some patients' ambivalent attitudes toward drugs often reflect the confusion about drug treatment that exists in the field of psychiatry. Patients often believe that taking a psychotherapeutic drug means that they are not in control of their

Table 33–4
Specific Instructions for Patients

- Name of the medication (brand name and generic name)
- Whether it is meant to treat the disease or the symptoms and, therefore, how important it is to take it
- How to tell if it is working and what to do if it appears not to be working
- When and how to take it—before or after meals
- What to do if a dose is missed
- How long to take it
- Side effects that are important for the patient and what to do about them
- Possible effects on driving, on work, and so on, and what precautions to take
- Interactions with alcohol and other drugs

Table adapted from N G Ward. In *Integrating Pharmacotherapy and Psychotherapy*, B D Beitman, G L Klerman, editors, p 87. American Psychiatric Press, Washington, 1991. Used with permission.

lives or that they may become addicted to the drug and have to take it forever. Psychiatrists should explain the difference between drugs of abuse that affect the normal brain and psychiatric drugs that are used to treat emotional disorders. Psychiatrists should also point out to patients that antipsychotics, antidepressants, and antimanic drugs are not addictive in the way that, for example, heroin is addictive. The psychiatrist's clear and honest explanation of how long the patient should take the drug will help the patient adjust to the idea of chronic maintenance medication if that is, indeed, the treatment plan. In some cases the psychiatrist may appropriately give the patient increasing responsibility for adjusting the medications as the treatment progresses. Doing so often helps the patient feel less controlled by the drug and in a collaborative role with the therapist.

COMBINED THERAPY IN SPECIFIC DISORDERS

Depression

Some patients and clinicians fear that medication will cover over the depression and that psychotherapy will be impeded. Medication should be viewed as a facilitator in overcoming the anergia that may inhibit a communication process between doctor and patient. The psychiatrist should also explain to the patient that depression interferes with interpersonal activity in a variety of ways. For instance, depression produces withdrawal and irritability, which alienates significant others who may otherwise gratify the strong dependency needs that make up much of depressive psychodynamics.

The psychiatrist should be alert for signs and symptoms of a recurrent depressive episode. Medication may have to be reinstituted. Before doing so, however, one should carefully review any stress, especially rejections, that may have precipitated the depressive episode. A depressive episode may also occur because the patient is in a stage of negative transference, and the psychiatrist must try to elicit negative feelings. In many cases the ventilation of angry feelings toward the therapist without an angry response can serve as a corrective emotional experience, and a severe depressive episode necessitating medication can thereby be forestalled. Depressed patients are generally maintained on their medication for six months after clinical improvement. The cessation of pharmacotherapy before that time is likely to result in a relapse.

Suicidal Behavior

The possibility of suicide must be considered in treating schizophrenic, bipolar disorder, depressed, and anxiety-disordered patients (especially those who have panic attacks). If the psychiatrist decides that the patient is in imminent risk for suicidal behavior, hospitalization is always indicated. If the patient can be managed outside a hospital, medication should be given to a responsible family member who can monitor the dosage and the frequency of the prescribed medication. As a further precaution, the psychiatrist may treat the patient with a drug known to have little or no lethal potential when taken in an overdose attempt—for example, fluoxetine (Prozac). Medication is almost always indicated in suicidally depressed patients.

Bipolar Disorder

Patients taking lithium (Eskalith) or other treatments for bipolar disorder are usually medicated for an indefinite period of time to prevent episodes of either mania or depression. Most psychotherapists insist that patients with bipolar disorder be medicated before starting any insight-oriented therapy. Without such premedication, most bipolar disorder patients are unable to make the necessary therapeutic alliance. When they are depressed, their abulia seriously disrupts their flow of thoughts, and the sessions are nonproductive. When they are manic, their flow of associations can be rapid and their speech so pressured that the therapist may be flooded with material and unable to make appropriate interpretations or unable to assimilate the material into the disrupted cognitive framework of the manic patient.

Anxiety Disorders

Anxiety disorders encompass obsessive-compulsive disorder, posttraumatic stress disorder, generalized anxiety disorder, phobic disorders, and panic disorder with or without agoraphobia. Many drugs are effective in managing distressing signs and symptoms. For example, obsessions and compulsions respond to clomipramine (Anafranil) and fluoxetine (Prozac); panic to alprazolam (Xanax) or clonazepam (Klonopin); generalized anxiety to diazepam (Valium); and posttraumatic stress disorder, depending on the symptoms, to tricyclics and antianxiety agents. As symptoms are controlled by medication, patients are reassured and develop confidence that they need not be incapacitated by the disorder. That effect is particularly so in panic disorder, which is often associated with anticipatory anxiety about the attack. Depression may also complicate the symptom picture in patients with anxiety disorders and has to be addressed both pharmacologically and psychotherapeutically.

Schizophrenia and Other Psychotic Disorders

Included in this group of disorders are schizophrenia, delusional disorder, schizoaffective disorder, schizophreniform disorder, and brief reactive psychosis. Drug treatment for those disorders is always indicated, and hospitalization is often necessary for diagnostic purposes, to stabilize medication, to prevent danger to self or others, and to establish a psychosocial treatment program that may include individual psychotherapy. In attempting individual psychotherapy, the therapist must establish a treatment relationship and a therapeutic alliance with the patient. The schizophrenic patient defends against closeness and trust and often becomes suspicious, anxious, hostile, or regressed in therapy. Before the advent of psychotropics, many psychiatrists were fearful for their own safety when working with such patients. Indeed, many assaults occurred.

Individual psychotherapy for schizophrenia is labor-intensive, expensive, and not often attempted. The recognition that combined psychotherapy-pharmacotherapy has a greater chance of success than does either type of therapy alone may reverse that situation. The psychiatrist who conducts such combined therapy must be especially empathetic and able to tolerate the bizarre manifestations of the illness. The schizophrenic patient is exquisitely sensitive to rejection, and individual psychotherapy should never be started unless the therapist is willing to make a total commitment to the process.

Psychoactive Substance Use

Patients who abuse alcohol or drugs present the most difficult challenge in combined therapy. They are often impulsive and, even though they promise not to abuse a substance, may do so repeatedly. In addition, they frequently withhold information from the psychiatrist about episodes of abuse. For that reason some psychiatrists do not prescribe any medication to such patients, especially not those substances with a high abuse potential, such as benzodiazepines, barbiturates, and amphetamines. Drugs with no abuse potential—such as thioridazine (Mellaril), amitriptyline (Elavil), and fluoxetine (Prozac)—have an important role in treating the anxiety or depression or both that almost always accompanies psychoactive substance use disorders. The psychiatrist conducting psychotherapy with such patients should have no reservations about sending the patient to a laboratory for random urine toxicological tests. As in all forms of insight-oriented psychotherapy, the psychological significance of such tests should be examined.

An overview of the medication issues in the combined therapy approach is given in Table 33–5.

ETHICAL AND LEGAL ISSUES

Informed Consent

Informed consent is a legal term indicating that the patient has agreed to a particular treatment program—for example, a drug trial—after having been advised of the potential benefits of treatment, the risks of treatment, and alternative treatments. Some states require patients to sign a document stating that they have given informed consent, and some clinicians have adopted that practice in states that do not require such a form. In either case the psychiatrist should make a notation in the patient's chart that the issue has been discussed. Clearly, the capacity of a psychiatric patient to understand the information is often difficult to assess. The

Table 33–5
The Stages of Individual Psychotherapy: A Medication Emphasis

Stage	Engagement	Pattern Search	Change	Termination
Goals	Trust Credibility Self-observer alliance	To define problem patterns that, if changed, would lead to a desirable outcome	1. Relinquish old pattern(s) 2. Initiate new pattern(s) 3. Practice new pattern(s)	To separate efficiently
Techniques	Convey empathic understanding Effective suggestions Effective medications	Questionnaires Homework—idiosyncratic meanings ascribed to medication	Interpretation Reframing Behavioral suggestion Medication-induced change	Mutually agreed Patient initiates Therapist initiates Medication-influenced
Content	Medication responsive Diagnosis	Does response to medication reflect a problem pattern?	Medication effects or insight around medication use accelerates change	Medications may prolong termination
Resistance	Are excessive side effects resistance to treatment?	Does pattern of nonadherence to medication regimen reflect a problem pattern?	Do new side effects suggest resistance to change?	Symptom reoccurrence not necessarily indication for medication change
Transference	Physician seen as malevolent or all-powerful	Is key interpersonal pattern reflected in meaning of medication?	Unresolved distortions may be signaled by a new medication issue inhibiting change	Desire for new or more medication reflects desire to hold therapist
Countertransference	Physician failure to prescribe appropriately	Medication prescription reflects distorted response to patient	Sudden change in regimen reflects an attempt to undermine change	New medication reflects desire to keep contact

Table by B D Beitman. In *Integrating Pharmacotherapy and Psychotherapy*, B D Beitman, G L Klerman, editors, p 22. American Psychiatric Press, Washington, 1991. Used with permission.

problem represents an ethical dilemma that can best be met by psychiatrists' attempting to meet the letter and the spirit of the law to the best of their abilities. When in doubt about a patient's ability to make such a decision, the psychiatrist should consult the patient's family, friends, or legal counsel.

Hospital Care

In hospitals, especially hospitals in the public sector, medication is often the major form of treatment offered. The shortage of psychiatrists and the excessive number of patients in the city and state mental hospital system prevent the use of psychotherapy for patients who are, for the most part, either psychotic or demented. Those patients unwilling to take medication can be forced to do so under certain circumstances. For example, if they are imminently dangerous to themselves or others, medication can be given against their will and forcibly, if necessary.

Treatment Records

In addition to making any process notes regarding psychotherapy, the psychiatrist should keep detailed records of prescription dates, dosages, directions, warnings about side effects, and physical and psychological responses to the drug.

Most malpractice cases against psychiatrists have been brought because of the adverse effects of psychotropic drugs, but some suits have been brought because doctors withheld medication. In one case a severely depressed patient was treated with insight-oriented psychotherapy and long-term hospitalization. The patient's attorney argued that, if psychotropic medication had been prescribed, the patient's depression would have lifted more rapidly than it did and his stay in the hospital would have been shortened. The parties settled the case out of court.

DURATION OF MEDICATION USE

The length of time a patient is expected to take medication depends on several factors: (1) the purpose of the medication (for example, symptom removal), (2) the disorder being treated (for example, depression or schizophrenia), (3) the type of associated psychotherapeutic program (for example, psychoanalysis), and (4) the characteristics of the drug (for example, whether it is associated with adverse effects, such as withdrawal symptoms). In some cases medication can and should be taken indefinitely, and in others it is used only as a short-term adjuvant.

Antidepressants and Antimanics

A wide range of antidepressant compounds are used to treat depression, and clinical improvement can occur in more than 50 percent of depressed patients so treated. Lithium and the anticonvulsants are the mainstays of treatment for mania.

Depression. An untreated depressive episode lasts 6 to 12 months on average. Because of that, the withdrawal of antidepressant medication before three months almost always results in the return of symptoms. Most psychiatrists keep giving medication to a depressed patient for six months after clinical improvement occurs. Long-term antidepressant drug treatment is often indicated as a prophylactic measure in patients with a history of recurrent serious depression. However, a relapse or a recurrence of depressive symptoms may occur. For that reason, combined drug therapy and psychotherapy is the treatment of choice.

Mania. Although most patients with manic episodes also experience depressive intervals, lithium is most often the drug of choice in mania. An untreated manic episode lasts about three months, and it is unwise to discontinue drugs before that time. As the illness progresses, the amount of time between manic episodes decreases, and most patients with bipolar disorder keep taking lithium indefinitely. As with all pharmacological agents, the risk of adverse effects must be considered—for example, lithium is contraindicated in pregnancy. Patients in psychotherapy who are observed by a psychiatrist frequently (once or twice a week) may be treated with lithium on an intermittent basis because the physician is able to assess an impending manic episode on the basis of his or her ongoing assessment of the patient.

Antipsychotic Drugs

Antipsychotic medication is the mainstay of treatment for schizophrenia and related disorders. Antipsychotic drugs are relatively safe and are prescribed indefinitely for most patients. Maintenance dosages of antipsychotics are usually lower than dosages for acute episodes. Schizophrenic patients receiving combined drug and psychosocial therapy do better than those treated with medication alone and are less likely to relapse.

Antianxiety Drugs

The most frequently used class of drugs in the treatment of anxiety disorders are the benzodiazepines. Most patients with generalized anxiety disorder are treated for about two to three months for their acute symptoms, at which point the drug is gradually withdrawn. Some patients require long-term administration of benzodiazepines. There is no evidence of tolerance or a need to increase the dosage of the drug when such patients are receiving concomitant individual psychotherapy. Long-term treatment is especially useful in patients with hyperactive autonomic nervous systems or with autonomic nervous system arousal syndromes. The risk of abuse in such patients is minimal when the drugs are used in an integrated therapy program.

Sympathomimetics

The sympathomimetics include dextroamphetamine (Dexedrine), methylphenidate (Ritalin), and pemoline (Cylert). They are used mainly in attention-deficit hyperactivity disorder in children and in adults when residual symptoms of attention-deficit hyperactivity disorder are present. The drugs are also useful in certain patients with chronic depressive states, even though psychostimulants are not labeled for that use by the Food and Drug Administration (FDA). Because sympathomimetics are subject to abuse if not used judiciously, they should always be prescribed in conjunction with a course of psychotherapy. Many patients with anhedonia, low energy levels, and abulia can be maintained with small dosages of amphetamines (5 to 15 mg a day) for long periods of time in such combined treatment without risk of abuse or tolerance. Chapter 26 discusses the use of sympathomimetics further.

References

Akiskal H S: Chronic depression. Bull Menninger Clin *55*: 156, 1991.

Beitman B D, Klerman G L, editors: *Integrating Pharmacotherapy and Psychotherapy*. American Psychiatric Press, Washington, 1991.

Chalfin R M, Altieri J: Supervised treatment of an obsessional patient by a psychiatric resident utilizing psychotherapy and pharmacotherapy. Am J Psychother *45*: 43, 1991.

Howland R H: Pharmacotherapy of dysthymia: A review. J Clin Psychopharmacol *11*: 83, 1991.

Hyland J M: Integrating psychotherapy and pharmacotherapy. Bull Menninger Clin *55*: 205, 1991.

Krull F: The problem of integrating biological and psychodynamic views in psychotherapeutic training of physicians. Psychother Psychosom *53*: 115, 1990.

Sautter F J, Heaney C, O'Neill P: A problem-solving approach to group psychotherapy in the inpatient milieu. Hosp Community Psychiatry *42*: 814, 1991.

Sotsky S M, Glass D R, Shea M T, Pilkonis P A, Collins J F, Elkin I, Watkins J T, Imber S D, Leber W R, Moyer J: Patient predictors of response to psychotherapy and pharmacotherapy: Findings in the NIMH Treatment of Depression Collaborative Research Program. Am J Psychiatry *148*: 997, 1991.

34

Laboratory Tests and Drug Therapy

Before initiating psychiatric treatment, the clinician should undertake a routine medical evaluation for the purposes of screening for concurrent disease, ruling out organicity, and establishing baseline values of functions to be monitored. Such an evaluation includes a medical history and routine medical laboratory tests, such as a complete blood count (CBC); hematocrit and hemoglobin; renal, liver, and thyroid function; electrolytes; and blood sugar (Table 34–1).

Thyroid disease and other endocrinopathies may present as a mood disorder or psychosis; cancer or infectious disease may present as depression; infection and connective tissue diseases may present as acute changes in mental status. In addition, a range of organic mental or neurological conditions may present initially to the psychiatrist. Those conditions include multiple sclerosis, Parkinson's disease, Alzheimer's disease, Huntington's chorea, acquired immune deficiency syndrome (AIDS) dementia, and temporal lobe epilepsy. Any suspected medical or neurological condition should be thoroughly evaluated with appropriate laboratory tests and consultation.

LABORATORY TESTS AND MEDICATION

Nonpsychiatric Drugs

The initial evaluation must always include a thorough assessment of prescribed and over-the-counter medications that the patient is taking. Many psychiatric syndromes can be iatrogenically caused by medications—for example, depression due to antihypertensives, delirium due to anticholinergics, and psychosis due to steroids. Often, if clinically possible, a washout of medications may help in diagnosis.

Psychiatric Drugs

Benzodiazepines. No special tests are needed before prescribing benzodiazepines, although liver function tests are often useful. The drugs are metabolized in the liver by either oxidation or conjugation. Impaired hepatic function increases the elimination half-life of benzodiazepines that are oxidized, but it has less effect on benzodiazepines that are conjugated (oxazepam [Serax], lorazepam [Ativan], and temazepam [Restoril]). Benzodiazepines can also precipitate porphyria.

Dopamine receptor antagonists. No special tests are needed, although it is good to have baseline liver function tests and CBC. Dopamine receptor antagonists are metabolized primarily in the liver, with metabolites excreted primarily in the urine. Many metabolites are active. Peak plasma level is reached usually two to three hours after an oral dose. Elimination half-life is 12 to 30 hours but may be much longer. Steady state requires at least a week at a constant dosage (months

Table 34–1
Routine Admission Workup

1. Complete blood count (CBC) with differential
2. Complete blood chemistry tests (including electrolytes, glucose, calcium, magnesium, hepatic, and renal function tests)
3. Thyroid function tests (TFTs)
4. Rapid plasma reagin (RPR) or Venereal Disease Research Laboratory (VDRL) test
5. Urinalysis
6. Urine toxicology screen
7. Electrocardiogram (ECG)
8. Chest X-ray (for patients over 35)
9. Plasma levels of any drugs being taken, if appropriate

at a constant dosage of depot antipsychotics). Dopamine receptor antagonists acutely cause elevation in serum prolactin (because of tuberoinfundibular activity). A normal prolactin level often indicates either noncompliance or nonabsorption.

Side effects include leukocytosis, leukopenia, impaired platelet functioning, mild anemia (both aplastic and hemolytic), and agranulocytosis. Bone marrow and blood element side effects can occur abruptly, even when the dosage has remained constant. Low-potency dopamine receptor antagonists are most likely to cause agranulocytosis, which is the most common bone marrow side effect. They can also cause electrocardiogram (ECG) changes (not as frequently as with tricyclic antidepressants) including a prolonged QT interval; flattened, inverted, or bifid T waves; and U waves. Large differences are seen among patients in dose-plasma level relations. High plasma levels probably offer no clinical benefit and increase the risk of side effects.

Side effects include hypotension, sedation, lowering of the seizure threshold, anticholinergic effects, tremor, dystonia, cogwheel rigidity, rigidity without cogwheeling, akathisia, akinesia, rabbit syndrome, and tardive dyskinesia.

Clozapine. Because of the risk of agranulocytosis (1 to 2 percent), patients who are being treated with clozapine (Clozaril) must have a baseline white blood cell (WBC) and differential count before the initiation of treatment, a WBC count every week throughout treatment, and a WBC count for four weeks after the discontinuation of clozapine.

Cyclic antidepressants. An ECG should be given before starting cyclic antidepressants to assess for conduction delays, which may lead to heart block at therapeutic levels. Some clinicians believe that all patients receiving prolonged cyclic antidepressant therapy should have an annual ECG. At therapeutic levels, the drugs suppress arrhythmias through a quinidinelike effect. Trazodone (Desyrel), an antidepressant unrelated to cyclic antidepressants, has been reported to cause ventricular arrhythmias and priapism, mild leukopenia, and neutropenia.

Blood levels are often tested routinely when using imipramine (Tofranil), desipramine (Norpramin), or nortriptyline (Pamelor) in the treatment of depression. Taking blood levels may also be of use in patients in whom there is a poor response at normal dose ranges and in high-risk patients for whom there is an urgent need to know whether a therapeutic or toxic plasma level of drug has been reached. Blood level tests should also include measurement of active metabolities (for example, imipramine is converted to desipramine, amitriptyline [Elavil] to nortriptyline). Some characteristics of tricyclic drug plasma levels are as follows:

1. *Imipramine*. The percentage of favorable responses correlates with plasma levels in a linear manner between 200 and 250 ng/mL, but some patients may respond at a lower level. At levels over 250 ng/mL, there is no improved favorable response, and side effects increase.
2. *Nortriptyline*. The *therapeutic window* (the range within which a drug is most effective) is between 50 and 150 ng/mL. There is a decreased response rate at levels over 150 ng/mL.
3. *Desipramine*. Levels greater than 125 ng/mL correlate with a higher percentage of favorable responses.
4. *Amitriptyline*. Different studies have produced conflicting results with regard to blood levels.

Procedure. The procedure for taking blood levels is as follows: The physician should draw the blood specimen 10 to 14 hours after the last dose, usually in the morning after a bedtime dose. Patients must be on a stable daily dosage for at least five days for the test to be valid. Some patients are unusually poor metabolizers of cyclic antidepressants and may have levels as high as 2,000 ng/mL while taking normal doses and before showing a favorable clinical response. Such patients must be monitored very closely for cardiac side effects. Patients with levels greater than 1,000 ng/mL are generally at risk for cardiotoxicity.

Monoamine oxidase inhibitors. Patients taking monoamine oxidase inhibitors (MAOIs) are instructed to avoid tyramine-containing foods (Table 24–2 in Chapter 24) because of the danger of a potential hypertensive crisis. A baseline normal blood pressure (BP) must be recorded, and the BP must be followed during treatment. MAOIs may also cause orthostatic hypotension as a direct drug side effect unrelated to diet. Other than their potential for causing elevated BP when taken with certain foods, MAOIs are relatively free of other side effects. There are no clinical blood level values available for MAOIs, although a research test involves correlating therapeutic response with the degree of platelet monoamine oxidase inhibition.

Lithium. Patients receiving lithium (Eskalith) should have baseline thyroid function tests, electrolytes, a white blood cell count (WBC), and renal function tests (specific gravity, blood urea nitrogen [BUN], and creatinine), and a baseline ECG. The rationale for those tests is that lithium can cause renal concentrating defects, hypothyroidism, and leukocytosis; sodium depletion can cause toxic lithium levels; and approximately 95 percent of lithium is excreted in the urine. Lithium has also been shown to cause ECG changes, including various conduction defects.

Lithium is most clearly indicated in the prophylactic treatment of mania (direct antimanic effect may take up to two weeks) and is commonly coupled with antipsychotics for the treatment of acute mania. Lithium itself may have antipsychotic activity as well. The maintenance level is 0.6 to 1.2 mEq per L, although acutely manic patients can tolerate up to 1.5 to 1.8 mEq per L. Some patients may respond at lower levels, whereas others may require higher levels. A response below 0.4 mEq per L is probably placebo. Toxic reactions may occur with levels over 2.0 mEq per L. Regular lithium monitoring is essential, since there is a narrow therapeutic range beyond which cardiac problems and central nervous system (CNS) effects can occur.

Table 34–2
Therapeutic and Toxic Blood Levels

Drug	Therapeutic Level	Toxic Level
Amitriptyline	>120 ng/mL	500 ng/mL
Bromide	20–120 mg/dL	150 mg/dL
Carbamazepine	8–12 μg/mL	15 μg/mL
Desipramine	>125 ng/mL	500 ng/mL
Imipramine	200–250 ng/mL	500 ng/mL
Lithium	0.6–1.5 mEq/L	2.0 mEq/L
Meprobamate	10–20 μg/mL	30–70 μg/mL
Nortriptyline	50–150 ng/mL	500 ng/mL
Phenobarbital	15–30 μg/mL	40 μg/mL
Phenytoin	10–20 μg/mL	30 μg/mL
Primidone	5–12 μg/mL	15 μg/mL
Propranolol	40–85 ng/mL	>200 ng/mL
Valproic acid	50–100 μg/mL	200 μg/mL

Lithium levels are drawn 8 to 12 hours after the last dose, usually in the morning after the bedtime dose. The level should be measured at least twice a week while stabilizing the patient and may be drawn monthly thereafter.

Carbamazepine (Tegretol).   A pretreatment CBC, including platelet count, should be done. Reticulocyte count and serum iron are also desirable. The tests should be repeated weekly during the first three months of treatment and monthly thereafter. Carbamazepine can cause aplastic anemia, agranulocytosis, thrombocytopenia, and leukopenia. Because of the minor risk of hepatotoxicity, liver function tests should be done every three to six months. The medication should be discontinued if there are any signs of bone marrow suppression as measured with periodic CBCs. The therapeutic level of carbamazepine is 8 to 12 μg/mL, with toxicity most often reached at levels of 15 μg/mL. Most clinicians report that levels as high as 12 μg/mL are hard to achieve.

Therapeutic and toxic blood levels.   Plasma levels of various drugs can help the clinician ascertain a variety of factors: (1) *compliance*—an absent blood level is found in noncompliant patients; (2) *pharmacodynamics*—blood levels may be abnormally high or low because of metabolic inhibition (for example, enzyme defects or liver damage), medical illness, and drug-drug interaction; (3) *therapeutic levels of drug*—this can correlate with clinical improvement; and (4) *toxic level of drug*—this can account for adverse side effects. Table 34–2 lists common therapeutic and toxic blood levels of some drugs used in psychiatry.

NEUROENDOCRINE TESTS

Thyroid Function Tests

Several thyroid function tests are available, including tests for thyroxine (T_4) by competitive protein binding (T_4 [D]) and by radioimmunoassay (T_4 [RIA]) involving a specific antigen-antibody reaction. Over 90 percent of T_4 is bound to serum protein and is responsible for thyroid-stimulating hormone (TSH) secretion and cellular metabolism. Other thyroid measures include the free T_4 index (FT$_4$I), triiodothyronine uptake, and total serum triiodothyronine measured by radioimmunoassay (T_3 [RIA]). Those tests are used to rule out hypothyroidism, which can present with symptoms of depression. In some studies, up to 10 percent of patients complaining of depression and associated fatigue had incipient hypothyroid disease. Lithium can cause hypothyroidism and more rarely hyperthyroidism. Neonatal hypothyroidism results in mental retardation and is preventable if the diagnosis is made at birth.

Thyrotropin-releasing hormone stimulation test.   The thyrotropin-releasing hormone (TRH) stimulation test is indicated in patients who have marginally abnormal thyroid test results with suspected subclinical hypothyroidism, which may account for clinical depression. It is also used in patients with possible lithium-induced hypothyroidism. The procedure entails an intravenous (IV) injection of 500 mg of TRH, which produces a sharp rise in serum TSH when measured at 15, 30, 60, and 90 minutes. An increase in serum TSH of from 5 to 25 μIU/mL above the baseline is normal. An increase of less than 7 μIU/mL is considered a blunted response, which may correlate with a diagnosis of depression. Eight percent of all patients with depression have some thyroid illness.

Dexamethasone-Suppression Test

Dexamethasone is a long-acting synthetic glucocorticoid with a long half-life. Approximately 1 mg of dexamethasone is equivalent to 25 mg of cortisol. The dexamethasone-suppression test (DST) is used to help confirm a diagnostic impression of major depression with melancholia (revised third edition of *Diagnostic and Statistical Manual of Mental Disorders* [DSM-III-R] classification) or endogenous depression (Research Diagnostic Criteria [RDC] classification).

Procedure.   The patient is given 1 mg of dexamethasone by mouth at 11 PM, and plasma cortisol is measured at 8 AM, 4 PM, and 11 PM. Plasma cortisol above 5 μg/dL (known as nonsuppression) is considered abnormal (that is, positive). Suppression of cortisol indicates that the hypothalamic-adrenal-pituitary axis is functioning properly. Since the 1930s, dysfunction of that axis has been known to be associated with stress.

The DST can be used to follow the response of a depressed person to treatment. Normalization of the DST, however, is not an indication to stop antidepressant treatment, because the DST may normalize before the depression resolves.

There is some evidence that patients with a positive DST (especially 10 μg/dL) will have a good response to somatic treatment, such as electroconvulsive therapy (ECT) or cyclic antidepressant therapy. The problems associated with the DST include varying reports of sensitivity and specificity. False-positive and false-negative results are common and are listed in Table 34–3. The sensitivity of the DST is considered to be 45 percent in major depression and 70 percent in psychotic mood disorders. The specificity is 90 percent compared with controls and 77 percent compared with other psychiatric diagnoses.

Other Endocrine Tests

A variety of other hormones affect behavior. Exogenous hormonal administration has been shown to affect behavior, and known endocrine diseases have associated psychiatric disorders.

Table 34–3
Medical Conditions and Pharmacological Agents That May Interfere with Results of the Dexamethasone-Suppression Test

False-positive results are associated with
  Phenytoin
  Barbiturates
  Meprobamate
  Glutethimide
  Methyprylon
  Methaqualone
  Carbamazepine
  Cardiac failure
  Hypertension
  Renal failure
  Disseminated cancer and serious infections
  Recent major trauma or surgery
  Fever
  Nausea
  Dehydration
  Temporal lobe disease
  High-dosage estrogen treatment
  Pregnancy
  Cushing's disease
  Unstable diabetes mellitus
  Extreme weight loss (malnutrition, anorexia nervosa)
  Alcohol abuse
  Benzodiazepine withdrawal
  Tricyclic antidepressant withdrawal
  Dementia
  Bulimia nervosa
  Acute psychosis
  Advanced age
False-negative results are associated with
  Hypopituitarism
  Addison's disease
  Long-term synthetic steroid therapy
  Indomethacin
  High-dosage cyproheptadine treatment
  High-dosage benzodiazepine treatment

Table from M Young, J Stanford: The dexamethasone suppression test for the detection, diagnosis, and management of depression. Arch Intern Med *100*: 309, 1984. Used with permission.

In addition to thyroid hormones, the hormones include the anterior pituitary hormone prolactin, growth hormone, somastatin, gonadotrophin-releasing hormone (GnRH), and the sex steroids—luteinizing hormone (LH), follicle-stimulating hormone (FSH), testosterone, and estrogen. Melatonin from the pineal gland has been implicated in seasonal affective disorder.

Catecholamines

The serotonin metabolite 5-hydroxyindoleacetic acid (5-HIAA) is elevated in the urine of patients with carcinoid tumors and at times in patients who take phenothiazine medication or in persons who eat foods high in serotonin (for example, walnuts, bananas, avocados). The amount of 5-HIAA in cerebrospinal fluid is low in some persons who are in a suicidal depression and in those who have committed suicide in particularly violent ways. Low cerebrospinal fluid 5-HIAA is associated with violence in general. Norepinephrine and its metabolic products—metanephrine, normetanephrine, and vanillylmandelic acid (VMA)—can be measured in the urine, blood, and plasma. Plasma catecholamines are markedly elevated in pheochromocytoma, which is associated with anxiety, agitation, and hypertension. Some cases of chronic anxiety may share elevated blood norepinephrine and epinephrine levels. Some depressed patients have a lower urinary norepinephrine to epinephrine ratio (NE:E).

High levels of urinary norepinephrine and epinephrine have been found in some patients with posttraumatic stress disorder. The norepinephrine metabolite 3-methoxy-4-hydroxyphenylglycol (MHPG) level is decreased in patients with severe depressive disorders, especially in those patients who attempt suicide.

Renal Function Tests

Creatinine clearance detects early kidney damage and can be serially monitored to follow the course of renal disease. Blood urea nitrogen (BUN) is also elevated in renal disease. Lithium may cause renal damage, and the serum BUN and creatinine are followed in patients taking lithium. If the serum BUN or creatinine is abnormal, the patient's two-hour creatinine clearance and ultimately the 24-hour creatinine clearance are tested.

Liver Function Tests

Total bilirubin and direct bilirubin are elevated in hepatocellular injury and intrahepatic bile stasis that can occur with phenothiazine or tricyclic medication and with alcohol and drug abuse. Certain drugs (for example, phenobarbital) may decrease serum bilirubin. Liver damage or disease, which is reflected by abnormal findings in liver function tests, may present with signs and symptoms of an organic mental syndrome, including disorientation and delirium. Impaired hepatic function may increase the elimination half-lives of certain drugs, including some of the benzodiazepines, so that the drug may stay in the system longer than it would under normal circumstances.

BLOOD TESTS FOR SEXUALLY TRANSMITTED DISEASES

The Venereal Disease Research Laboratory (VDRL) test is used as a screening test for syphilis. If positive, the result is confirmed by using the more specific fluorescent treponemal antibody-absorption test (FTA-ABS test), which uses the spirochete *Treponema pallidum* as the antigen. Central nervous system VDRL is measured in patients with suspected neurosyphilis. A positive human immunodeficiency virus (HIV) test result indicates that the person has been exposed to infection with the virus that causes AIDS.

URINE TESTING FOR DRUGS OF ABUSE

A number of drugs may be detected in a patient's urine if the urine is tested within a specific (and variable) period of time after ingestion. Knowledge of urine

Table 34–4
Drugs of Abuse That Can Be Tested in Urine

Drug	Length of Time Detected in Urine
Alcohol	7–12 hours
Amphetamine	48 hours
Barbiturate	24 hours (short-acting)
	3 weeks (long-acting)
Benzodiazepine	3 days
Cocaine	6–8 hours (metabolites 2–4 days)
Codeine	48 hours
Heroin	36–72 hours
Marijuana	3 days to 4 weeks (depending on use)
Methadone	3 days
Methaqualone	7 days
Morphine	48–72 hours
Phencyclidine (PCP)	8 days
Propoxyphene	6–48 hours

drug testing is becoming crucial for practicing physicians as the controversial issue of mandatory or random drug testing becomes prevalent. Table 34–4 provides a summary of drugs of abuse that can be tested in urine.

OUTLINE OF OTHER TESTS

A. Polysomnography

1. Measures many aspects of sleep: ECG, electroencephalogram (EEG), electro-oculography (EOG), electromyography (EMG), chest expansion, penile tumescence, blood oxygen saturation, body movement, body temperature, galvanic skin response (GSR), gastric acid
2. Indications—to assist in the diagnosis of
   a. Sleep disorders—insomnias, hypersomnias, parasomnias, sleep apnea, nocturnal myoclonus, and bruxism
   b. Childhood sleep-related disorders—functional enuresis, somnambulism (sleepwalking), and sleep terror disorder (pavor nocturnus)
   c. Other disorders—impotence, seizure disorders, migraine and other vascular headaches, drug abuse, gastroesophageal reflux, and major depression
   d. Comments
      i. Correlation between decreased rapid eye movement (REM) latency and major depression, with degree of decreased REM latency correlating with degree of depression
      ii. Shortened REM latency as a diagnostic test for major depression seems to be slightly more sensitive than DST
      iii. Use with DST or TRH stimulation test can improve sensitivity; preliminary data indicate that depressed DST nonsuppressors show extremely high rate of having shortened REM latency
3. Polysomnographic findings in major depression
   a. Most depressed patients (80 to 85 percent) show hyposomnia
   b. Depressed patients have decreased slow wave (delta wave) sleep and shorter sleep stages 3 and 4

    c. Depressed patients have a shortened time between onset of sleep and onset of the first REM period (REM latency)

    d. Depressed patients have a greater percentage of their REM sleep early in the night (the opposite is true for nondepressed controls)

    e. Depressed patients have been found to have more REMs over the entire night (REM density) than do nondepressed controls

B. Electroencephalography (EEG)

1. First clinical application was by the psychiatrist Hans Berger in 1929
2. Measures voltages between electrodes placed on skin
3. Gives gross description of electrical activity of central nervous system (CNS) neurons
4. Each person's EEG is unique, like a fingerprint
5. For decades, researchers have attempted to correlate specific psychiatric conditions with characteristic EEG changes but have been unsuccessful
6. Changes with age
7. Normal EEG does not rule out seizure disorder or organic disease; yield is higher with sleep-deprived studies and also with nasopharyngeal leads
8. Uses
    a. General organic mental syndrome (OMS) workup
    b. Part of routine workup for any first-break psychosis
    c. Can diagnose specific seizure disorders
    d. Helpful in diagnosing CNS lesions—space-occupying lesions, vascular lesions, and encephalopathies, among others
    e. Characteristic changes caused by specific drugs
    f. EEG is exquisitely sensitive to drug changes
    g. Diagnose brain death
9. EEG waves
    a. Beta 14 to 30 Hz (cycles per second)
    b. Alpha 8 to 13 Hz
    c. Theta 4 to 7 Hz
    d. Delta 0.5 to 3 Hz
10. Grand mal seizures—onset characterized by epileptic recruiting rhythm of rhythmic synchronous high-amplitude spikes between 8 and 12 Hz; after 15–30 seconds, spikes may become grouped and may be separated by slow waves (correlates with clonic phase); finally, a quiescent phase of low-amplitude delta (slow) waves
11. Petit mal seizures—sudden onset of bilaterally synchronous generalized spike and wave pattern with high amplitude and characteristic 3 Hz frequency

C. Lactate Provocation of Panic Attacks

1. Indications
    a. Possible diagnosis of panic disorder
    b. Lactate-provoked panic confirms presence of panic attacks

    c. Up to 72 percent of panic patients will have a lactate-provoked attack

    d. Has been used to induce flashbacks in patients with posttraumatic stress disorder

2. Procedure

    a. Inject a 5 percent dextrose in water solution intravenously slowly for 28 minutes, then rapidly for 2 minutes

    b. Infuse 0.5 M racemic sodium lactate (total 10 mL/kg of body weight) over a 20-minute period or until panic occurs

3. Physiological changes from lactate infusion include hemodilution, metabolic alkalosis (metabolized to bicarbonate), hypocalcemia (calcium bound to lactate), and hypophosphatemia (caused by increased glomerular filtration rate [GFR])

4. Comments

    a. Effect is a direct response to lactate or its metabolism and occurs peripherally

    b. Simple hyperventilation has not been as sensitive in inducing panic attacks

    c. Lactate-induced panic is not blocked by peripheral β-blockers but is blocked by alprazolam (Xanax) and by tricyclic antidepressants

    d. CO_2 inhalation precipitates panic attacks, but mechanism is thought to be central and related to CNS concentrations of CO_2, possibly as a locus ceruleus stimulant (CO_2 crosses blood-brain barrier [BBB] but bicarbonate does not)

    e. Lactate crosses BBB through an easily saturated active transport system

    f. L-Lactate is metabolized to pyruvate

D. Amytal Interview

Amobarbital—a medium half-life barbiturate with a half-life of 8 to 42 hours

1. Diagnostic indications—catatonia; hysterical stupor; unexplained muteness; differentiating functional and organic stupors (organic conditions should worsen, and functional conditions should improve because of decreased anxiety)

2. Therapeutic indications (as an interview aid for disorders of repression and dissociation)

    a. Abreaction of posttraumatic stress disorder

    b. Recovery of memory in psychogenic amnesia and fugue

    c. Recovery of function in conversion disorder

3. Procedure

    a. Have patient recline in an environment in which cardiopulmonary resuscitation is readily available should hypotension or respiratory depression develop

    b. Explain to patient that medication should help him or her relax and feel like talking

    c. Insert narrow-bore needle into peripheral vein

    d. Inject 5 percent solution of sodium Amytal (500 mg dissolved in 10 cc of sterile water) at a rate no faster than 1 cc a minute (50 mg a minute)

e. Conduct interview by using frequent suggestion and beginning with neutral topics; often helpful to prompt patient with known facts about his or her life

f. Continue infusion until either sustained lateral nystagmus or drowsiness is noted

g. To maintain level of narcosis, continue infusion at a rate of 0.5 to 1.0 cc/5 minutes (25 to 50 mg/5 minutes)

h. Have·patient remain in reclining position for at least 15 minutes after the interview is terminated and until patient can walk without supervision

i. Use the same method every time to avoid dosage errors

4. Contraindications

a. Presence of upper respiratory infection or inflammation

b. Severe hepatic or renal impairment

c. Hypotension

d. History of porphyria

e. Barbiturate addiction

E. Brain Imaging

1. Computed tomography (CT) scan (formerly computerized axial tomography [CAT] scan)

a. Clinical indications—dementia or depression, general OMS workup, and routine workup for any first-break psychosis

b. Research

  i. Differentiating subtypes of Alzheimer's disease

  ii. Cerebral atrophy in alcohol abusers

  iii. Cerebral atrophy in benzodiazepine abusers

  iv. Cortical and cerebellar atrophy in schizophrenia

  v. Increased ventricle size in schizophrenia

2. Magnetic resonance imaging (MRI) (formerly nuclear magnetic resonance)

a. Measures radiofrequencies emitted by different elements in the brain after application of an external magnetic field and produces slice images

b. Measures structure, not function

c. Technique has been available to other sciences for 30 years

d. Much higher resolution than CT scan, particularly in gray matter

e. No radiation involved; minimal or no risk to patients from strong magnetic fields

f. Can image deep midline structures well

g. Does not actually measure tissue density; measures density of particular nucleus being studied

h. A major problem is time needed to make a scan (5 to 10 minutes)

i. May offer information about cell function in the future, but stronger magnetic fields are needed

j. The ideal technique for evaluating multiple sclerosis and other demyelinating diseases

3. Positron emission tomography (PET) scan

a. Positron emitters—for example, carbon-11 and fluorine-18—are used to label glucose, amino acids, neurotransmitter precursors, and many other molecules—particularly high-affinity ligands, such as N-methylpiperone—which are used to measure receptor densities

b. Can follow the distribution and fate of the molecules

c. Produces slice images like CT scan

d. Labeled antipsychotics—for example, N-methylpiperone—can map out location and density of dopamine receptors

e. It has been shown (through PET scans) that dopamine receptors decrease with age

f. Can assess regional brain function and blood flow

g. 2-Deoxyglucose (a glucose analog) is absorbed into cells as easily as glucose but is not metabolized; can be used to measure regional glucose uptake

h. Measures brain function and physiology

i. Potential for developing understanding of brain functioning and sites of action of drugs

j. Research

   i. Usually compare laterality, anteroposterior gradients, and cortical-subcortical gradients

   ii. Findings reported in schizophrenia

      (a) Cortical hypofrontality (was also found in depressed patients)

      (b) Steeper subcortical to cortical gradient

      (c) Decreased uptake in left compared with right cortex

      (d) Higher activity in left temporal lobe

      (e) Lower metabolism in left basal ganglia

      (f) Higher density of dopamine receptors (only one study, which was not replicated)

      (g) Higher increase in metabolism in anterior brain regions in response to unpleasant stimuli, but the finding not specific to patients with schizophrenia

4. Brain electrical activity mapping (BEAM)

   a. Topographic imaging of EEG and evoked potentials (EPs)

   b. Shows areas of varying electrical activity in the brain through scalp electrodes

   c. New data processing techniques produce new ways of visualizing massive quantities of data produced by EEG and EP

   d. Each point on the map is given a numerical value representing its electrical activity

   e. Each value is computed by linear interpolation among the three nearest electrodes

   f. Some preliminary results show differences in schizophrenic patients; EPs differ spatially and temporally; increased asymmetric beta wave activity in certain regions; increased delta wave activity, most prominent in frontal lobes

5. Regional cerebral blood flow (rCBF)

   a. Yields a two-dimensional cortical image, which represents blood flow to different brain areas

   b. Blood flow believed to correlate directly with neuronal activity

    c. Xenon-133 (low-energy gamma-ray-emitting radioisotope) is inhaled; crosses BBB freely but is inert

    d. Detectors measure rate at which xenon-133 is cleared from specific brain areas and compare with calculated control, yielding a mean transit time for the tracer

       i. Gray matter—clears quickly

      ii. White matter—clears slowly

    e. rCBF may have great potential in studying diseases that have a decrease in the amount of brain tissue—for example, dementia, ischemia, atrophy

    f. Highly susceptible to transient artifacts—for example, anxiety → hyperventilation → low pCO_2 → high CBF

    g. Test is fast, equipment relatively inexpensive ($140,000)

    h. Low radiation

    i. Compared with PET, has less spatial resolution but better temporal resolution

    j. Preliminary data show that schizophrenic patients may have decreased dorsolateral frontal lobe and increased left hemisphere CBF when activated—for example, Wisconsin Card-Sorting Test

    k. No differences found in resting schizophrenic patients

    l. Still under development

  6. Single photon emission computed tomography (SPECT)

    a. Adaptation of rCBF techniques to obtain slice tomograms, rather than two-dimensional surface images

    b. Presently can get tomograms at 2, 6, and 10 cm above and parallel to the canthomeatal line

F. Other Laboratory Tests

    Laboratory tests listed in Table 34–5 have application for clinical and research psychiatry. Standard textbooks of medicine give the laboratory values. The psychiatrist must always know the normal values of the particular laboratory performing the test, because those values vary from one laboratory to another. Two types of measurements are currently in use—the conventional and the Système International (SI) units. The latter, now the more commonly accepted type, is an international language of measurement calculated by multiplying the conventional unit by a

Table 34–5
Other Laboratory Tests

Test	Major Psychiatric Indications	Comments
Acid phosphatase	Organic mental syndrome (OMS) workup	Increased in prostate cancer, benign prostatic hypertrophy, excessive platelet destruction, bone disease
Adrenocorticotropic hormone (ACTH)	OMS workup	Increased in steroid abuse; may be increased in seizures, psychoses, or Cushing's disease or in response to stress Decreased in Addison's disease

Table 34–5
Other Laboratory Tests (Continued)

Test	Major Psychiatric Indications	Comments
Alanine aminotransferase (ALT) (formerly called serum glutamic-pyruvic transaminase [SGPT])	OMS workup	Increased in hepatitis, cirrhosis, liver metastases Decreased in pyridoxine (vitamin B_6) deficiency
Albumin	OMS workup	Increased in dehydration Decreased in malnutrition, hepatic failure, burns, multiple myeloma, carcinomas
Aldolase	Eating disorders Schizophrenia	Increased in patients who abuse ipecac (e.g., bulimic patients), schizophrenia (60–80%)
Alkaline phosphatase	OMS workup Use of psychotropic medications	Increased in Paget's disease, hyperparathyroidism, hepatic disease, hepatic metastases, heart failure, phenothiazine use Decreased in pernicious anemia (vitamin B_{12} deficiency)
Amylase, serum	Eating disorders	May be increased in bulimia nervosa
Aspartate aminotransferase (AST) (formerly SGOT)	OMS workup	Increased in heart failure, hepatic disease, pancreatitis, eclampsia, cerebral damage, alcoholism Decreased in pyridoxine (vitamin B_6) deficiency or terminal stages of liver disease
Bicarbonate, serum	Panic disorder Eating disorders	Decreased in hyperventilation syndrome, panic disorder, and anabolic steroid abuse May be elevated in patients with bulimia nervosa, in laxative abuse, and in psychogenic vomiting
Bilirubin	OMS workup	Increased in hepatic disease
Blood urea nitrogen (BUN)	Delirium Use of psychotropic medications	Elevations associated with lethargy, delirium If elevated, can increase toxic potential of psychiatric medications, especially lithium and amantadine (Symmetrel)
Bromide, serum	Dementia Psychosis	Bromide intoxication can cause psychosis, hallucinations, delirium Part of dementia workup, especially when serum chloride is elevated
Caffeine level, serum	Anxiety	Evaluation of patients with suspected caffeinism
Calcium (Ca), serum	OMS workup Mood disorders Psychosis Eating disorders	Increased in hyperparathyroidism, bone metastases Increase associated with delirium, depression, psychosis Decreased in hypoparathyroidism, renal failure Decrease associated with depression, irritability, delirium, chronic laxative abuse
Carotid ultrasound	Dementia	Occasionally included in dementia workup, especially to rule out multi-infarct dementia Primary value is in search for possible infarct causes
Cerebrospinal fluid (CSF)	OMS workup	Increased protein and cells in infection, positive VDRL in neurosyphilis, bloody CSF in hemorrhagic conditions
Ceruloplasmin, serum; copper, serum	OMS workup	Low in Wilson's disease (hepatolenticular disease)
Chloride (Cl), serum	Eating disorders Panic disorder	Decreased in patients with bulimia and psychogenic vomiting Mild elevation in hyperventilation syndrome and panic disorder

Table 34–5
Other Laboratory Tests (Continued)

Test	Major Psychiatric Indications	Comments
Cholecystokinin (CCK)	Eating disorders	Compared with controls, blunted in bulimic patients after eating meal (may normalize after treatment with antidepressants)
CO_2 inhalation; sodium bicarbonate infusion	Anxiety	Panic attacks produced in subgroup of patients
Coombs' test, direct and indirect	Hemolytic anemias secondary to psychotropic medications	Evaluation of drug-induced hemolytic anemias, such as those secondary to chlorpromazine, phenytoin, levodopa, and methyldopa
Copper, urine	OMS workup	Elevated in Wilson's disease
Cortisol (hydrocortisone)	OMS workup Mood disorders	Excessive level may indicate Cushing's disease associated with anxiety, depression, and a variety of other conditions
Creatine phosphokinase (CPK)	Use of antipsychotics Use of restraints Substance abuse	Increased in neuroleptic malignant syndrome, intramuscular injection, rhabdomyolysis (secondary to substance abuse) patients in restraints, patients experiencing dystonic reactions; asymptomatic elevations seen with use of antipsychotics
Dopamine (L-dopa stimulation of dopamine)	Depression	Inhibits prolactin Test used to assess functional integrity of dopaminergic system, which is impaired in Parkinson's disease, depression
Doppler ultrasound	Impotence OMS workup	Carotid occlusion in organic mental syndrome (OMS), transient ischemic attack (TIA), reduced penile blood flow in impotence
Echocardiogram	Panic disorder	10–40% of patients with panic disorder show mitral valve prolapse
Electroencephalogram (EEG)	OMS workup	Seizures, brain death, lesions; shortened REM latency in depression High-voltage activity in stupor; low-voltage fast activity in excitement; in functional nonorganic cases (e.g., dissociative states), alpha activity is present in the background, which responds to auditory and visual stimuli Biphasic or triphasic slow bursts seen in dementia of Creutzfeldt-Jakob disease
Epstein-Barr virus (EBV); cytomegalovirus (CMV)	OMS workup Chronic fatigue Mood disorders	Part of herpes virus group EBV is causative agent for infectious mononucleosis, which can present with depression and personality change CMV can produce anxiety, confusion, mood disorders EBV associated with chronic mononucleosislike syndrome associated with chronic depression and fatigue. May be association between EBV and major depression
Erythrocyte sedimentation rate (ESR)	OMS workup	An increase in ESR represents a nonspecific test of infectious, inflammatory, autoimmune, or malignant disease
Estrogen	Mood disorder	Decreased in menopausal depression and premenstrual syndrome; variable changes in anxiety
Ferritin, serum	OMS workup	Most sensitive test for iron deficiency

Table 34–5
Other Laboratory Tests (Continued)

Test	Major Psychiatric Indications	Comments
Folate (folic acid), serum	Alcohol abuse Use of specific medications Dementia	Usually measured with vitamin B_{12} deficiencies associated with psychosis, paranoia, fatigue, agitation, dementia, and delirium Associated with alcoholism, use of phenytoin, oral contraceptives, and estrogen
Follicle-stimulating hormone (FSH)	Depression	High normal in anorexia nervosa, higher values in postmenopausal women; low levels in patients with panhypopituitarism
Glucose, fasting blood (FBS)	Panic attacks Anxiety Delirium Depression	Very high FBS associated with delirium Very low FBS associated with delirium, agitation, panic attacks, anxiety, depression
Glutamyl transaminase, serum	Alcohol abuse OMS workup	Increase in alcohol abuse, cirrhosis, liver disease
Gonadotrophic-releasing hormone (GnRH)	Depression Anxiety Schizophrenia	Decrease in schizophrenia; increase in anorexia; variable in depression, anxiety
Growth hormone (GH)	Depression Schizophrenia	Blunted GH responses to insulin-induced hypoglycemia in depressed patients; increased GH responses to dopamine agonist challenge in schizophrenic patients; increased in some cases of anorexia
Hematocrit (Hct); hemoglobin (Hb)	OMS workup	Assessment of anemia (anemia may be associated with depression and psychosis)
Hepatitis A viral antigen (HA Ag)	Mood disorders OMS workup	Less severe, better prognosis than hepatitis B; may present with anorexia, depression
Hepatitis B surface antigen (HBsAg); hepatitis Bc antigen (HBcAg)	Mood disorders OMS workup	Active hepatitis B infection indicates greater degree of infectivity and of progression to chronic liver disease May present with depression
Holter monitor	Panic disorder	Evaluation of panic disordered patients with palpitations and other cardiac symptoms
Homovanillic acid, plasma (pHVA)	OMS workup	Metabolite of dopamine reduced with antipsychotic medication
Human immunodeficiency virus (HIV)	OMS workup	CNS involvement: AIDS dementia, organic personality disorder, organic mood disorder, acute psychosis
17-Hydroxycorticosteroid	Depression	Deviations detect hyperadrenocorticalism, which can be associated with major depression Increased in steroid abuse
5-Hydroxyindoleacetic acid (5-HIAA)	Depression Suicide Violence	Decrease in CSF in aggressive or violent patients with suicidal or homicidal impulses Low level may be indicator of decreased impulse control and predictor of suicide
Iron, serum	OMS workup	Iron-deficiency anemia; found in 30% of geriatric patients
Lactate dehydrogenase (LDH)	OMS workup	Increased in myocardial infarction, pulmonary infarction, hepatic disease, renal infarction, seizures, cerebral damage, megaloblastic (pernicious) anemia, factitious elevations secondary to rough handling of blood specimen tube

Table 34–5
Other Laboratory Tests (Continued)

Test	Major Psychiatric Indications	Comments
Lupus anticoagulant (LA)	Use of phenothiazines	An antiphospholipid antibody, which has been described in some patients using phenothiazines, especially chlorpromazine
Lupus erythematosus (LE) test	Depression Psychosis Delirium Dementia	Positive test associated with systemic LE, which may present with various psychiatric disturbances, such as psychosis, depression, delirium, and dementia; also tested for with antinuclear antibody (ANA) and antiDNA antibody tests
Luteinizing hormone (LH)	Depression	Low in patients with panhypopituitarism; decrease associated with depression
Magnesium, serum	Alcohol abuse OMS workup	Decreased in alcoholism; low levels associated with agitation, delirium, seizures
MAO, platelet	Depression	Low in depression
MCV (mean corpuscular volume) (average volume of a red blood cell)	Alcohol abuse	Elevated in alcoholism and vitamin B_{12} and folate deficiency
Melatonin	Seasonal affective disorder	Produced by light and pineal gland and decrease in seasonal affective disorder
Metal (heavy) intoxication (serum or urinary)	OMS workup	Lead—apathy, irritability, anorexia, confusion Mercury—psychosis, fatigue, apathy, decreased memory, emotional lability, "mad hatter" Manganese—manganese madness, Parkinson-like syndrome Aluminum—dementia Arsenic—fatigue, blackouts, hair loss
3-Methoxy-4-hydroxyphenyglycol (MHPG)	Depression Anxiety	Most useful in research; decreases in urine may indicate decreases centrally; lower in bipolar disorder depressed patients than in unipolar depressed patients
Myoglobin, urine	Phenothiazine use Substance abuse Use of restraints	Increased in neuroleptic malignant syndrome; in PCP, cocaine, or lysergic acid diethylamide (LSD) intoxication; and in patients in restraints
Nicotine	Anxiety Nicotine addiction	Anxiety, smoking
Nocturnal penile tumescence (NPT)	Impotence	Quantification of penile circumference changes, penile rigidity, frequency of penile tumescence Evaluation of erectile function during sleep Erections associated with rapid eye movement (REM) sleep Helpful in differentiation between organic and functional causes of impotence
Parathyroid (parathormone) hormone	Anxiety OMS workup	Low level causes hypocalcemia and anxiety Dysregulation associated with wide variety of organic mental disorders
Phosphorus, serum	OMS workup Panic disorder	Increased in renal failure, diabetic acidosis, hypoparathyroidism, hypervitamin D; decreased in cirrhosis, hypokalemia, hyperparathyroidism, panic attack, hyperventilation syndrome
Platelet count	Use of psychotropic medications	Decreased by certain psychotropic medications (carbamazepine, clozapine, phenothiazines)

Table 34–5
Other Laboratory Tests (Continued)

Test	Major Psychiatric Indications	Comments
Porphobilinogen (PBG)	OMS workup	Increased in acute porphyria
Porphyria synthesizing enzyme	Psychosis OMS workup	Acute panic attack or OMS can occur in acute porphyria attack, which may be precipitated by barbiturates, imipramine
Potassium (K), serum	OMS workup Eating disorders	Increased in hyperkalemic acidosis; increase is associated with anxiety in cardiac arrhythymia Decreased in cirrhosis, metabolic alkalosis, laxative abuse, diuretic abuse; decrease is common in bulimic patients and in psychogenic vomiting, anabolic steroid abuse
Prolactin, serum	Use of antipsychotic medications Cocaine use Pseudoseizures	Antipsychotics, by decreasing dopamine, increase prolactin synthesis and release, especially in women Elevated prolactin levels may be seen secondary to cocaine withdrawal Lack of prolactin rise after seizure suggests pseudoseizure
Protein, total serum	OMS workup Use of psychotropic medications	Increased in multiple myeloma, myxedema, lupus Decreased in cirrhosis, malnutrition, overhydration Low serum protein can result in greater sensitivity to conventional doses of protein-bound medications (lithium is not protein-bound)
Prothrombin time (PT)	OMS workup	Elevated in significant liver damage (cirrhosis)
Reticulocyte count (estimate of red blood cell production in bone marrow)	OMS workup Use of carbamazepine	Low in megaloblastic or iron deficiency anemia and anemia of chronic disease Must be monitored in patient taking carbamazepine
Salicylate, serum	Organic hallucinosis Suicide attempts	Toxic levels may be seen in suicide attempts and may cause organic hallucinosis
Serine hydroxymethyl-transferase (SHMT)	Psychosis	Low in some schizophrenic patients
Sodium (NA$^+$), serum	OMS workup Use of lithium	Increased with excessive salt ingestion; decreased with excessive diaphoresis Decreased in hypoadrenalism, myxedema, congestive heart failure, diarrhea, polydipsia, use of carbamazepine, anabolic steroid Low levels associated with greater sensitivity to conventional dose of lithium
Testosterone, serum	Impotence Inhibited sexual desire	Increase in anabolic steroid abuse May be decreased in organic workup of impotence Decrease may be seen with inhibited sexual desire
Thyroid function	Depression	10 percent of patients with depression and fatigue have thyroid disease
Tryptophan	Depression	Low plasma levels in depression and schizophrenia
Urinalysis	OMS workup Pretreatment workup of lithium Drug screening	Provides clues to cause of various OMSs (assessing general appearance, pH, specific gravity, bilirubin, glucose, blood, ketones, protein, etc.); specific gravity may be affected by lithium
Urinary creatinine	OMS workup Substance abuse Lithium use	Increased in renal failure, dehydration Part of pretreatment workup for lithium

Table 34-5
Other Laboratory Tests (Continued)

Test	Major Psychiatric Indications	Comments
Venereal Disease Research Laboratory (VDRL)	Syphilis	Positive (high titers) in secondary syphilis (may be positive or negative in primary syphilis) Low titers (or negative) in tertiary syphilis
Vitamin A, serum	Depression Delirium	Hypervitaminosis A is associated with a variety of mental status changes
Vitamin B_{12}, serum	OMS workup Dementia	Part of workup of megaloblastic anemia and dementia B_{12} deficiency associated with psychosis, paranoia, fatigue, agitation, dementia, delirium, mania Often associated with chronic alcohol abuse
White blood cell (WBC)	Use of psychotropic medications	Leukopenia and agranulocytosis associated with certain psychotropic medications, such as phenothiazines and carbamazepine, clozapine Leukocytosis associated with lithium and neuroleptic malignant syndrome

number factor being adopted by many laboratories. The SI measurement system uses *moles* as the basic unit for the amount of a substance, *kilograms* for its mass, and *meters* for its length.

References

Arana G W, Baldessarini R J, Ornsteen M: The dexamethasone suppression test for diagnosis and prognosis in psychiatry. Arch Gen Psychiatry *42*: 1193, 1985.

Carroll B J: Dexamethasone suppression test: A review of contemporary confusion. J Clin Psychiatry *46*: 13, 1985.

Evans L: Some biological aspects of panic disorder. Int J Clin Pharmacol Res 9: 139, 1989.

Galen R S, Gambino S R: *Beyond Normality: The Predictive Value and Efficiency of Medical Diagnoses.* Wiley, New York, 1975.

Garattini S, Tognoni G, editors: Biological markers in mental disorders (symposium). J Psychiatr Res *18*: 327, 1984.

Gold M S, Pottash A L C: *Diagnostic and Laboratory Testing in Psychiatry.* Plenum, New York, 1986.

Griner P F, Glaser R J: Misuse of laboratory tests and diagnostic procedures. N Engl J Med *307*: 1336, 1982.

Hall R C W, Beresford T P, editors: *Handbook of Psychiatric Diagnostic Procedures*, vols 1, 2. SP Medical and Scientific Books, New York, 1984, 1985.

Kirch D G: Medical assessment and laboratory testing in psychiatry. In *Comprehensive Textbook of Psychiatry*, ed 5, H I Kaplan, B J Sadock, editors, p 525. Williams & Wilkins, Baltimore, 1989.

Koranyi E K: Morbidity and rate of undiagnosed physical illnesses in a psychiatric clinic population. Arch Gen Psychiatry *36*: 414, 1979.

Lake C R, Ziegler M G, editors: *The Catecholamines in Psychiatric and Neurologic Disorders.* Butterworth, Boston, 1985.

Martin R L, Preskorn S H: Use of the laboratory in psychiatry. In *The Medical Basis of Psychiatry*, G Winokur, P Clayton, editors, p 522. Saunders, Philadelphia, 1986.

Norman T R, Burrows G D, Judd F K, McIntyre I M: Serotonin and panic disorders: A review of clinical studies. Int J Clin Pharmacol Res 9: 151, 1989.

Perry J C, Jacobs D: Overview: Clinical applications of the Amytal interview in psychiatric emergency settings. Am J Psychiatry *139*: 552, 1982.

Rosse R B, Giese A A, Deutsch S I, Morihisa J M: *Laboratory and Diagnostic Testing in Psychiatry.* American Psychiatric Press, Washington, 1989.

Usdin E, Hanin I, editors: *Biological Markers in Psychiatry and Neurology.* Pergamon, New York, 1982.

Weinberger D R: Brain disease and psychiatric illness: When should a psychiatrist order a CAT scan? Am J Psychiatry *141*: 1521, 1984.

35

Investigational Drugs

The past decade of neuroscience research has produced an explosion of knowledge regarding neurotransmitter receptors and their subtypes. The most recent advances in the field can be attributed to the techniques of molecular genetics, which have allowed investigators to discover ever more subtypes. The key beneficial effect of the knowledge will be the development of psychiatric drugs that affect receptors responsible for beneficial therapeutic effects but not other receptors responsible for adverse effects. Although only a small fraction of the basic science knowledge has already been used in the development of new central nervous system (CNS) compounds, a huge variety of new candidate drugs are in the pharmaceutical industry development pipeline (Table 35–1).

STAGES OF DRUG DEVELOPMENT

The first stage of drug development involves the identification of a compound that for theoretical reasons may be effective in treating some disorder. The compound is then studied in a wide variety of in vitro and in vivo tests that are somewhat predictive of clinical drug effects. Compounds found to be of potential importance in those tests then undergo studies of their toxicity and pharmacokinetics in animals. If those preliminary preclinical tests are thought to merit the costs of further drug development, a pharmaceutical company in the United States files an Investigational New Drug (IND) application with the Food and Drug Administration (FDA). If the application is granted, the compound can then be used in humans for research purposes. The first such experiments are called phase I experiments, in which the drug is administered to normal persons to assess its pharmacokinetics and its potential to cause adverse effects. Phase I studies are conducted primarily to determine the safety and the tolerability of a new compound. The information from the phase I studies is then used to help decide on a dosage of the drug to use in phase II trials, which involve the use of the new compound in a patient population. The primary purpose of phase II trials is to assess the efficacy of the new drug in the treatment of specific disorders. If the phase II trials indicate that a drug is efficacious, safe, and well-tolerated, much larger phase III trials are conducted to validate the findings of the phase II studies. Phase III studies also gather detailed information regarding the optimum dosage schedules and the use of the drug in elderly and young populations and in persons with impaired renal or hepatic function. At some time between the phase II trials and the phase III trials, the pharmaceutical company can apply to the FDA for a New Drug Application (NDA), which, if granted, allows the drug company to market the drug commercially.

Table 35–1
Status of CNS Compounds in Clinical Development by Manufacturer*

Company	Compound	Category	Phase of Clinical Development
Abbott	Idebenone	Nootropic†	II
	Sertindole	Antipsychotic	II
	A75200	Antidepressant	II
	Tiagabine	Anticonvulsant	III
American Home Products	Venlafaxine	Antidepressant	NDA approved
	Vinpocetine	Nootropic	NDA filed
	WY-47846	Anxiolytic	I
	AHR-11748	Anticonvulsant	I
	Enciprazine	Anxiolytic	II
	Guanfacine	Nootropic	II
Angelini	Etoperidone	Antidepressant	III
Bayer	Ipsapirone	Anxiolytic	III
Biocodex	Stripentol	Anticonvulsant	I
Boehringer Ingelheim	Brotizolam	Hypnotic	II
	Talipexole	Antiparkinsonism	II
Boots	Dosulepine	Antidepressant	NDA filed
	Sibutramine	Antidepressant	II
Bristol-Myers Squibb	NKT-01	Multiple sclerosis	I
	Gepirone	Anxiolytic	II
	BMY-21502	Nootropic	II
	Nefazodone	Antidepressant	III
Burroughs Wellcome	Lamotrigine	Anticonvulsant	III
Ciba-Geigy	CGS-15873A	Antipsychotic	I
	CGS-18416A	Antipsychotic	I
	CGS-11361	Anxiolytic	I
	Brofaromine	Antidepressant	II
	Oxacarbazepine	Anticonvulsant	III
Dainippon	Zonisamide	Anticonvulsant	III
Dow	MDL-72974A	Antiparkinsonism	I
	Vigabatrin	Anticonvulsant	III
Du Pont	DUP-996	Nootropic	III
	DUP-734	Antipsychotic	I
	DUP-750	Antipsychotic	I
Erbamont	Reboxetine	Antidepressant	I
Fidia	Bros	Nootropic	III
Fisons	Remacemide	Anticonvulsant	II
Forest	Synapton	Nootropic	III
Glaxo	Sumatriptan	Antimigraine	NDA filed
	Fluparoxan	Antidepressant	I
	Odansetron	Antipsychotic	II
Gruenthal	Orotirelin	Psychostimulant tranquilizer	I
Hoechst	Suronacrine malcate	Nootropic	I
	Velnacrine	Nootropic	III
Hoffmann-La Roche	Moclobemide	Antidepressant	III
	Bretazenil	Antipsychotic	II
ICI	ICI-204636	Antipsychotic	II
Johnson & Johnson	Loreclezole	Anticonvulsant	I
	Topiramate	Anticonvulsant	III
	Bromperidol	Antipsychotic	III
	Risperidone	Antipsychotic	III
	Flunarizine	Antimigraine	III
	Ritanserin	Antidepressant-anxiolytic	III

Table 35–1
Status of CNS Compounds in Clinical Development by Manufacturer* (Continued)

Company	Compound	Category	Phase of Clinical Development
Kabi-Pharmacia	Nicotine transdermal	Antismoking	NDA filed
Kissei	Cabergoline	Antiparkinsonism	I
Kodak	Napamezole	Antidepressant	I
Eli Lilly	LY-210448	Anoretic	I
	LY-277359	Antimigraine	I
	Sergolexole	Antimigraine	II
	LY-053857	Antimigraine	II
	Quinelorane	Antimigraine	III
	Tomoxetine	Antidepressant	III
Macrochem	Eterobarb	Anticonvulsant	NDA filed
Martec	Femoxitine	Antidepressant	II
Medicis	TRH	Neuroprotectant	III
Merck	MK-912	Antidepressant	I
	Eptastigmine	Nootropic	I
	Devazepide	Obesity	I
	Raclopride	Antipsychotic	II
	Remoxipride	Antipsychotic	III
Novo Nordisk	Boxeprazine	Antidepressant	II
	FG-7516	Anxiolytic	III
Organon	Mirtrazapine	Antidepressant	III
Orion	Dexmedetomidine	Hypnotic	I
Pfizer	Tandospirone	Anxiolytic	II
Reckitt and Coleman	Idazoxan	Antidepressant	II
Recordati	Nicotine transdermal	Antismoking	II
Rhone-Poulenc Rorer	Zopiclone	Hypnotic	II
	Suriclone	Anxiolytic	III
Rugby	Propranolol	Antimigraine	II
Sandoz/Novo Nordisk	Abecarnil	Anxiolytic	I
Scarle	BTG-1501	Anxiolytic	II
	SC-49088	Nootropic	II
	Alpidem	Anxiolytic	III
Schering AG	Lormetazepam	Hypnotic	NDA filed
	Rolipram	Antidepressant	I
Schering-Plough	SCH-39166	Antipsychotic	I
Sigma-Tau	ST-200	Nootropic	III
SmithKline Beecham	Paroxetine	Antidepressant	NDA filed
	Oxiracetam	Nootropic	II
	Ropinerole	Antiparkinsonism	II
Solvay	Eltoprazine	Antipsychotic	II
Syntex	Fibroblast growth factor	Nootropic	III
Synthelabo	Zolpidem	Hypnotic	NDA filed
Upjohn	Adinazolam	Antidepressant	NDA filed
	U-78875	Anxiolytic	I
	Tirilizad methylate	Nootropic	III
	Deracyn	Antipsychotic	II
Upjohn-Solvay	Fluvoxamine	Antidepressant	NDA filed
Wallace	Felbamate	Anticonvulsant	II

Table 35–1
Status of CNS Compounds in Clinical Development by Manufacturer* (Continued)

Company	Compound	Category	Phase of Clinical Development
Warner-Lambert	Tacrine	Nootropic	NDA filed
	Nicotine patch	Antismoking	NDA filed
	CI-966	Anticonvulsant	I
	Pramiractam	Nootropic	II
	CI-933	Nootropic	II
	CI-943	Antipsychotic	II
	CI-844	Nootropic	II
	Gabapentin	Anticonvulsant	III
	Fosphenytoin	Anticonvulsant	III
Whitby	N-0437	Antiparkinsonism	I
Yeda	Autoimmune vaccine	Multiple sclerosis	I

Table from The Neuroscience Market Intelligence Service. The Wilkerson Group, New York, 1992. Used with permission.
*Some compounds were discovered and patented by one company (usually a small one) but are being developed for clinical application by another company (usually a larger one).
†A nootropic is a drug that helps improve memory and cognition (from the Greek *noesis*, meaning to know).

DRUGS UNDER DEVELOPMENT

Table 35–1 lists an impressive roster of CNS compounds under development for clinical application. Indeed, 10 years from now the psychopharmacotherapy armamentarium will be almost completely different from today's armamentarium. For a variety of reasons, it is difficult to predict which new drugs will come to market in the United States. First, for commercial reasons, pharmaceutical companies are somewhat secretive about their drugs under development. Second, a candidate drug may be well into phase III development before its association with a particularly severe adverse effect is noted, resulting in the termination of the development of that compound. Third, a candidate drug may be well into phase III development before an assessment of its efficacy results in a determination that it is not significantly better than competing compounds to merit the cost of introducing the drug commercially. Nevertheless, one can attempt to predict which antipsychotic and antidepressant compounds will be introduced into the United States soon.

Antipsychotics

The major reasons to develop new antipsychotic compounds are (1) the association of current compounds with serious or undesirable adverse effects (for example, extrapyramidal symptoms, tardive dyskinesia, anticholinergic activity, and adverse cardiovascular effects); (2) the existence of many treatment-resistant patients; and (3) the general lack of efficacy of the standard antipsychotics for the treatment of negative symptoms.

Many new antipsychotic compounds have been labelled atypical, although no precise definition of what constitutes an atypical antipsychotic agent has been agreed on. Compounds are variously classified as atypical antipsychotics if they have one or more of the following characteristics: (1) serotonin antagonism, (2) no dopamine type 2 (D_2) antagonism as their primary pharmacodynamic effect, and (3) less association with extrapyramidal symptoms than the standard antipsychotic. Clozapine (Clozaril) is the classic atypical antipsychotic; in fact, it meets all three of the above criteria.

Candidate antipsychotics. After the recent introduction of clozapine, it is a reasonable guess that the next two compounds to be introduced to the United States drug market as antipsychotics will be risperidone and remoxipride. Risperidone (Johnson & Johnson) is a combined dopamine type 2 (D_2) receptor-serotonin (5-HT_2) receptor antagonist. Remoxipride (Merck) is a D_2 antagonist that appears to be associated with fewer extrapyramidal symptoms than are the standard D_2 antagonists, such as haloperidol (Haldol).

In general, most new antipsychotics that will be introduced in the next five years will be in one of three categories: first, D_2 receptor antagonists that are associated with fewer extrapyramidal symptoms than are conventional drugs, perhaps because they actually act on non-D_2 receptors as well; second, combined D_2-5-HT_2 receptor antagonists; third, serotonin antagonists without dopamine antagonist activity, such as odansetron (Glaxo) and ritanserin (Johnson & Johnson), although it is not clear yet whether those drugs will be effective antipsychotics. In addition, other drugs will not fit into those categories, including benzodiazepine receptor antagonists (for example, deracyn [Upjohn], bretazenil [Hoffman-La-Roche]), sigma receptor antagonists (for example, DUP-734 and DUP-750 [Du Pont]), and drugs with as yet unknown mechanisms of actions (for example, ICI-204636 [ICI]).

Antidepressants

The major reasons to develop new antidepressant compounds are (1) the fact that 50 to 70 percent of the depressed patients do not respond to currently available antidepressants, (2) the three- to six-week delay in the therapeutic effects, and (3) the presence of many cardiovascular and other adverse effects (for example, high lethality in overdose). Fluoxetine (Prozac) was the first of the dramatically new antidepressants to be introduced in the United States. Sertraline (Zoloft), which was introduced in 1991, also has the specific blockade of serotonin reuptake as a primary mechanism of action. Both drugs are associated with fewer adverse effects than the standard antidepressants and appear not to be lethal when taken alone in overdose attempts.

Candidate antidepressants. The next six antidepressant compounds to be introduced in the United States will probably be paroxetine (SmithKline Beecham), fluvoxamine (Upjohn-Solvay), venlafaxine (American Home Products), gepirone (Bristol-Myers Squibb), ipsapirone (Bayer), and nefazodone (Bristol-Myers Squibb). Paroxetine and fluvoxamine share with fluoxetine and sertraline a primary mechanism of action of the specific blockade of serotonin reuptake. Venlafaxine blocks serotonin reuptake but also blocks norepinephrine and dopamine reuptake. Gepirone and ipsapirone are 5-HT_{1A} agonists that are similar to buspirone (BuSpar), the currently available antianxiety agent. Nefazodone blocks serotonin reuptake and is a 5-HT$_2$ agonist.

Many additional candidate antidepressant compounds are under development. Many have novel mechanisms of action, including α_2-adrenergic antagonists, phosphodiesterase inhibitors, adenosine agonists, acetylcholinesterase inhibitors, and N-methyl-D-aspartate (NMDA) inhibitors.

References

Gelders Y G, Heylen S L E, Vanden Bussche G, Reyntjens A J M, Janssen P A J: Pilot clinical investigation of risperidone in the treatment of psychotic patients. Pharmacopsychiatry *23*: 206, 1990.

Jenkins S W, Robinson D S, Fabre L F, Andory J J, Messina M E, Reich L A: Gepirone in the treatment of major depression. J Clin Psychopharmacol *10* (3, Suppl): 77S, 1990.

Schweizer E, Weise C, Clary C, Fox I, Rickels K: Placebo-controlled trial of venlafaxine for the treatment of major depression. J Clin Psychopharmacol *11*: 233, 1991.

Walinder J, Holm A-C: Experiences of long-term treatment with remoxipride: Efficacy and tolerability. Acta Psychiatr Scand *82* (Suppl 338): 158, 1990.

36

Intoxication and Overdose

Drug	Toxic or Lethal Dose*	Signs and Symptoms	Treatment†
β-Adrenergic receptor antagonists	Propranolol 1 g	Hypotension, bradycardia, seizures, loss of consciousness, bronchospasm, cardiac failure	Supportive care; emesis or gastric lavage after acute ingestion. If needed (comatose, seizures, absent gag), lavage with endotracheal tube with inflated cuff in place; intravenous (IV) atropine for symptomatic bradycardia, IV isoproterenol for persistent cases, a pacemaker if refractory; norepinephrine or dopamine for severe hypotension; IV diazepam for seizures; glucagon may be useful for hypotension and myocardial depression, theophylline or β_2-agonist for bronchospasm, a diuretic or cardiac glycoside for heart failure
Amantadine	2.5 g	Disorientation, visual hallucinations, confusion, aggressive behavior, minimally reactive and slightly dilated pupils, urinary retention, acid-base disturbances, coma	Induce emesis or use gastric lavage in recent overdose; supportive measures, including airway maintenance, cardiovascular monitoring, control of respiration and oxygen administration, monitoring urine pH, urinary output, serum electrolytes; acidifying agents can increase the rate of excretion, force fluids (IV if needed); observe for hypotension, seizures, psychosis, urinary retention, arrhythmias, hyperactivity, which should be treated appropriately; physostigmine may be useful in treating central nervous system (CNS) toxicity; chlorpromazine may be useful for toxic psychosis; adrenergic agents may predispose the patient to ventricular arrhythmias
Amphetamine	100 mg	Elation, irritability, hyperactivity, rapid speech, anorexia, hyperreflexia, insomnia, dry mouth, chest pain, arrhythmia, heart block, poor concentration, restlessness, psychotic symptoms	Emesis or lavage can be effective long after ingestion because of recycling through gastric mucosa; reduce external stimuli; treat cerebral edema and hyperthermia; peritoneal dialysis; sedate with chlorpromazine 0.5–1 mg/kg intramuscular (IM) or by mouth every 30 minutes as needed; use ½ the dose for mixed amphetamine-barbiturate overdose

Drug	Toxic or Lethal Dose*	Signs and Symptoms	Treatment†
Anti-cholinergics	700 mg–7 g, (doses vary, depending on agent involved)	Hot, dry, flushed skin; unreactive dilated pupils; blurred vision; dry mucous membranes; foul breath; difficulty in swallowing; urinary retention; decreased bowel sounds; tachycardia; nausea; vomiting; rash; anticholinergic delirium with delusions, hallucinations, disorientation	Supportive and symptomatic therapy; continuous electrocardiograph (ECG) monitoring; empty stomach immediately by inducing emesis if patient is conscious, has gag reflex and no seizures; otherwise, gastric lavage and activated charcoal can be used with endotracheal tube with inflated cuff in place; saline cathartics may be used; exchange transfusions can be considered in extreme cases; fluid therapy should be used for shock; cold packs, mechanical cooling devices, or sponging with tepid water can be used for hyperthermia; diazepam can be used for agitation; 1 mg can reverse adverse effects of physostigmine; IV propranolol may be useful for supraventricular tachyarrhythmias; avoid dopamine receptor antagonists
Antihistamines	2.8 g (diphenhy-dramine), 1,750–17,500 mg (hydroxyzine)	Disorientation, drowsiness, excitation or depression, hallucinations, anxiety, delirium, hyperthermia, tachycardia, arrhythmias, seizures	Empty stomach with ipecac emesis or gastric lavage; support cardiorespiratory function; physostigmine may be useful for anticholinergic effects, diazepam for seizures; sponge baths with tepid water (not alcohol) or cold packs for hyperthermia
Barbiturates	10 times the daily therapeutic dose (e.g., 1–2 g of secobarbital)	Delirium, confusion, excitement, headache, CNS and respiratory depression from somnolence to coma, areflexia, circulatory collapse	Supportive treatment, including maintaining airway and respiration and treating shock as needed; within 30 minutes of ingestion, use activated charcoal; gastric lavage and aspiration can be used within 4 hours of ingestion; nasogastric administration of charcoal in multiple doses can shorten coma; maintain vital signs, fluid balance; alkalinizing the urine increases the excretion of mephobarbital, aprobarbital, phenobarbital; forced diuresis may be of use if renal function is normal; hemodialysis or peritoneal dialysis may be useful in severe cases
Benzo-diazepines	Toxic dose: diazepam: 2 g; chlordiaze-poxide: 6 g	Slurred speech, incoordination, somnolence, confusion, coma, hyporeflexia, hypotension	General supportive care; induce emesis for recent ingestions in fully conscious patients; gastric lavage with endotracheal tube with inflated cuff if comatose; after above, use a saline cathartic and activated charcoal; maintain airway, monitor vital signs, give IV fluids; norepinephrine or metaraminol can be used for hypotension; flumazenil can be used with extreme caution (see Chapter 21)

Drug	Toxic or Lethal Dose*	Signs and Symptoms	Treatment†
Bromocriptine	Survival of 225 mg dose reported	Severe hypotension, nausea, vomiting, psychosis	Empty stomach by lavage and aspiration; IV fluids for hypotension
Bupropion	Ingestions of 850–4,200 mg have been survived; deaths have been reported in massive overdoses	Seizures, loss of consciousness, hallucinations, tachycardia	Ipecac emesis if conscious; gastric lavage with endotracheal tube with inflated cuff if there are seizures or a decreased level of consciousness; during first 12 hours after ingestion, use activated charcoal every 6 hours, provide fluids; electroencephalogram (EEG) and ECG monitoring for 48 hours; seizures can be treated with IV benzodiazepines
Buspirone	Toxic dose of 375 mg (used in studies); lethal dose unknown	Dizziness, drowsiness, nausea, vomiting, miosis, gastric distension	Symptomatic and supportive care; empty stomach with emesis or lavage in acute ingestions; if needed, perform lavage with endotracheal tube in place with cuff inflated; monitor vital signs
Calcium channel inhibitors	9.6 g of verapamil has resulted in death; patients have survived ingestion of 8 to 10 g of diltiazem and 9 g of nifedipine (case reports)	Confusion, headache, nausea, vomiting, seizures, flushing, constipation, bradycardia, hypotension, atrioventricular block, hyperglycemia, metabolic acidosis	Emesis followed by gastric lavage with activated charcoal; calcium gluconate or calcium chloride 10–20 mg/kg in 10% solution with normal saline IV given over 30 minutes and repeated as needed; atropine or isoproterenol for atrioventricular block; a pacemaker may be needed
Carbamazepine	Lowest known lethal dose in adults: 60 g; highest known doses survived: children 10 g, adults 30 g	Drowsiness, stupor, dizziness, restlessness, ataxia, agitation, nausea, vomiting, involuntary movements, abnormal reflexes, adiadochokinesis, nystagmus, mydriasis, flushing, cyanosis, urinary retention, hypotension or hypertension, coma, cardiac arrhythmias	Induce emesis or gastric lavage; supportive measures; ECG monitoring
Carisoprodol	Patients have recovered from 3.4 g and 9.45 g ingestions	Stupor, shock, coma, respiratory depression, headache, diplopia, dizziness, drowsiness, nystagmus	Supportive treatment; induce emesis or use gastric lavage with endotracheal tube with cuff inflated if clinically indicated; activated charcoal after emptying stomach; maintain airway, respiration, and blood pressure; pressor agents can be used with caution if necessary; elimination may be enhanced by forced diuresis with hemodialysis, peritoneal dialysis, or osmotic diuresis; avoid overhydration; monitor neurological status, electrolytes, and vital signs;

Drug	Toxic or Lethal Dose*	Signs and Symptoms	Treatment†
			continue monitoring for relapse secondary to delayed absorption and incomplete gastric emptying
Chloral hydrate	4–10 g	Coma, confusion, drowsiness, respiratory depression, hypotension, hypothermia, vomiting, miosis, gastric necrosis and perforation, esophageal stricture, hepatic injury, renal injury	General supportive measures; gastric lavage with endotracheal tube with inflated cuff in place; maintain airway, oxygenation, cardiorespiratory function, and body temperature; hemodialysis or peritoneal dialysis may be of use; saline enema if drug was administered rectally
Clonidine	No known deaths from overdoses of clonidine alone; 100 mg is the largest known overdose survived; 2 known deaths from mixed overdoses that included clonidine	Hypotension, hyporeflexia or areflexia, vomiting, weakness, irritability, sedation, coma, lethargy, hypothermia, constricted pupils, dry mouth, hypoventilation, seizures, arrhythmia, cardiac conduction defects	Induce emesis or lavage followed by activated charcoal and a saline cathartic; lavage is preferred in patients with decreased levels of consciousness and should be used with endotracheal tube with inflated cuff in place if patient is comatose, has seizures, or lacks gag reflex; supportive and symptomatic measures; establish airway, IV fluids, and Trendelenburg position for hypotension; if persistent, use dopamine; atropine IV for symptomatic bradycardia; tolazoline 10 mg IV every 30 minutes may reverse cardiovascular effects of clonidine; IV furosemide, α-blockers, or diazoxide for hypertension; IV benzodiazepines can be used for seizures
Clozapine	Lethal dose: >2.5 g, although patients have survived ingestions of >4 g	Delirium, drowsiness, coma, respiratory depression, tachycardia, arrhythmias, hypotension, hypersalivation, seizures	Symptomatic and supportive care; establish and maintain airway, ventilation, and oxygenation; activated charcoal with sorbitol (may be as effective or more effective than lavage or emesis); monitor and adjust acid-base and electrolyte balance; physostigmine may be a useful adjunct for anticholinergic toxicity but is not for routine use; epinephrine, quinidine, procainamide are to be avoided; patient should be observed for several days for delayed effects
Dantrolene	No data available	Speech and visual disturbances, gastrointestinal (GI) upset or bleeding, liver damage, nausea, vomiting, CNS depression	Supportive measures; immediate gastric lavage; ECG monitoring; large quantities of IV fluids; maintain airway; have artificial respiratory measures available; observe patient
Disulfiram	6 or more fatalities have occurred with	Headache, rash, peripheral or optic neuropathy, mucous	Supportive treatment, gastric lavage or aspiration

Drug	Toxic or Lethal Dose*	Signs and Symptoms	Treatment†
	ingestions of 0.5–1 g of disulfiram with blood alcohol levels of 1 mg/mL; a 30 g ingestion would produce serious toxicity	membrane injury, psychotic behavior	
L-Dopa	Dose should not exceed 8 g a day in therapeutic use	Palpitations, arrhythmias, spasm or closing of eyes, psychosis	Symptomatic treatment; maintain airway; lavage; ECG monitoring; IV fluids; treat arrhythmias as necessary
Dopamine receptor antagonists	Fatal doses reported: chlorpromazine: 26 g (in an adult), 350 mg in a child; thiothixene: 2.5–4 g; phenothiazines: 1,050 mg– 10.5 g	Sedation, hypotension, severe extrapyramidal symptoms, confusion, excitement, CNS depression, coma, arrhythmias, miosis, tremor, spasm, rigidity, seizures, dry mouth, ileus, difficulty in swallowing, muscular hypotonia, difficulty in breathing, hypothermia, vasomotor or respiratory collapse, sudden apnea	Symptomatic and supportive care; if clinically indicated, lavage may be performed with endotracheal tube with inflated cuff in place; emesis should not be induced; saline cathartic may be helpful; hypotension should be treated as necessary (avoid epinephrine); anticholinergics may be useful for extrapyramidal symptoms; exchange transfusions may be useful; oversedation and hypothermia should be treated as appropriate
Ethchlorvynol	6 g has been lethal; overdoses of 50 g and in one case 100 g have been survived	Hypotension, hypothermia, severe respiratory depression, apnea, deep coma (can last days to weeks), areflexia, mydriasis, bradycardia	Supportive treatment; gastric lavage with endotracheal tube with inflated cuff in place; maintain airway; give oxygen; maintain cardiorespiratory function and body temperature; monitor blood gases; provide pulmonary care; hemoperfusion with Amberlite XAD-4 resin hastens drug elimination; hemodialysis or peritoneal dialysis may be beneficial
Fenfluramine	2 g (460 mg in a child) was lowest reported fatal dose; 1.8 g in an adult is the highest reported nonfatal dose	Drowsiness, agitation, flushing, tremor, confusion, shivering, hyperventilation, dilated nonreactive pupils, tachycardia, hyperpyrexia, coma, seizures, cardiac arrest	Symptomatic and supportive care; gastric lavage; activated charcoal; endotracheal tube placement in consultation with an anesthesiologist is needed if trismus is present and lavage is to be performed; maintain cardiorespiratory function; cardiac monitoring; defibrillation, cardioversion, ventilatory support if needed; phenobarbital or diazepam for seizures or muscle hyperactivity; propranolol for severe tachycardia; lidocaine for ventricular extrasystoles; chlorpromazine may be useful for hyperthermia; forced acid diuresis

Drug	Toxic or Lethal Dose*	Signs and Symptoms	Treatment†
			with ammonium chloride may increase excretion rate
Fluoxetine	Lethal dose unknown (one death reported)	Restlessness, insomnia, agitation, tremor, hypomania, tachycardia, seizures, nausea, vomiting, hypertension, drowsiness, coma, nystagmus	Supportive and symptomatic care; keep airway open; maintain oxygenation and ventilation; monitor ECG and vital signs; gastric lavage (if clinically indicated, have endotracheal tube with cuff inflated during lavage) or emesis in recent ingestion, or use activated charcoal; IV diazepam for ongoing seizures; consider phenobarbital or phenytoin if refractory to diazepam
Glutethimide	5 g: severe intoxication; 10–20 g: often lethal	Hypotension, prolonged coma (up to days), shock, respiratory depression, hypothermia, fever, inadequate ventilation, apnea, cyanosis, fixed and dilated pupils, ileus, bladder atony, dry mouth, hyporeflexia, areflexia, intermittent spasticity or flaccidity	Supportive treatment; gastric lavage using 1 to 1 mixture of castor oil and water (may be more effective than aqueous lavage); perform with endotracheal tube in place with inflated cuff; leave 50 mL castor oil in stomach as a cathartic; activated charcoal may be of use; maintain airway and cardiorespiratory function; hemodialysis may be useful in severe cases (particularly with activated charcoal or soybean dialysate); hemoperfusion with Amberlite XAD-2 resin may be more effective than hemodialysis; charcoal hemoperfusion may be useful; continue drug removal procedures for at least 2 hours after the patient regains consciousness; maintain urinary output but avoid overhydration
Lithium	Lethal dose produces serum levels of >3.5 mEq/L 12 hours after ingestion	Diarrhea, vomiting, confusion, drowsiness, tremor, apathy, giddiness, nausea, ataxia, muscle rigidity, vertical nystagmus, impaired consciousness, cogwheel rigidity, coma, seizures, cardiovascular collapse	Induce emesis or lavage (lavage with endotracheal tube in place with cuff inflated if indicated); infuse 0.9% sodium chloride IV if toxicity is due to sodium depletion; hemodialysis for 8–12 hours if fluid and electrolyte imbalance does not respond to supportive measures; if level is >3 mEq/L or if level is 2–3 mEq/L and patient is deteriorating or if level has not decreased 20% in 6 hours, repeated courses of dialysis are often needed; goal is level of <1 mEq/L 8 hours after dialysis is completed
Meprobamate	12 g is usually lethal; 40 g overdoses have been survived	Stupor, drowsiness, lethargy, ataxia, coma, respiratory depression, hypotension	Supportive treatment; induce emesis or use gastric lavage with endotracheal tube with cuff inflated if clinically indicated; use activated charcoal after emptying stomach; maintain airway, respiration, and blood pressure; pressor agents can be used with

Drug	Toxic or Lethal Dose*	Signs and Symptoms	Treatment[†]
			caution if necessary; elimination may be enhanced by forced diuresis with hemodialysis, peritoneal dialysis, or osmotic diuresis
Methadone	Lethal dose: 40–60 mg in nontolerant persons	CNS depression (stupor to coma), pinpoint pupils, shallow respiration, bradycardia, hypotension, hypothermia, cold and clammy skin, apnea, cardiac arrest, mydriasis in severe hypoxia or terminal narcosis	Establish and maintain airway and respiration; gastric lavage; supportive care with IV fluids; naloxone may be used to treat respiratory depression; initial adult dose is 0.4–2 mg IV every 2–3 minutes if needed; if there is no response after a total of 10 mg has been given, other diagnoses should be considered; repeated doses of naloxone may be needed, as narcotic-induced respiratory depression may return as the effects of naloxone diminish; dosage regimes for continuous naloxone infusions are not well established and should be titrated to the patient's response; patients should be observed for sustained improvement after treatment
Methylphenidate hydrochloride	2 g	Delirium, confusion, psychosis, agitation, hallucinations, palpitations, arrhythmias, hypertension, vomiting, hyperpyrexia, mydriasis, sweating, tremors, muscle twitching, seizures, coma	Emesis or lavage in mild cases; if patient is conscious, careful use of a short-acting barbiturate may be required before lavage in severe cases; supportive measures, including maintenance of respiratory and circulatory function; isolation to reduce external stimuli; protection against self-harm; external cooling procedures for hyperpyrexia
Methyprylon	Toxic blood concentration: 30 μg/mL	Confusion, somnolence, hypotension, tachycardia, edema, coma, shock, respiratory depression	Induce emesis or gastric lavage with endotracheal tube in place with cuff inflated if clinically indicated; support cardiorespiratory function; barbiturates can be used with caution to control seizures and agitation
Monoamine oxidase inhibitors (MAOIs)	Single doses of 1.75–7 g have been fatal	Dizziness, drowsiness, irritability, ataxia, restlessness, insomnia, headache, tachycardia, hypotension, arrhythmia, confusion, fever, diaphoresis, hyporeflexia or hyperreflexia, respiratory depression, chest pain, shock, hypertension (rare)	Symptomatic and supportive care; induce emesis or use gastric lavage with endotracheal tube with inflated cuff if clinically indicated; maintain normal vital signs; correct fluid and electrolyte abnormalities with conservative measures; volume expansion for hypotension (pressor amines may be potentiated by MAOIs and may be of limited value); evaluate liver function immediately and 4–6 weeks later; barbiturates may relieve myoclonic reactions, but MAOIs may prolong their effect; phenothiazines can be used for agitation. Hypertensive crisis

Drug	Toxic or Lethal Dose*	Signs and Symptoms	Treatment†
			mainly occurs in conjunction with tyramine. Discontinue MAOIs and treat with phentolamine (5 to 10 mg by slow IV injection)
Pemoline	2 g	Excitement, agitation, restlessness, hallucinations, tachycardia, rhabdomyolysis, choreoathetosis	Gastric lavage in mild cases; symptomatic treatment; maintain respiratory and circulatory function; monitor cardiac function; reduce stimulation; haloperidol or chlorpromazine for psychosis and agitation; IV benzodiazepines can control choreoathetosis; hemodialysis may be of value
Sertraline	3 known overdoses at 750–2,100 mg; no deaths reported	Possible symptoms include confusion, ataxia, incoordination, hypotension, hypertension, seizures, arrhythmias, serotonin syndrome, coma, mydriasis	General symptomatic and supportive measures; establish and maintain airway; ensure adequate oxygenation and ventilation; use activated charcoal with sorbitol; monitor vital signs and cardiac function
Thyroid hormones	0.3 g/kg desiccated thyroid has caused severe toxicity (with recovery)	Nervousness, sweating, palpitations, abdominal cramps, diarrhea, tachycardia, hypertension, headache, arrhythmias, tremors, cardiac failure	Symptomatic and supportive treatment; induce emesis or use gastric lavage with endotracheal tube in place with cuff inflated if clinically indicated; control fluid loss, fever, hypoglycemia; give oxygen and maintain ventilation; β-adrenergic receptor antagonists can be used to counteract increased sympathetic activity
Trazodone	Patients have survived overdoses of 7.5 g and 9.2 g	Lethargy, vomiting, drowsiness, headache, orthostasis, dizziness, dyspnea, tinnitus, myalgias, tachycardia, incontinence, shivering, coma	Symptomatic and supportive treatment; induce emesis or use gastric lavage; forced diuresis may enhance elimination; treat hypotension and sedation as appropriate
Tricyclics and tetracyclics	700–1,400 mg: moderate to severe toxicity; 2.1–2.8 g: often fatal; one patient survived ingestion of 10 g amitriptyline; lowest known fatal dose of amitriptyline: 500 mg; average lethal dose of imipramine: 30 mg/kg (fatalities occurred with 500 mg)	Initial CNS stimulation, confusion, agitation, hallucinations, hyperpyrexia, hypertension, nystagmus, hyperreflexia, parkinsonian symptoms, mydriasis, ileus, constipation, seizures, CNS depression (follows stimulation), hyperthermia, areflexia, respiratory depression, cyanosis, hypotension, coma, cardiac conduction abnormalities, tachycardia, quinidinelike effects (QRS prolongation,	Symptomatic and supportive care; monitor ECG and vital signs; support vital functions; establish and maintain airway; treat and correct fluid, electrolyte, acid-base, and temperature abnormalities; minimize stimulation; gastric lavage with activated charcoal or ipecac emesis if gag reflex is present and patient is awake; treat hypotension supportively; IV diazepam (with caution) for seizures; lidocaine, phenytoin, propranolol for life-threatening arrhythmias, sodium bicarbonate IV to achieve pH of 7.4–7.5 to help treat arrhythmias and hypotension; use of multiple antiarrhythmics or pacemaker may be needed in some cases; physostigmine has been used for anticholinergic symptoms, but its

Drug	Toxic or Lethal Dose*	Signs and Symptoms	Treatment[†]
		the degree of which may be the best indication of the severity of the overdose)	use is controversial because of serious adverse effects, and it should be used only for life-threatening treatment-refractory anticholinergic toxicity
Valproic acid	One adult survived an ingestion of 36 g valproic acid as part of a polydrug overdose	Somnolence, coma	Supportive measures; lavage may be of limited value because of drug's rapid absorption; the value of emesis or lavage varies with time since ingestion if delayed-release preparations are ingested; maintain adequate urinary output; naloxone may reverse CNS depressant effects of overdose but may also reverse anticonvulsant effects and should be used with caution

*The toxic dose is the amount of the drug capable of producing signs and symptoms of an overdose. The same dose may also have lethal effects, depending on such factors as the rate of administration, the rate of absorption, and the age and health of the patient. A toxic dose for one patient may be lethal for another. The ranges given in this table are approximate, based on available scientific literature.

   The clinician should always consult Physician's Desk Reference *(PDR) or contact the manufacturer of the drug for the latest information on toxicity and lethality.*

[†]A patient may have ingested more than one substance, and the signs and symptoms may represent polysubstance abuse or overdose. Treatment must be adjusted accordingly, and a careful history (from other persons, if necessary) and an inspection of all drugs should be obtained. The psychotherapeutic drug identification guide (shown in the front of the book) can be of help in that regard.

•Chapter by Eugene Rubin, MD, Benjamin Sadock, MD, and Harold Kaplan, MD.

Index

Page numbers in **boldface** type indicate major discussions; those followed by an "f" or a "t" denote figures or tables, respectively.